Commission on Systemic Interoperability

Ending the Document Game

Connecting and Transforming Your Healthcare Through Information Technology

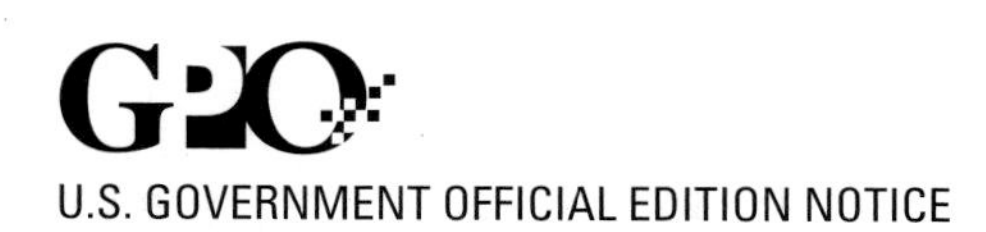

U.S. GOVERNMENT OFFICIAL EDITION NOTICE

NOTICE: This report was approved and produced by the Commission on Systemic Interoperability, whose members were appointed by the President of the United States of America and members of the United States Congress. Support for this report was provided by the National Library of Medicine and the Department of Health and Human Services. Any opinions, findings, conclusions, or recommendations expressed in this material are those of the authors and do not necessarily reflect the views of the sponsors.

This is the Official U.S. Government edition of this publication and is herein identified to certify its authenticity. Use of the 0-16 ISBN prefix is for U.S. Government Printing Office Official Editions only. The Superintendent of Documents of the U.S. Government Printing Office requests that any reprinted edition clearly be labeled as a copy of the authentic work with a new ISBN.

Additional copies of this report are available for sale from the U.S. Government Printing Office/Superintendent of Documents, 732 North Capitol Street, NW, Washington, DC 20401. Call (866) 512-1800 or (202) 512-1800 (in the Washington metropolitan area), or e-mail at ContactCenter@gpo.gov, or visit the GPO Access web page at **http://bookstore.gpo.gov/**

First published in 2005
Printed in the United States of America
First Edition

ISBN 0-16-072711-1

U.S. Government Printing Office
732 North Capitol St. NW
Washington, DC 20401
www.gpo.gov

COMMISSION MEMBERS

Scott Wallace, J.D., M.B.A.
Chair

Donald A.B. Lindberg, M.D.
Designated Federal Official

Simon P. Cohn, M.D., M.P.H.

Herbert Pardes, M.D.

Don E. Detmer, M.D.

Thomas M. Priselac, M.P.H.

Vicky B. Gregg

Ivan Seidenberg, M.B.A.

C. Martin Harris, M.D., M.B.A.

Fredrick Slunecka

Gary A. Mecklenburg, M.B.A.

William W. Stead, M.D.

COMMISSION STAFF

Dana Haza
Director

Michael Long
Senior Writer

Amanda Smith
Senior Policy Analyst

KaLea Kunkel
Policy Analyst

Raymond Sass
Policy Analyst

Carolyn Wise
Policy Analyst

Research Team
Noah Frank
Steven Genson
Chelsea Phillips
Lauren Levy

Foreword

Healthcare is a huge part of our economy, a dynamic topic of national debate, a focal point of enormous scientific and technical endeavor. But those large-scale issues don't change the fact that much of healthcare has always been innately personal—one person seeking and receiving help from another person.

Today the financial relationship between doctor and patient has grown complex, with a massive industry of professionals who negotiate prices, transfer reams of paperwork, and insulate individuals from the costs of their care. Politically, healthcare is volatile, encompassing issues spanning conception and birth to the ending of life and death. Major parts of our relationships with our doctors are not governed by us or our physicians, but by laws and regulations. Modern medical miracles have reduced many terminal diseases to chronic conditions and made multi-organ transplants a matter of routine. But delivering miracles is a complex undertaking that in many ways resembles a shuttle launch more than a house call, with teams of anonymous clinicians and technicians replacing the black bag-toting family doctor from across town.

The shift from black bag to transplants has been gradual. Almost without notice, we have allowed the complexity of healthcare to blossom without developing and deploying tools to manage it. The structures we have built to create, pay for, and govern the medical miracles we seek have led to a depersonalization of care. We have, in many ways, disconnected ourselves from healthcare, from physicians, from those to whom we turn for help. But when a child is sick, or a parent's health is failing, when we've taken ill or been injured, national issues fade into irrelevant obscurity, and we desire medicine to immediately become entirely personal again.

In the face of robotic gamma knives and sophisticated medical imaging devices, it might seem that what is affecting healthcare is too much technology, not too little. But the reality is different. The only way to manage the complexity of healthcare is to start managing information using connected computer systems.

We have the potential to ensure that all Americans get the healthcare they need. But to do so, we must put consumers in control of their care and allow them to make informed choices about what will be done to them and to those for whom they care. We must provide timely, accurate, and complete information to doctors and nurses, to public health officials, and to scientists. We must be efficient in the ways we use our healthcare dollars.

This report is all about people and using computers to connect them and their healthcare information. It is a report about how we get consumers and clinicians to use these tools, how we pay for them, and what we want the computers to do. But computers are only a tool, a means to an end. We have focused this report on computers because they seem to be the best tool—and maybe the only tool—that will allow the nation to change the way healthcare works.

While this report is about computers and the information they manage, make no mistake: it is a report for people—for Americans who want and need better and more efficient care, for policy makers and political leaders who are seeking ways to help improve care delivery, and for providers and staff who want to give Americans the best healthcare possible.

Healthcare's Crisis. Despite medical miracles and dramatic increases in life expectancy in recent decades, healthcare in America has been diagnosed with a seemingly baffling, unconnected series of problems. Critics characterize the problems in simple terms: healthcare is unsafe, ineffective, inefficient, and inconvenient. They point to a staggering array of studies and commission reports—like this one—cataloguing the problems.

In 1999, the Institute of Medicine shook the medical community—and the nation—when it reported that as many as 98,000 Americans are killed each year through preventable medical errors. A similarly shocking report by The Rand Corporation in 2004 concluded that the people they studied had received only 55 percent of recommended care. Estimates of the financial costs of healthcare's inefficiency vary but run as high as $300 billion to $500 billion a year. While precision of the statistics continues to be hotly debated, the conclusions are clear. No one needs to be told healthcare is inconvenient. There is no other area of our economy where consumers are so consistently frustrated, their time so carelessly wasted. From scheduling appointments to waiting room delays, from waiting for test results to resolving billing problems, healthcare lags behind almost every other field in customer convenience.

Systematic problems in healthcare waste consumers' time and money, leave doctors and nurses without the critical information they need to deliver the right care, and sometimes cause well-meaning caregivers to inflict life-ending injuries on patients.

An Information Problem. The problems of healthcare have many causes but they share a single characteristic—they result from a lack of information. Clinicians make mistakes not because they are careless, but most often because they lack information necessary to make better decisions. Critical information may exist somewhere in the system, but healthcare information isn't connected and can't move where it is needed to deliver safer and better care, or to reduce inefficiency and improve effectiveness.

The lack of information about the care a patient receives creates additional costs for the people who create and who pay medical bills. The bureaucracies within healthcare translate information from medical records into billing records, then go back into those medical records to defend the bills before they are paid.

Healthcare communicates by phone and by fax. Consumers spend interminable hours on phones to book appointments. Physicians and their staffs call other physicians' offices to relay information or confirm the receipt or explain the fax. Doctors, whose poor handwriting has been lampooned for generations on late night television, are responsible for much of what is written. It all takes time and it all wastes money.

Creating the Solution. We need to do better. Healthcare must be safe; there is no excuse for a preventable death due to medical error. Healthcare must also be more effective, efficient, and convenient. The losses in suffering, time, and money are just too great.

The solution is to connect healthcare information electronically. The concept is fairly simple: information relevant to a person's healthcare should be available wherever and whenever it is needed and authorized. It's not a pie in the sky technical dream. We have the ability to connect people's information, to move it where they want it, to put it in the hands of trusted physicians and caregivers, and to guard it from prying eyes and accidental disclosures.

We have the technical ability, but we haven't taken the steps to make connectivity a reality. We have created a healthcare system that pays for visits and procedures, but doesn't reward quality and therefore lacks incentives for quality improvement. We have created a patchwork of incomprehensibly complex state privacy laws making it almost impossible for our healthcare information to follow us as we travel. As a nation, we have fixated on concerns about our privacy without paying attention to the real costs—in lives, dollars, and time—that a lack of connected information imposes on us.

This report articulates a vision of an information-connected healthcare system, where consumers' privacy is protected and their convenience facilitated, where doctors and nurses have the information they need to efficiently deliver safe and effective care, where our public health and homeland security can be protected while still guarding each individual's privacy. The report recommends specific actions and broader policy objectives, all with the goal of allowing healthcare to effectively use computers and information technology. If followed, the Commission's recommendations will accelerate healthcare's transformation.

There is a great deal to be done. Consumers must understand and embrace the healthcare dimension of information technology, declaring not just a willingness for their clinicians to use computers, but a desire for the many benefits of connected healthcare information. Physicians and hospitals must embrace and adopt the technology as well, overcoming challenges inherent in changing the way things are done and seeking to improve the care given patients. Employers, insurance companies, and federal agencies paying for healthcare must recognize that the benefits of safer, more efficient, and more effective care will aid them as well, and they must step forward to help with the investment needed to transform care.

While we have focused much of this report on consumers and clinicians, there are many other constituencies with an interest in and a commitment to improving healthcare. Each is critical to the successful transformation of healthcare. In particular, companies making computer systems must recognize that the nation needs connected systems; standardized systems working seamlessly together are the only possible future. There are models of success around the world. Our everyday experience with banking, cell phones, and e-mail demonstrates that information can be connected, moved, and effectively protected.

This Commission came together for the first time in January 2005 and its members have met and worked diligently over these past 10 months. In addition to echoing the acknowledgments on the following page, I am indebted to my fellow Commissioners who share a vision, one many of them have been contributing to their entire careers. I am grateful to each of them, for their selflessness, their openness, and their commitment to this project and to the country.

I undertook this project as a memorial to my father, Thom Wallace, who suffered through a host of preventable medical errors that severely compromised the quality of his last years of life. What I learned is my father's experience was all too typical, his unnecessary suffering all too common. Instead of a static memorial, I hope this report will guide, cajole, inspire, or compel action to transform care. We can transform healthcare, for ourselves and for those we love. We can, and we must.

Scott Wallace
Chair

Acknowledgments

This Commission on Systemic Interoperability was authorized by the Medicare Modernization Act. The commissioners were appointed by the President, Senate Majority Leader Bill Frist, Former Senate Minority Leader Tom Daschle, Speaker of the House Dennis Hastert, and House Minority Leader Nancy Pelosi. We have sought to fulfill the promise of this Commission, to change and improve healthcare by offering concrete recommendations for connecting Americans' health information. We are honored by and grateful for the trust of those who nominated us.

Health and Human Services Secretary Mike Leavitt put our work at the top of his own priorities. His personal commitment to our deliberations helped guide our extensive examination of connectivity and interoperability. We are grateful to the Secretary and his staff for their support of our work and for keeping this issue a national priority. We are grateful as well to Secretary Leavitt's predecessor, Secretary Tommy Thompson, who convened the Commission and launched our endeavors.

Dr. Donald Lindberg, Director of the National Library of Medicine, contributed significantly to our understanding of the challenges of interoperability and its centrality in the wide range of issues confronting medicine. Dr. Lindberg, along with the Library's Deputy Director, Betsy Humphreys, and the entire NLM staff have been gracious hosts, providing the Commission and its staff with office space and ready counsel. We thank them for their tireless efforts and flexibility.

Dr. David Brailer, National Health Information Technology Coordinator, has made enormous strides in defining the framework for healthcare information technology in the United States and shared generously his insights and perspectives. Dr. Brailer consistently matched his sage advice with humor and creativity. We are grateful for his assistance and leadership on this issue, and to the Office of the National Coordinator's staff for their assistance.

The many patients, doctors, and experts who testified before the Commission and sat for interviews with Commissioners and staff provided us with firsthand knowledge of the real-world problems caused by the lack of connected health information and interoperability. We appreciate their willingness to share their stories of inconvenience and challenge, heartbreak, and tragedy caused by the lack of connecting health information technology. Healthcare is ultimately a personal experience, and credit for its transformation will go largely to those willing to share their personal stories and to insist on change.

Members and staff of the U.S. House of Representatives and Senate counseled us on how to create change. We are grateful for their guidance and hope that this report gives them the tools they need to make a difference.

Finally, we offer a note of thanks to the Commission's staff. Dana Haza, our Director, has mixed diligent project management with a constant infusion of new ideas, delivering it all with Southern charm and wit that is disarming and effective. In a remarkably short time, she assembled a staff and created the structure by which this Commission operated. We are all in her debt. The Commission's staffers—Michael Long, Amanda Smith, Raymond Sass, Carolyn Wise, KaLea Kunkel, Chelsea Phillips, Steven Genson, Noah Frank, and Lauren Levy—are a remarkable group of professionals who personally invested themselves in gathering patient and provider stories and undertaking comprehensive research and writing. The energy, creativity, and enthusiasm each member of the team brought into this project helped bring the story of interoperability to life. Without a doubt, their dedication made this report a reality. Our appreciation for this team knows no bounds.

Ending the Document Game

Department of Health and Human Services
Secretary Mike Leavitt's Remarks for the Commission on Systemic Interoperability

August 29, 2005

I recently had a surgical procedure that is recommended for men my age. I made my appointment four weeks in advance, talked with colleagues about what to expect, followed the instructions about what to eat and when, and then went dutifully to my local hospital, where I proceeded to fill out my contact and insurance information seven times.
SEVEN times!

I cannot imagine doing this in any other business, yet we do it in healthcare without a second thought. Just think of it: seven different people will enter my information into seven different and incompatible databases, seven different times.

Making the medical clipboard a thing of the past is what *Ending the Document Game* is all about. It's about moving away from filing cabinets and clipboards, and moving toward mouse clicks and memory sticks. It will mean higher quality, lower costs, and less hassle.

During the same hospital visit, when the doctor asked me about my medical history, I nearly forgot to mention that I have sleep apnea—a condition that can be serious if not treated but that I've been managing, with the help of my doctor, for several years. Sleep apnea is not a big problem for me, but it is something a doctor should know about if you are going to be anesthetized, as I was. The omission was my fault; I simply forgot to tell the doctor.

When our health practitioners do not have compatible data, they order tests and procedures we don't need. This makes healthcare more expensive. Even worse, with incomplete data, practitioners can make medical errors that may cause complications, or even cost us our lives.

We live in the digital age, and yet in healthcare we settle for the paper age, even though there is considerable evidence that interoperable electronic health records will reduce errors, improve quality, and save money.

Up to a third of healthcare spending—more than half a trillion dollars every year—is wasted on wrong or redundant care or other problems. Even more serious, more people die each year in this country because of medical errors than from motor vehicle accidents, breast cancer, or AIDS.

We can do better than this.

Our Nation has an economic and humanitarian imperative: get more efficient or face losing our economic prosperity and more human lives. Nothing short of the transformation of our healthcare system will do.

President Bush is resolved to transform the healthcare system by putting information technology to work. He has set a national goal to have most Americans using electronic health records within 10 years. He has asked us to ensure that the privacy and security of those records are protected.

The cornerstone of this effort is the American Health Information Community. The Community is a private/public collaboration to help develop standards and interoperability in a smooth, market-led way.

I congratulate the Commission on Systemic Interoperability for its work and pledge to move forward with expedience. We will move our healthcare system to the plug-and-play world. As a result of this move, we will see fewer medical mistakes, lower costs, better care, and less hassle.

Table of Contents

Recommendations

There is no single step that, if taken, would create a connected nationwide system of health information. This Commission has organized the steps needed to create such a system into three categories: adoption, interoperability, and connectivity. These categories were formed acknowledging the obvious overlap, but recognizing a need to structure recommendations to facilitate understanding.

Adoption focuses on the challenge of getting clinicians and consumers to use computer programs and information networks to maintain healthcare records, access relevant information about patient's background and illness, and offer support for safer, better decisions. Adoption includes the need to train doctors and other caregivers to ensure they are able to adopt these technologies effectively in their practices, provide technical support so clinicians do not need to become computer technicians, and make clinicians and consumers aware of the benefits and the privacy safeguards of these systems. The issues of adoption also require addressing the difficult economic and regulatory issues slowing investment and use of connected computer systems and the growing gaps between communities' access to these technologies.

Information is valuable when it is available as needed. **Interoperability** focuses on the need for healthcare information to be connected so information is accessible whenever and wherever it is needed and authorized. Interoperability issues often become exceedingly technical, focusing on the rules for how information is created, stored, and moved among computer systems.

Finally, there must be physical networks and operating rules for actually moving information around. **Connectivity** focuses on the networks providing the conduits for moving healthcare information seamlessly. A major obstacle to connectivity is creating a mechanism to connect an individual with his or her healthcare information. Connectivity also encompasses the major issue of consumer confidentiality—providing uniform privacy laws across the country and punishing those who seek to violate them.

In crafting these recommendations, the Commission focused on providing actionable advice. While the recommendations will possibly provoke debate in some circles, the Commissioners, reflecting consensus and compromise, as well as a commitment toward action and the transformation of healthcare, present them with unanimous support.

To advance progress of the **adoption** of health information technology, the following actions should be taken:

1. **Adoption Incentives.** The Department of Health and Human Services (HHS) should implement, or seek authorization from Congress as necessary to implement, financial and other incentives for participation in a standards-based healthcare information network. These incentives should be directed toward individuals and organizations including healthcare providers, medical institutions, purchasers, and health plans. Incentives should include broad-based approaches such as pay-for-performance, as well as targeted approaches that include grants directed at small, safety net, and financially challenged providers. These incentives should begin to be implemented within two years. Employers and other private sector healthcare payers who will benefit from the adoption of interoperable healthcare information systems should be encouraged to provide similar incentives.

2. **Regulatory Reform.** The Secretary of HHS should act with urgency to revise or eliminate regulations that prevent healthcare entities, networks, hospitals, and clinicians from working together to create and adopt interoperable healthcare information systems, while promoting competition and maintaining reasonable protections against inurement and kickbacks. To ensure that healthcare providers can be confident in the legality of their actions, the Secretary should clearly state in the regulations those actions that are permissible and should direct the Centers for Medicare and Medicaid Services and the Office of the Inspector General to provide effective guidance to accelerate legally compliant activities that advance adoption of healthcare information technology. This effort should begin with 42 U.S.C. 1395nn, known as the Physician Self-Referral or Stark Law, and 42 U.S.C. 1320a-7b, known as the Federal Anti-Kickback Law, and regulations issued pursuant to those laws.

3. **Reporting on Adoption Gaps.** To ensure that the benefits of healthcare information technology are equally available to all the nation's citizens, HHS should monitor and annually issue a public report on gaps in the adoption

and effective implementation of interoperable healthcare information technology systems across all sectors of the nation's health system. The report should specifically identify types of gaps and should propose public and private sector policies to address and close those gaps.

4. **Workforce Needs and Impacts.** The Departments of Labor and Commerce, in concert with HHS, should identify and quantify deficiencies in healthcare workforce knowledge and skills that must be addressed in order to secure maximum benefit from healthcare information technology. The effects of healthcare information technology on the use of labor and the upward mobility of workers in the healthcare system should also be considered. Based on these findings, these Departments should create a plan to meet such workforce needs and better estimate the financial impact of workforce changes that occur as a result of effectively adopting healthcare information technology.

5. **Public Awareness.** HHS should develop and execute a public awareness campaign that helps educate consumers, providers, and other interested constituencies of the benefits of using interoperable health information technology and the steps they can take to realize those benefits. HHS should implement the campaign in conjunction with the Department of Commerce and other government and private-sector organizations.

The adoption of healthcare information technology has been hindered by the economics of healthcare. The Commission's recommendations seek to provide an incentive for adoption by rewarding the desired outcomes through pay-for-performance programs. In addition, direct financial and other support will be needed by small providers who get less direct benefit from use of the technology than larger providers and by safety net and other healthcare providers whose lack of financial resources have prevented their adoption of information technology.

Much of existing provider-based healthcare information technology is found inside hospitals. However, existing laws and regulations prevent hospitals from sharing those resources with other clinicians in the community. While these laws serve to protect competition among healthcare providers and to prohibit inappropriate payments to doctors, changes should be made to facilitate the sharing of information technology systems.

Information technology promises to help bring about an extraordinary transformation in healthcare. The Commission recognizes three foundational areas where these changes are not being adequately addressed. The use of information technology adds another dimension to the gaps in both healthcare's availability and quality. The first step in closing the gaps is to identify and quantify them. Using information technology effectively will require considerable changes in the way doctors, nurses, and other healthcare professionals practice medicine and approach their jobs. The Commission recommends a new focus on those changes, as well as on quantifying the benefits to healthcare workers from the implementation of information technology.

The second step is to deal directly with workforce issues. A shift to connected health information requires changes in practice by caregivers. It enables shifts in roles within the care team resulting in increased effectiveness and efficiency. It creates new roles for informatics experts and technical support personnel. The Commission recommends planning for these changes so that work force availability does not block adoption.

Finally, a critical dimension of this report is its focus on consumers. Consistent with the Commission charter, we recommend a concerted public education campaign to inform consumers and caregivers of the value and security of interoperable healthcare information systems.

To advance progress of the **interoperability** of health information technology, the following actions should be taken:

1. **Product Certification.** Purchasers of healthcare information technology products must have a reliable source of information about the interoperability, functionality, and security of these products; and vendors must be able to compete by differentiating their products beyond minimum standards. HHS should support a single, voluntary, private-public process to certify that products meet minimum standards. To ensure continual improvement in the products available to the healthcare community, the scope of certification activities should aggressively be expanded to include additional healthcare information technology products, and the minimum performance specifications should be augmented over time as technology and standards progress.

2. **Data Standards.** HHS, advised by the American Health Information Community (AHIC) and in consultation with the National Committee for Vital and Health Statistics (NCVHS), should ensure broad acceptance, effective implementation, and ongoing maintenance of a complete set of interoperable, non-overlapping data standards that function to assure data in one part of the health system is, when authorized, available and meaningful across the complete range of clinical, administrative, payment system, public health, and research settings. Additionally, AHIC should build upon the Health Insurance Portability and Accountability Act of 1996 (HIPAA) to develop national standards for authentication, authorization, and security that will permit the necessary infrastructure for consumers' confident adoption of healthcare information technology.

3. **Standard Product Identifiers and Vocabulary.** Standardizing data at the point of its creation will greatly accelerate the creation of an interoperable healthcare information network. HHS should work with manufacturers of drugs, devices, and test kits to achieve standardized identifiers and vocabulary in labels and packaging, and in all data outputs of devices and test kits.

4. **Drug Records.** Interoperable healthcare information technology will ensure that all providers have access, when authorized, to their patients' medication records and will establish a robust capability for post-marketing surveillance of drugs. AHIC should, in its early activities, take a phased approach to developing a fully interoperable drug record for every American by 2010.

Interoperability of healthcare information can be achieved, but it will take more than good intentions or favorable marketing statements. Ensuring clinicians, hospitals, and other providers can purchase information technology systems enabling interoperability and appropriate functionality while protecting confidentiality requires an independent entity that can offer reliable product certifications. Certification depends upon the use of comprehensive, commonly accepted data, and technology standards—a critical infrastructure component not existing today but ready to be put into place rapidly through the work of AHIC. The Commission strongly endorses the creation of AHIC and the leadership demonstrated by HHS Secretary Mike Leavitt to chair and lead that entity.

Other industries have achieved interoperability by attaching computer readable information at the point of product manufacture. Manufacturers of retail products include a bar code with all the information needed to manage the product. Downstream participants in the supply chain use this information within their local systems. In healthcare, it is not yet practical to attach a physical tag to every drug or lab result with all the needed information. It is practical to identify the product with a standard identifier, to include that identifier in a national database, and to link it to all relevant information according to the appropriate terminology standard. The Commission recommends manufacturers of drugs, devices, and test instruments and kits identify the drug or result with standard identifiers and relay information in a standard vocabulary. The standardization of these items is the starting point to ensuring interoperability throughout the information supply chain.

Finally, we recommend, and in the body of the report provide the framework for an interoperable drug record for all Americans. This roadmap provides a management dashboard and coordinates choices, shows what needs to be done, and when each step needs to be completed to achieve this goal in a reasonable time. While this Commission could not, in 10 months, complete a roadmap for every dimension of healthcare information technology, the specific roadmap recommended for drug records can serve as a model for the development of other interoperable healthcare modules, such as a laboratory record, in the coming months.

To advance progress of the **connectivity** of health information technology, the following actions should be taken:

1. **Patient Authentication Standard.** Correctly aggregating and exchanging information about a specific person is essential and requires a uniform mechanism for authenticating the patient's identity. Congress should authorize HHS to develop a national standard for determining patient authentication and identity.

2. **Federal Privacy Standard.** Congress should authorize the Secretary of HHS to develop a uniform federal health information privacy standard for the nation, based on HIPAA and pre-empting state privacy laws, which anticipates and enables data interoperability across the nation.

3. **Nationwide Health Information Network.** A national healthcare information network is part of the critical infrastructure of national security. Therefore, HHS and its relevant agencies should coordinate and seek Congressional approval to coordinate, as necessary, with the Department of Homeland Security (DHS) and other cabinet Departments to ensure the nationwide health information network is created and receives funding commensurate with its contribution to the safety and security of the American public.

4. **Criminal Sanctions for Privacy Violations.** To augment the protections provided by HIPAA, Congress should authorize Federal criminal sanctions against individuals who intentionally access protected data without authorization.

5. **Consumer Protections.** Patients should be protected from the consequences of unauthorized access to or release of their healthcare information. Therefore HHS should study and recommend to Congress actions to prohibit discrimination based on data obtained in that way.

A uniform national approach to patient authentication was part of HIPAA. Creating a single, unique patient identifier would be the most direct way to establish patient authentication, and this approach is used throughout Europe. However, no approach to personal authentication in computer systems is free of financial costs, management issues, and privacy concerns. A direct approach would involve an administrative infrastructure that may be unacceptable to some at this time for a variety of reasons, including privacy concerns.

This approach could be modified to allow individuals to opt out of the uniform patient identifier. This compromise would let the nation provide a system benefiting individuals who recognize that their need for connected health information exceeds their privacy concerns while not penalizing those who find privacy more valuable. However, such a compromise would sharply reduce the administrative savings because the system would have to accommodate both sets of individuals. It would also present new liability challenges, specifically involving the potential liability of providers who lacked information in the treatment of a consumer whose information was not available.

An alternative to creating unique personal identification for everyone is to define a national standard set of authenticating information required to receive healthcare. This set of data could be captured when an individual first enters the healthcare system. Such information could include a set of data such as date of birth, school, employment, and insurance policy number.

Each of these approaches has strengths and weaknesses. The National Academies' Computer Science and Telecommunications Board's 2002 report, "IDs—Not That Easy," is a learned, post-9/11 look at the options from the perspective of national security. For purposes of healthcare and of national security, the time has come to select an alternative and eliminate the unacceptable cost of unconnected healthcare.

Much like the huge variety in patient authentication mechanisms, the variety and contradictions within the patchwork of state privacy laws also prevents the nation from connecting healthcare information. HIPAA set a minimum national privacy standard, but many states have augmented that standard. The resulting cacophony of state laws is fundamentally inconsistent: what is mandated in one state is prohibited in another. Congress must enact a uniform national privacy standard for the nation to realize the benefits of connected healthcare information.

The networks that will allow connected healthcare information are a critical national infrastructure, promoting the safe, efficient, and effective delivery of care; the protection of public health; the defense of the nation; and the promotion of rapid medical advancement. Without a connected health information network, the nation is slower in detecting epidemics of natural or man-made viruses and compromised in its ability to detect and recall defective drugs or medical devices. The healthcare field alone cannot carry the full burden of establishing the networks and infrastructure to connect healthcare information, and the Commission calls on DHS and other appropriate Federal agencies to assist in this essential task.

Finally, the Commission recognizes that no system of confidentiality and security protections will protect against all malicious attacks. To ensure the nation's reliance on the confidentiality of connected healthcare information, the Commission calls upon Congress to enact stiff criminal sanctions against individuals who purposefully access protected data without authorization. We also recommend providing clear and comprehensive safeguards against discrimination to protect anyone whose personal data were improperly released.

Executive Summary

Addressing Healthcare Connectivity as a Matter of Life and Death

Americans need a connected system of electronic healthcare information available to all doctors and patients whenever and wherever necessary.

In 2000, the Institute of Medicine (IoM) estimated that between 44,000 and 98,000 Americans die each year from preventable medical errors.[1] Subsequent studies have estimated that the number may be twice as high.[2] Medical errors are killing more people per year, in America, than breast cancer, AIDS, or motor vehicle accidents.[3] This pain and suffering is compounded by the knowledge that many of these errors could have been avoided.

The lack of immediate access to patient healthcare information is the source of one-fifth of these errors.[4]

One of every seven primary care visits is affected by missing medical information.[5] In a recent study, 80 percent of errors were initiated by miscommunication, including missed communication between physicians, misinformation in medical records, mishandling of patient requests and messages, inaccessible records, mislabeled specimens, misfiled or missing charts, and inadequate reminder systems.[6]

Under the current paper-based system, patients and their doctors lack instant, constant access to medical information. As a result, when a patient sees more than one doctor, no doctor knows exactly what another doctor is doing, or even that another doctor is involved. The consequences range from inconvenient to critical or even fatal. Each time an individual encounters a new healthcare

[1] Kohn, L., J. Corrigan, and M. Donaldson. *To Err Is Human: Building a Safer Health System.* Committee of Health Care in America, Institute of Medicine. 2000.

[2] HealthGrades. *In-Hospital Deaths from Medical Errors at 195,000 per Year, HealthGrades Study Finds.* July 27, 2004.

[3] Institute of Medicine and Centers for Disease Control and Prevention. *National Center for Health Statistics: Preliminary Data for 1998 and 1999.* 2000.

[4] Health Research Institute & Global Technology Center. *Reactive to Adaptive: Transforming Hospitals with Digital Technology*, PriceWaterhouseCoopers. 2005.

[5] Smith, Peter, et. al. "Missing Clinical Information During Primary Care Visits," *The Journal of the American Medical Association.* February 2005. <http://murphy.house.gov/UploadedFiles/HealthCareFYI_5a.pdf>

[6] *Annals of Family Medicine.* July/August 2004. <http://annalsfm.highwire.org/cgi/content/astract/2/4/317>

provider, that patient must retell his or her medical history. Not only is this redundant, it can introduce error and imprecision, ensuring that no two copies of a personal medical record will be exactly alike. In an emergency, delay and a lack of information can be deadly.

In the age of the Internet, this shortcoming is unacceptable.

Many other problems stem from the lack of connectivity. Since doctors often work independently, the lack of shared knowledge can cause duplicate tests to be ordered, resulting in unnecessary expense and, occasionally, risk, and pain. The same problem exists for prescriptions, which can conflict with one another to create life-threatening drug interactions.

Security and confidentiality are limited by the difficulty of tracking access to paper-based records. The paper-based system necessitates consultations via telephone calls, faxes, and e-mails without the benefit of complete medical records. Patients who want follow-up information on their conditions must schedule time with doctors, nurses, or staff, or conduct research independently—there is no networked access to supporting information.

Handwritten records—most notoriously, prescriptions—are easily misread, causing potentially life-threatening mistakes. Similarly, analysis of large numbers of paper records is impossible, denying the public the benefits of early warnings of dangerous trends in disease or bioterrorism, and other research-driven efforts.

The benefits of a connected system of healthcare information

These problems and others are well addressed by a connected system of healthcare information, one that is referred to in this report as interoperable. The benefits of this interoperable system will extend to both patients and healthcare providers and may be categorized as promoting convenience, confidentiality, access, and quality of care.

Interoperability creates convenience by allowing doctors and other healthcare providers to share medical history, lab results, and other pertinent information in a more timely and accurate way. It makes backups of data easier to maintain, so catastrophic data loss is more easily remedied. It provides improved support for adults who care for aging parents, especially from far away. Such systems enhance and ease post-diagnosis and post-treatment contact with doctors via on-line services.

By more effectively limiting unauthorized access, and tracking who views personal healthcare information, interoperability provides patients with more security and confidentiality.

Prescriptions and data are typed and stored electronically and not on paper, so they are always readable. Notification of drug or device recalls is faster and more thorough. And interoperability makes possible a powerful public-health resource against bioterrorism, the spread of disease, and other nationwide medical concerns by allowing national-level analysis of trends in disease and symptoms.

In short, interoperable healthcare information enhances the quality of care for all Americans.

The time patients and caregivers must spend filling out forms is dramatically reduced, affecting both cost and convenience. Similarly, the system improves continuity of care when treatment is ongoing and conducted among multiple healthcare providers, an especially important consideration for patients with chronic conditions. After patients move or when they travel, interoperable healthcare information helps ensure care consistent with treatment that is already under way.

In the field of obstetrics, contact with multiple healthcare providers is an almost universal facet of pregnancy and childbirth. Interoperability allows physicians and others to share medical records and to provide additional medical information for expectant mothers. Similar effects benefit rural residents and those who rely on community health centers, who can receive more consistent treatment across multiple providers, a reduction in the number of office visits required, and access to personalized information that can help them live healthier lives.

When all providers in the chain of healthcare are able to share information, it will be much more difficult to commit fraud and abuse. Connectivity will create new opportunities to ensure that prescriptions are valid and have not been duplicated, and the status of payment and reimbursement information will be better integrated and more frequently updated.

The first major manifestation of interoperability in people's lives will be electronic prescribing, also known as e-prescribing. Doctors will be able to file prescriptions without paper, bringing an end to the age-old problems of illegibly written prescriptions, lost prescriptions, delays in taking prescriptions to a pharmacy, and doubts about whether prescriptions have been filled correctly.

In addition to the recommendations made by the Commissioners, this report includes many other resources. There is a timeline in the chapter, *The Problem and The Solution*, that describes steps to create an electronic prescription drug record for every American. Patient and provider stories throughout the report document the challenges in a healthcare system without interoperability—and success stories of current implementations. The *Existing Efforts* chapter documents over 300 interoperability projects under way nationwide. Recommendations of previous commissions, dating back to 1978, digitize the healthcare system and are listed in Appendix C.

In order to make the information contained in this report available to the largest number of people, we have also chosen to make it electronically accessible, on-line (at www.EndingTheDocumentGame.gov) and on a CD-ROM (included with each hard copy of the report). The CD-ROM and Web versions will include such things as a video statement by Secretary Mike Leavitt of the Department of Health and Human Services, as well as interviews with the Commissioners and Dr. David Brailer (National Coordinator for Health Information Technology). There are also audio interviews that detail important ways in which connected health information and e-prescribing have helped save lives and improve the quality of life for patients and care providers.

The quality of our healthcare, on both societal and individual levels, is suffering from the lack of a connected system of healthcare information. The cost comes in injury, wasted resources, and lost lives. Much of the technology for such a system is already being applied to infinitely less critical concerns such as making travel plans on-line and checking bank balances at any ATM. Much of the world has addressed this lack of medical connectivity to a far greater extent than the United States has. Our problem is not a lack of technology, but a lack of attention and a lack of will.

This report describes what can be gained and what is required to achieve an interoperable system of electronic healthcare information. This goal can be reached, and its benefits are worth the effort that will be required.

The evidence cited in this report compels action to achieve an interoperable health information technology system in the United States.

Lives are in the balance.

The Problem and the Solution
Table of Contents

The Problem and the Solution

"The day is not far off when we can walk into a medical clinic and not be handed a clipboard to enter the same information you've filled out a hundred times."

Mike Leavitt, Secretary, Department of Health and Human Services

The Problem with the Paper System

The healthcare system: Did you know it could be better?

Your life should not depend on your ability to memorize. Yet to some extent today, it does.

On a business trip, you wake up with strange, painful symptoms in the middle of the night. You take a cab to the emergency room where doctors try to help you. They need to know your medical history.

And you … don't know. Or can't remember. Or never knew the details.

Although your airline ticket confirmation number, your rental car record, and even your cellular phone bills and calling history are available 24/7 on-line, your medical records are locked away in filing cabinets somewhere, partially hand-written and partially typed, stored in paper folders, and stacked alphabetically.

At four in the morning, that person with the key to your medical information is fast asleep and, in this case, a thousand miles away. How would you reach him or her? Would you call your doctor's answering service and hope someone will go down to the office? Perhaps it can wait until morning—but wouldn't it be better for the doctor treating you now to have that information now?

Meanwhile, that emergency room doctor is asking you to remember as much of your history as you can … while your stomach is in a knot … or your head pounds … or the pain in your chest begins to creep into your jaw and down your arm.

Scenes like this play out daily in America in emergency rooms, in the backs of ambulances, in doctors' offices and hospitals, in walk-in clinics and neighborhood health centers. Sometimes it's merely inconvenient, and a healthcare provider can contact another provider to get the necessary information—a few hours or days do not make a difference. But often there is no time for delay. Not after a serious car accident. Not during a stroke or heart attack. Not in a medical emergency far away from home. Not after a natural disaster or a terrorist attack.

Interoperability or connectivity—constant, instant access to your medical information—is the only answer. Although such access is available for everything from shopping to helping with homework, it is not available for medical records.

Yet it ought to be. And the technology to make it available already exists.

The most basic information about your health—medicines you take, tests you've had, doctors you've seen, vaccinations you've received, illnesses you've had—ought to be available at your fingertips. And at your doctors' fingertips.

But it isn't. Not for you. Not for your children. Not for your parents. Not for your wife, husband, partner, or best friend.

Not unless you carry it around yourself—and who carries copies of their own x-rays and medical charts? And even if you did, could you possibly carry them around wherever you go on the chance you might be injured and need them?

Individuals who rely on the medical system may find themselves in a dire situation: the most critical information about health and quality of life—the data that would and should guide future treatment—can't be accessed in a timely manner by many healthcare providers.

The cost comes in wasted time, diminished quality of care, duplicate testing, needless expense, unnecessary worry … and, worst of all, in lives lost.

"The learning and knowledge that we have, is, at most, but little compared with that of which we are ignorant."

Plato, Greek Philosopher

The paper-based system is not good enough anymore

Consumers don't realize how much benefit there is in having an interoperable system of medical information. Most people don't even realize such a thing is possible. And not knowing the need for such a system, people certainly don't know that the technological answer to the need is within reach. The public has accepted that medical records are kept in paper files in metal cabinets, and that's the way it is.

Making the connection. ATMs and on-line banking provide universal access to your financial records. Oil service centers keep service records on your car accessible nationwide. Airlines keep track of your flight history, your seat preference, your payment history, and your frequent-flyer miles—and you can access them yourself on-line, too.

This technology should be applied to healthcare immediately. It means more than convenience: this technology will save lives.

The paper-based system of medical information currently in use has no connectivity, no ease of access for either patients or providers, and limited security and tracking of access. It is a barrier to improved treatment, and it diverts critical resources to bureaucracy and administration when they could be put to better use for direct patient care.

The problems with paper

Problems with the paper-based system run the gamut. Some are just inconvenient: waiting for vaccination records before a parent can take a child to camp or enroll the child in school, or making a trip across town to take the child's records to another doctor. Others are critical: for example, treating a patient with a chronic condition or who is in a life-threatening situation far from home, but unable to supply the healthcare provider with detailed medical information.

"We live in the Information Age, but our healthcare industry is stuck in the Stone Age."

Senate Majority Leader Bill Frist

The problems affect both healthcare providers and patients. For instance, doctors must be sure that access to paper records is limited to authorized personnel and must keep track of physical files that can be inconvenient to move around. Patients suffer because there are health benefits available that a paper-based system cannot support: post-visit interaction with a doctor by electronic communication; the ability to track one's own health information and more closely follow detailed treatment plans; and, of course, the ability to provide a physician with instant access to critical information, especially in an emergency.

The inconvenience of paper-based systems

- **Difficulty sharing medical history and lab results with other doctors.** When doctors do consultations, accept new patients, or review lab results, paper-based information is almost always involved. That means information is transmitted via fax machine, telephone conversation, courier, or mail. All these methods have the potential for misread or misheard data, lost information, delay, and breaches of security.

- **Inconvenience of securing vaccination records for camp and school enrollment.** Almost every childhood activity outside the home requires proof of vaccination. That means a trip to the doctor's office for the patient or the parent. A paper-based system costs your family time.

- **Recounting medical history for every new doctor.** Nearly every new healthcare provider a patient sees will need to review his or her medical history. People move and travel more than ever, so this need is especially acute. No one can be expected to remember his or her entire medical history, and the record will be remembered even less accurately when a patient must see a new doctor in an emergency.

- **No support in caring for aging parents far away.** Many adults find themselves taking care of their aging parents, and they often have to do so from far away. Medical information is almost always written down or conveyed in conversation, leaving long-distance caregivers with an additional burden. They have no convenient way to keep track of prescriptions, interact with a physician, review test results, or be sure that the parent is following the doctor's treatment plan.

- **No easy way of getting quick answers to follow-up questions.** Doctors want to help patients as much as they can, especially with matters such as following the treatment plan, providing more details about a condition, or finding general information about lifestyle choices. But the lack of connectivity means that patients have to wait by the phone or play "telephone tag" with their healthcare providers instead of using e-mail or accessing on-line articles that physicians and others have made available.

“President Bush wants to maximize the benefits of information technology—electronic medical records—so that doctors and nurses can better monitor treatments and reduce errors and patients can go from doctor to doctor with their complete medical history.”

First Lady Laura Bush

The lack of confidentiality in a paper-based system

- **Confidentiality is hard to preserve using paper.** Patients do not want their sensitive, personal medical information stored in a way others can easily access. Doctors are committed to honoring the trust patients place in them, and they are bound by laws, regulations, and rules of ethics to protect confidentiality. But under today's paper-based system, privacy is most often a matter of locks and keys: paper records are kept in file cabinets on the premises of a healthcare provider, and older records may be stored off-site. When records are being accessed—when doctors and nurses are referring to them during an office visit, for instance—privacy is often a matter of trust: notes regarding patients are kept in file folders that rest in plastic trays attached to an exam-room door, or on a billing clerk's desk, or in a pile awaiting lab results.

- **No way to keep track of who sees paper records or to keep unauthorized people out.** Unlike electronic records, paper records can be examined without any record of who looked at them, when a person looked at them—or copied them—and why. While security is always a priority for administrative staff and medical librarians, a record casually left out for even a few moments can easily be examined or even copied by unauthorized persons.

“The single biggest problem in communication is the illusion that it has taken place.”

George Bernard Shaw, Winner of the Nobel Prize for Literature in 1925

Patients, especially those with serious illnesses or those who have confided compromising secrets to their doctors, understand that if their information is exposed, they could be irreparably harmed. They fear the loss of a job, embarrassment at home or work, bias, and the inability to get insurance coverage.

Lack of access in the paper-based world

- **No instant, constant access to your healthcare information.** Paper records have to be carried from place to place, faxed, or summarized in a phone call. The only way this transferred information is preserved is if it has successfully been received and placed in your medical file.

- **No guarantee for information backup.** Your paper-based records could be destroyed by fire, flood, or other catastrophe, like Hurricane Katrina, or they could be damaged or stolen. Unless the doctor has made copies of every paper in the filing cabinet, that part of your medical history is lost.

Possible compromises to quality of care from a paper-based system

- **Illegible handwriting in records and prescriptions.** Paper records are a mix of typed text and handwriting, and prescriptions are usually written completely by hand. Illegible handwriting in healthcare information can

The Document Game

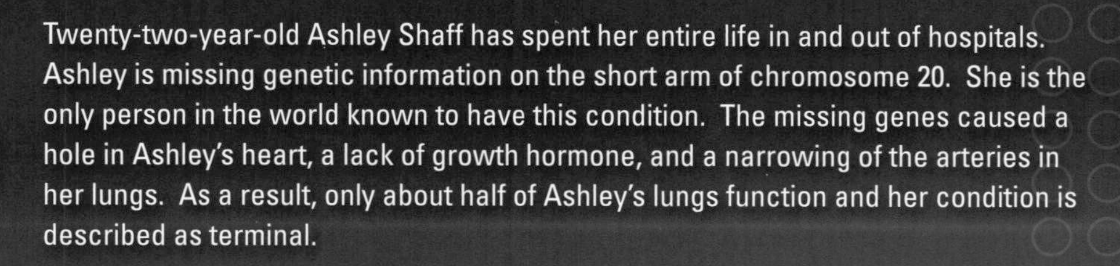

Twenty-two-year-old Ashley Shaff has spent her entire life in and out of hospitals. Ashley is missing genetic information on the short arm of chromosome 20. She is the only person in the world known to have this condition. The missing genes caused a hole in Ashley's heart, a lack of growth hormone, and a narrowing of the arteries in her lungs. As a result, only about half of Ashley's lungs function and her condition is described as terminal.

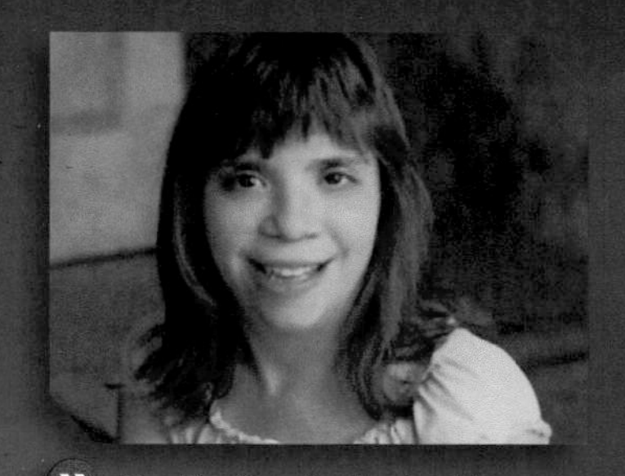

» PROFILE:

Ashley Shaff

CALIFORNIA

~ 22 Years Old, 35 Hospitalizations, a Terminal Diagnosis, and a Complicated Medical Journey ...

"I couldn't be left alone with my thoughts and pain; no, instead I was forced to regurgitate a horrific medical journey, once again."

– Peggy Frank

Ashley's mother, Peggy Frank, is Ashley's advocate and her librarian. Peggy has managed her daughter's care from the moment she was born. She keeps track of her extensive and complex medical records stored in boxes, binders, and personal memory, dating back to eye surgery at the age of nine months.

Ashley has been the patient of at least 36 doctors and has been hospitalized over 35 times in 12 different hospitals around the nation. Her list of medical procedures includes heart surgery, two adenoid surgeries, four cardiac catheterizations, and three pulmonary angioplasties. Keeping order in this jumble of critical information is a source of frustration and desperation for Peggy—and a danger for Ashley.

As the volume of Ashley's medical records grow, it becomes more challenging for Ashley and Peggy to play the "document game." Peggy is left to keep track of every detail in order to retell her daughter's medical history during even the most stressful times. She must recite it over and over—hundreds of times—because Peggy is the only source of information that follows Ashley around.

In addition to providing an oral history, Peggy transports binders filled with laboratory reports, x-rays, medication lists, and medical reports. Despite Peggy's best efforts to accumulate all the relevant data, she is always fearful she has forgotten or is missing crucial information. Hospitals and physicians are not accustomed to providing the detailed level of information that Peggy needs.

Peggy knows that even during the most critical times, she is the lifeline—the only source of information that connects Ashley's complicated medical history with her current care.

Did You Know?

~ 1 pulp tree (loblolly pine 8" (200 mm) diameter, 50 ft. (15 m tall, 20 years old) = .1 cord of wood (.2 cu. m of wood) = 10,000 pages = 1 file cabinet = 4 boxes/ drawers = .5 GB = 1 CD-ROM

~ 10 pulp trees (loblolly pine 8" (200 mm) diameter, 50 ft. (15 m) tall, 20 years old) = 1 lumber tree (20" (500 mm) diameter, 110 ft (35 m) tall, 50 years old) = 1 cord of wood (2 cu. m of wood) = 100,000 pages = 10 file cabinets = 40 file boxes/ drawers = 5 GB = 10 CD-ROMs

Source: Intergraph Solutions Group. "Data Integration, Interoperability, and Conversion Services for US Army Corps of Engineers Automated Document Conversion Strategy Initiative." US Army. Madison, 2003.

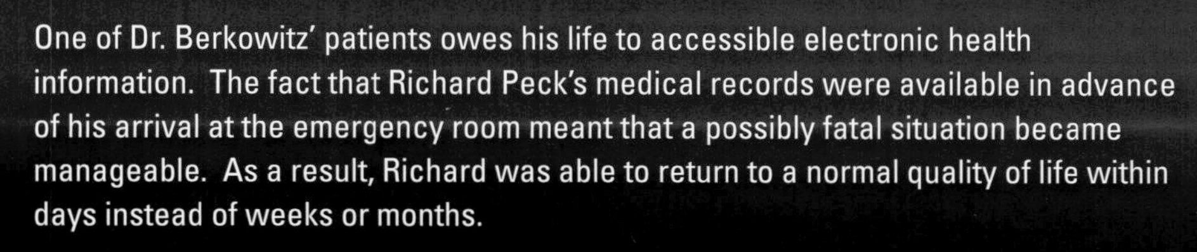

No Going Back

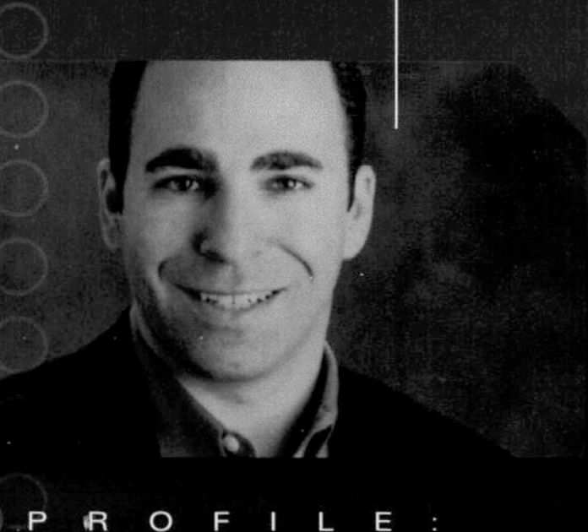

» PROFILE:

Lyle Berkowitz, M.D.

ILLINOIS

~ Chicago Doctor Helped Spearhead EHR Program in His Hospital

One of Dr. Berkowitz' patients owes his life to accessible electronic health information. The fact that Richard Peck's medical records were available in advance of his arrival at the emergency room meant that a possibly fatal situation became manageable. As a result, Richard was able to return to a normal quality of life within days instead of weeks or months.

Dr. Berkowitz can't imagine going back to the system of paper records he used just a few years ago. "There's no question it helps us improve the quality of care that we deliver. Just access to information that's legible significantly improves the care in a number of different ways. It decreases how much redundant care has to be done—and redundant care is a potential for risk. It also makes sure the right people have the right information at the right time."

"Now that there are thousands of drugs that often have similar-sounding names, you can't have any room for error. I can't imagine handwriting a prescription anymore. It seems so fundamentally wrong at this point. In our electronic health record, when we do prescription-writing there's a system of checks for allergies and drug interaction."

Dr. Berkowitz has also seen firsthand the barriers that need to be overcome in order to have a system truly work for patients. "One barrier to this is that we have to pay for the system without being compensated. Also, our current system compensates mainly on volume of care. So, in fact, if I do something that creates a mild error with a patient, or I can't find a lab value or a chest x-ray and have to repeat it, well, I make more money. Our system and the incentives are completely misaligned."

"Now that there are thousands of drugs that often have similar-sounding names, you can't have any room for error. I can't imagine handwriting a prescription anymore. It seems so fundamentally wrong at this point."

– Lyle Berkowitz, M.D.

"You can actually provide better healthcare if you have a well-functioning electronic medical record. You never have to worry about finding chart information. It's all there, and it's not going to get lost."

– David Levy, M.D.

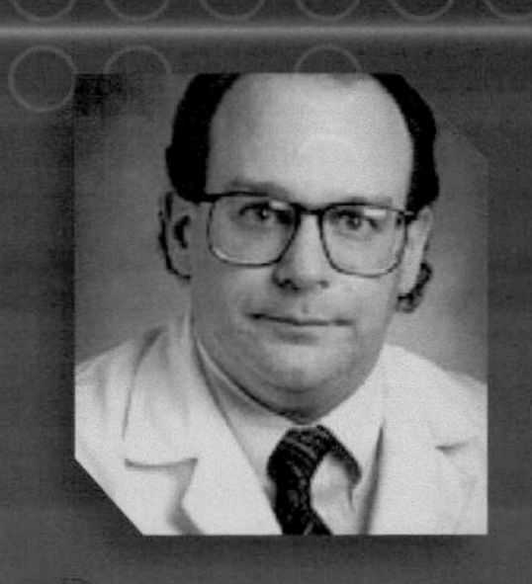

» PROFILE:

David Levy, M.D.
ILLINOIS

~ Taking Steps to Provide the Best Possible Care

Creating a Paperless Environment

Dr. David Levy wants the best for all his patients: to provide each of them with the best possible care he can give them. It's the reason his small practice went out on a limb to buy a new electronic medical records (EMR) system in 2004.

Dr. Levy's practice in Chicago is affiliated with a hospital in Berwin, Illinois. In 1994, the hospital started using an EMR, but the company that sold them the system went out of business shortly after, leaving them without the technical support they needed.

After dealing with a practically useless system for years, Dr. Levy and the other doctors in his practice decided to buy their own system. While it still may be too early to tell, he is optimistic about the positive effect the new EMR will have on his practice and for his patients.

"Practicing medicine, particularly in primary care, is very scary these days. No longer are we in a situation where we can feel reassured that if we come to work each day we're going to be able to pay for all we need to pay for." Malpractice costs have kept him and many doctors from implementing these systems, due to the up-front cost to their practice.

Their system also cannot access information from the hospital, and the hospital cannot access information from them. Even with his new EMR, if one of his patients goes to the hospital, there is no way for him to know what happened there unless they fax the chart to his office, since the hospital's system is still paper-based. Plus, Dr. Levy's EMR system does not allow him to search for information like a diagnosis for a patient with a certain set of problems, e-mail information to patients, or catch possibly harmful drug interactions.

Dr. Levy hopes one day to have the ability to fully utilize his system to provide all his patients with optimal care, while also being able to recover his costs with a more efficient system.

Mother Copes with Frustration

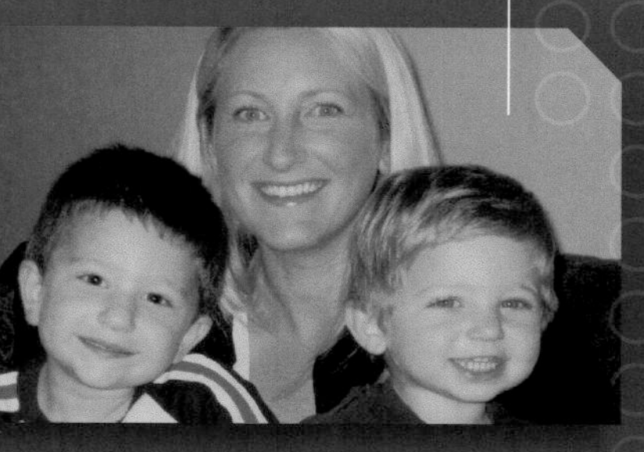

PROFILE:

Melissa Santini
FLORIDA

~ Mother with Chronically Ill Child Desperate for Electronic Health Records

"I constantly have to lug records around with me. Nobody is interacting. I'm so overwhelmed by all the information, paperwork, blood tests, hospital visits ... and I still don't have an answer. I am beyond frustrated."

– Melissa Santini

There are a lot of things that are difficult to understand about her son's health. Why his doctors can't see a simple list of his medications and test results should not be one of them.

Melissa Santini's two-year-old son, Rocco, has six doctors and counting—not to mention other healthcare providers. When he was just 10 months old, Rocco developed severe digestive problems. Since that time, he's been referred to several specialists. After exhaustive and repeated testing, doctors have ruled out certain diseases—but no one has been able to diagnose his condition, which continues unabated. He has also struggled with asthma since he was only a few months old.

Melissa is at the breaking point. She carries around an expandable file full of Rocco's records, x-rays, and test results. Every time Rocco goes to a new doctor or new medical facility she has to repeat the litany of his medical care and fill out the same forms numerous times while trying to hang onto two-year-old Rocco and her healthy and energetic four-year-old son. With the incredible volume of information she has been forced to memorize, she can barely remember what happened with Rocco just last week, let alone recount the chronology of his entire medical history.

She cannot understand why all his information is not available on one digital record, or why she has to fill out the same paper forms every time she takes Rocco in for an appointment. She is incensed that in today's world, a nurse writes Rocco's weight down on a yellow sticky note and loses it before it gets entered in his paper chart. She wants to be able to access her son's medical test results on-line, rather than wait for days for a doctor to call her back.

She is also concerned that her son has to repeat invasive tests. "They referred us to a pediatric GI doctor, and he basically did all of the same tests that the other doctor just did. I had to wait another two or three weeks for him to retest all of the things that had just been tested, even though I had copies of them that I had to pay for from my pediatrician's office. That just made me furious." She is concerned that there's no way for all the doctors to get together to review all the medical records. She is livid ... and her son is not getting any better.

A Life Threatening Close Call

"Having the information about my medical records on the computer might have saved my life."

– Richard Peck

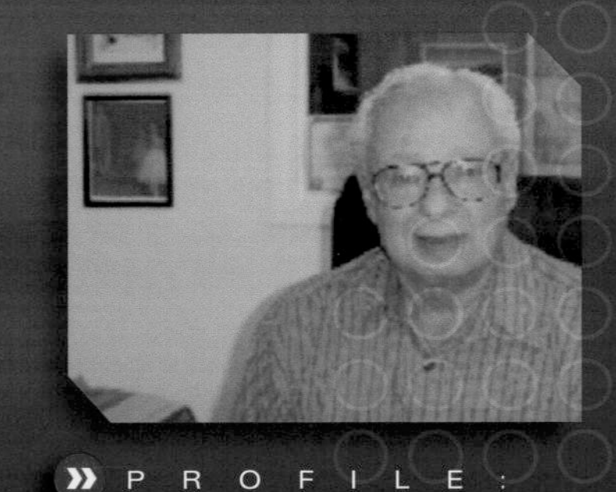

» PROFILE:

Richard Peck

ILLINOIS

~ 80-Year-Old Man Says Electronic Health Information Proved Useful in an Emergency

Richard Peck loves to enjoy life. That is why he was surprised when his health suddenly took a turn for the worse while he was changing doctors. Fortunately for him, his new doctor was able to transfer all his information from the previous doctor and created an electronic medical record for Richard.

Richard fell ill while visiting Florida in April 2005, following a major surgery in January. He started feeling unwell while still in Florida but decided to wait until he got back home to visit his doctor. By that time, he was quite ill with a fever and irregular heartbeat. "I was just in terrible shape, and my doctor called an ambulance service, printed out everything about my medical records, which he gave to the ambulance service. By the time I got to the emergency room they had already contacted the urologist who had done the surgery on me. The doctors had a course of action planned out. They did everything right."

Richard was later told that if he had delayed going to the doctor, he would have died within 24 hours. The fact that his entire medical history was available to the hospital and printed out for the ambulance crew allowed the emergency room to have the course of treatment available when he arrived, saving precious time. For him, it meant more than the convenience of having to repeat his medical history. Access to electronic information meant the difference between life and death for Richard.

mean the loss of potentially important data when someone returns later to find that he or she cannot read the information written. In addition, pharmacists may make mistakes filling prescriptions because of illegible handwriting, or may have to spend extra time calling the doctor's office to get clarification about a prescription. The Institute for Safe Medication Practices estimates that pharmacists make more than 150 million calls to physicians each year to clarify what was written on prescriptions.[1]

- **Patients with chronic conditions cannot easily get the information they need.** Short of conducting their own research in a medical library, patients have no way of learning how to take better care of themselves or better understand their condition in light of details from their medical test results and treatment.

- **Recalls are slowed or may be incomplete.** When medical devices and drugs are recalled, either by the Food and Drug Administration or by the companies that manufacture them, there is no system in place to quickly and efficiently contact physicians and their patients to advise them what to do.

- **We are missing out on powerful public health tools, especially against bioterrorism.** Healthcare monitoring based on information technology is crucial in fighting bioterrorism, tracking disease, and supporting medical research. This information should be available quickly, on a day-to-day basis, and accessible at our nation's hospitals and research facilities.

Americans Embracing Technology

People initially bought cell phones for emergencies only, but today they are in common use. We wonder how we got along without them. Consumers may initially demand connectivity because it seems like a vital element of a safe and efficient healthcare system—which it is. But once it is in place, the convenience and security it makes possible will make it hard for us to imagine what life was like before it.

Barriers to connecting health information

A connected healthcare system will overcome a lot of challenges, but implementing that system brings about challenges of its own:

- **Fear of change.** Doctors' methods and work habits are key to their ability to help patients. Doctors understand implicitly that changing those habits can affect the quality of care they deliver; but once a physician has embraced technology, he or she can help drive further interoperable efforts to improve healthcare.

[1] Institute for Safe Medication Practices. "Electronic Prescribing Can Reduce Medication Errors." August 2005. <http://www.ismp.org/msaarticles/whitepaper.html>

- **Cost.** A question from every healthcare provider is: Where will the money come from to pay for this? The answer is that some will come in the form of direct savings and some in the form of governmental and private incentives.

- **Connecting vendors.** Vendors—the companies that sell electronic health-care systems—often try to protect their market share by making sure their systems will not interact with anybody else's system. Vendors have financial incentives to work against each other, not with each other. But with the establishment of common standards, and as healthcare providers and the public realize that interoperable systems can save lives, pressure will grow for vendors to give their clients systems that can connect to one another. And, since the technology already exists, vendors will be able to provide connected systems faster and more easily than ever before.

- **Lack of standards.** Besides allowing vendors to create systems that don't "talk" to each other, the lack of standards discourages significant investment or effort toward an interoperable healthcare system. The Institute of Electrical and Electronics Engineers sets standards for computers and Underwriters Laboratories ensures that appliances meet safety specifications. Without an industry-recognized body for healthcare, the government will need to set those standards, coordinate their establishment among groups now pursuing them, or act as a catalyst for the creation of standards through some other method.

Legal considerations

Legal considerations are of special concern, especially regarding those laws that make it illegal to set up business deals that would promote interoperability. The Inspector General for the Department of Health and Human Services has addressed the Federal "anti-kickback" law:

> On the books since 1972, the Federal anti-kickback law's main purpose is to protect patients and the Federal healthcare programs from fraud and abuse by curtailing the corrupting influence of money on healthcare decisions. Straightforward but broad, the law states that anyone who knowingly and willfully receives or pays anything of value to influence the referral of Federal healthcare program business, including Medicare and Medicaid, can be held accountable for a felony. Violations of the law are punishable by up to five

years in prison, criminal fines up to $25,000, administrative civil money penalties up to $50,000, and exclusion from participation in Federal healthcare programs.[2]

Changes in the law created "safe harbors":

> Because the law is broad on its face, concerns arose among healthcare providers that some relatively innocuous—and in some cases even beneficial—commercial arrangements are prohibited by the anti-kickback law. Responding to these concerns, Congress in 1987 authorized the Department to issue regulations designating specific "safe harbors" for various payment and business practices that, while potentially prohibited by the law, would not be prosecuted....
>
> Safe harbors immunize certain payment and business practices that are implicated by the anti-kickback statute from criminal and civil prosecution under the statute. To be protected by a safe harbor, an arrangement must fit squarely in the safe harbor. Failure to comply with a safe harbor provision does not mean that an arrangement is per se illegal. Compliance with safe harbors is voluntary, and arrangements that do not comply with a safe harbor must be analyzed on a case-by-case basis for compliance with the anti-kickback statute.[3]

Safe harbors such as those addressing investments in large, publicly held healthcare companies or investments in small healthcare joint ventures, referral services, and certain settings in managed care need revisiting to remove roadblocks that discourage physicians, hospitals, other healthcare providers, and payers from working together to invest in interoperability.[4]

In addition, the "Stark Law" merits adjustment, either by statute or by regulatory clarification. By prohibiting referral of Medicare patients between physicians who have a financial relationship, the law not only cuts down on kickbacks—a desirable goal—but also makes it impossible for doctors and hospitals to join

[2] Office of Inspector General, Office of Public Affairs. *Fact Sheet: Federal Anti-Kickback Law and Regulatory Safe Harbors.* DHHS. November 1999.
[3] Ibid.
[4] Ibid.

together to acquire interoperable systems at anything but considerable financial sacrifice.[5] Greater precision is needed.

Connecting around the world

- **The United States is far behind other countries.** Several countries have already invested in electronic tools to reduce costs and improve healthcare. Many countries are now developing strategies and investing in interoperable tools to connect their health systems and reap even greater benefits from information technologies. Although the United States leads the world in healthcare spending per capita, our technology lags far behind other nations.

“Americans are spending $1.7 trillion on healthcare every year, accounting for 15.3 percent of our gross domestic product, at an average cost of $5,670 per person. Our lagging health IT infrastructure compounds the problem, contributing to fragmentation, waste, and inefficiency.”

Statement by Senate Majority Leader Bill Frist and Senator Hillary Rodham Clinton

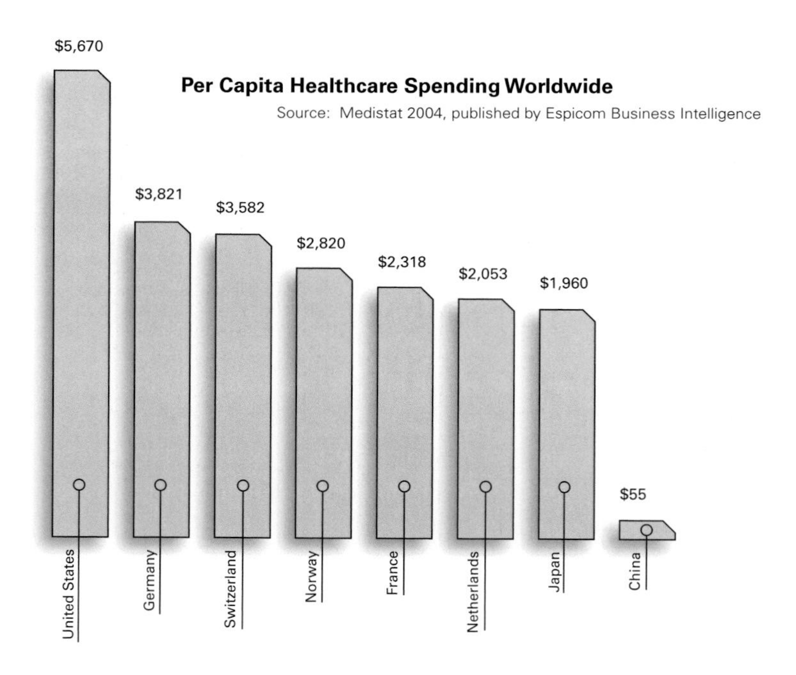

- **The United States leads the world in healthcare spending per capita.** Germany, in second place, spends roughly 60 percent of what the United States spends. France, in fifth place, spends about 40 cents per person for every dollar spent in America.[6]

[5] American Academy of Physical Medicine and Rehabilitation. *Stark II Analysis and Summary: Introduction.* 2005. <http://www.aapmr.org/hpl/pmrprac/starkb.htm>

[6] Information from Medistat 2004, published by Espicom Business Intelligence.

Deaths Due to Mistakes in Surgical and Medical Care

Deaths/100,000 Pop.
(Standardized Rate)

Source:
OECD HEALTH DATA 2005,
June 2005

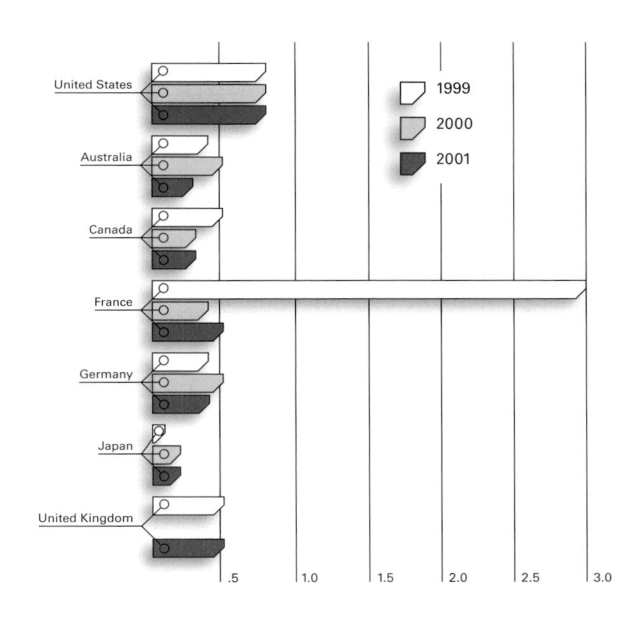

We're Not the Best

(Rank in Surveys of 1,400 Adults and 750 Sicker Adults; Ranking of 0 is the Worst, Ranking of 5 is the Best)

Data:
2004 Commonwealth Fund International Health Policy Survey of Adults Experiences with Primary Care

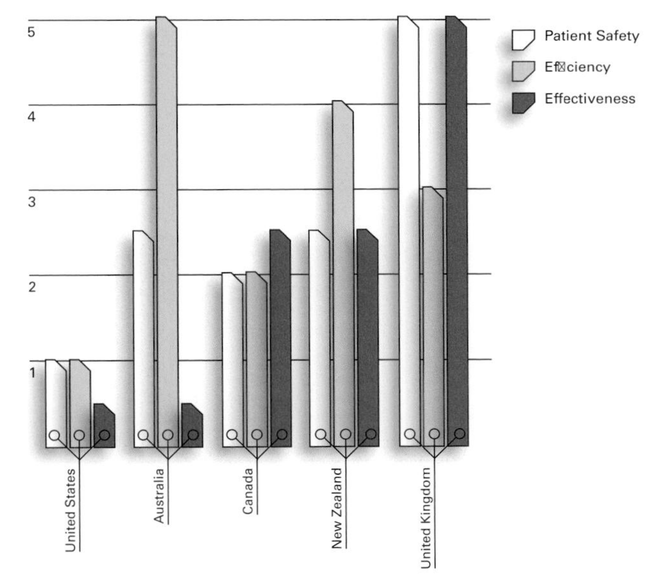

❝It may seem a strange principle to enunciate as the very first requirement in a hospital that it should do the sick no harm.❞

Florence Nightingale, Founded Modern Nursing and Helped Improve the Care Provided by Hospitals (1820 – 1910)

- **Yet the United States is far behind the world in quality of care and has the highest death rate due to medical error.** The Nation is behind the United Kingdom, Australia, Canada, and New Zealand in patient safety and efficiency of treatment.[7]

[7] 2004 Commonwealth Fund International Health Policy Survey of Adults Experiences with Primary Care, conducted March through May 2004.
<http://www.cmwf.org/surveys/surveys_show.htm?doc_id=24540>

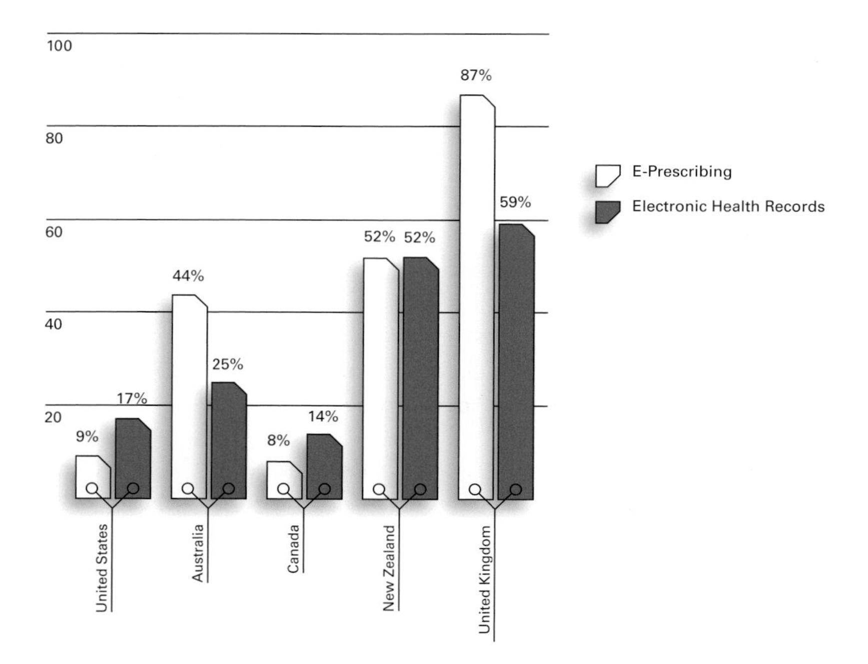

- **One reason for all the spending and the lack of success may be that the U.S. healthcare system lacks connectivity.** Only 17 percent of physicians in America use electronic healthcare records, and only nine percent use electronic prescription systems (e-prescribing). Yet in the United Kingdom, nearly six out of 10 physicians use electronic health records, as do about half of the physicians in New Zealand and Australia.[8]

Nations on their way to interoperability

- **United Kingdom:** The United Kingdom uses electronic healthcare records, but interoperability is limited. Successes in interoperability include exchanging pathology reports and sharing emergency information.[9] The common care record enables all of England to link up health information and produce integrated information about a person's state of well-being.[10]

[8] Information from the Harris Interactive Survey. 2001.

[9] British Computer Society. "Comprehensive Computerised Primary Care Records Are an Essential Component of Any National Health Information Strategy: Report from an International Consensus Conference." *Informatics in Primary Care* 12 (2004): 255–64.

[10] United Kingdom Department of Health. "A Guide to the National Program for Information Technology." *NHS Connecting for Health* <http://www.connectingforhealth.nhs.uk/>

- **New Zealand:** New Zealand uses electronic healthcare records, but interoperability is limited. Yet "New Zealand has many of the ... components [necessary for interoperability]: secure health information networking ... a unique patient identifier, well-developed privacy and security legislation, and a national standards organization."[11] "The New Zealand health sector ... is second only to the United Kingdom in terms of primary care use of electronic healthcare records, double that achieved to date in Australia (25 percent) and triple that of the U.S. (17 percent).[12]

- **Sweden:** Sweden's healthcare system is widely digitized, but not able to freely exchange information. Still, more than 90 percent of general practitioners use electronic healthcare records.[13]

- **Canada:** Canada has committed over a billion dollars to the development and implementation of interoperable electronic health records, and aims to have infrastructure solutions in place in half of Canadian jurisdictions by 2010.[14]

- **Denmark:** Demark has had an interoperable system since the late 1980s. Currently, the majority of general practitioners, laboratories, and hospitals are connected to one another, although patient referrals and a few other types of messages are still sent on paper.[15]

[11] Karolyn Kerr. "The Electronic Health Record in New Zealand–Part 1." *Health Care and Informatics Review Online.* 8, no. 1. March 2004. <http://www.enigma.co.nz/hcro/website/index.cfm?fuseaction=articledisplay&featureid=040304 >

[12] Ibid.

[13] "Increasing use of electronic prescriptions in Sweden." *European eGovernment News.* April 27, 2005. <www.europa.eu.int/idabc/en/document/4221/353>

[14] "About Infoway." *Canada Health Infoway, 2004.* August 2005. <http://www.infoway-inforoute.ca/aboutinfoway/index.php?lang=en>

[15] ACCA and Medcom, in collaboration with the European Commission Information Society Directorate-General. *The Cost of Electronic Patient Referrals in Denmark Summary Report.* 2004.

The Solution—Interoperability

"The first rule of any technology used in business is that automation applied to an efficient operation will magnify the efficiency. The second is that automation applied to an inefficient operation will magnify the inefficiency."

Bill Gates

A System for Biosecurity

The Center for Biosecurity at the University of Pittsburgh Medical Center (UPMC) is a model for preparing for outbreaks of disease. Its system is an inbound call center for medical information. The call center allows UPMC to know what hospitals within the network have open beds or other resources that can be shared. All 7,000 physicians in the UPMC system can call a number and speak to an expert within minutes. Such a system can also serve as a command and control center should a disaster occur, having been tested in emergencies including fires, floods, and breakdowns in hospital ventilation systems. Western Pennsylvania healthcare providers, public health officials, and law enforcement officers can access the system.[16]

Don't reform! Transform instead

Healthcare must always be about people, not about a system. Even though people working in the healthcare system have great concern for patients, there are not always ways built into the system to encourage personalized attention and "second looks" at difficult choices. However, a connected system of health information would make that more possible by creating new and better ways to personalize information and interact with medical information. How? By making critical information more readily available for review on an individual basis.

A connected system of healthcare information will be a major shift—but it will come about through incremental change. Those changes will be more than automated or more efficient versions of what we already do. There will be new ways to support and even provide healthcare: replacements and refinements for existing processes, procedures, and work habits that will improve outcomes.

An interoperable system will enable faster and more efficient care by connecting the healthcare providers who take care of you with critical, personalized information. It will better integrate research, new best practices, and pharmaceutical information into the common practice of medicine. As new technology makes your health more a part of the decision of treatment, an interoperable system will make your information available in a timely way. And the concept of evidence-based care will become a more integral part of the practice of medicine.

The push for making medical records systems "talk" to one another is focused on the needs of patients, doctors, nurses, and others involved in treatment, allowing for personalization, adaptability, and individual choice on all parts.

[16] Fred Baldwin. "Nine Tech Trends." *Healthcare Informatics Online* (February 2005): 13.

Views from the Floor - The Nurse Perspective

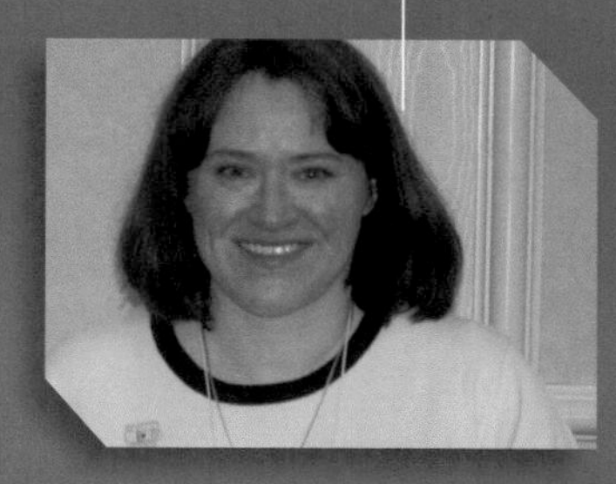

PROFILE:

Holly Sox
RN, RAC-C
SOUTH CAROLINA

~ Long-Term Care Nurse at a County-Owned Rural Facility, and Devoted Mother of an Epileptic Child

"The lack of electronic information exchange has hindered or delayed long-term healthcare. At the facility I work in, a high percentage of the residents have dementia and are thus unable to give reliable health history. Approximately one-fourth of the residents have no close family members available to give medical history to providers. Thus, upon admission, the facility is often left with only the records that are sent from the hospital. One new resident went for three weeks without medication for glaucoma because the diagnosis could not be confirmed upon her admission. Another resident underwent unnecessary blood draws for lab tests that had already been performed, but the results were unavailable and care had to be given. I often will spend hours trying to find the records that are needed for care planning and delivery. How nice it would be if I didn't have to do that and could devote that time to patient care instead.

Also, as the mother of a child with epilepsy, my concern about this issue is multiplied exponentially. My son has been on four different seizure medications and has had three different types of seizures. He has been transported by ambulance with prolonged seizures twice. It frightens me to think of him being taken to a different hospital where he is unknown to the staff. A delay in appropriate treatment for him could be life-threatening."

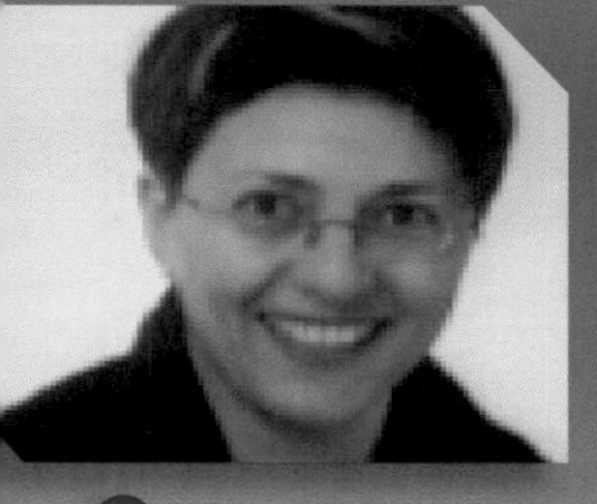

PROFILE:

Helga Bragadóttir
PhD, RN
IOWA

~ Working with the Parents of Children with Cancer

"For four months a group of 17 mothers and fathers whose children had been diagnosed with cancer participated in a support group using their e-mail. Parents enjoyed being able to communicate with other parents who were going through the same experience. They felt less isolated and less alone with their problems. They felt like they were 'all in the same boat.' Some of these parents lived far away from other families of children diagnosed with cancer, and for these families the support group seemed very important."

Views from the Floor - The Nurse Perspective

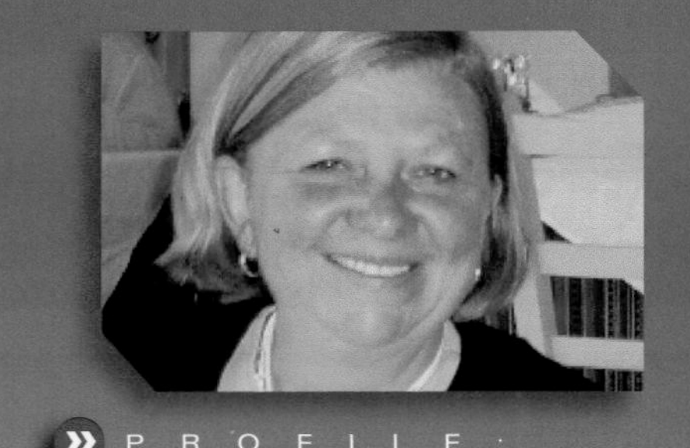

PROFILE:

Nancy Gorsha
BSN, MBA
PENNSYLVANIA

~ Emergency Department Nurse Testifies to Life-changing Patient Care Through Electronic Health Information

"A patient electronic health record went live at our hospital on September 11, 2004. Almost immediately we recognized improvements. A patient record could be viewed by multiple healthcare providers simultaneously and from different areas of the hospital. The physicians were instantly alerted to patient allergies, and a multidisciplinary plan of care could be initiated and later updated as the patient's condition warranted.

Our Emergency Department (ED) has multiple integrated software applications that help us deliver quality care for the urgent and emergent patient. These applications include a patient and staff locating system, a patient tracking board, a telephone system that connects the patient's call bell to his nurse's portable phone, and cardiac monitors with individualized alarms. The ED tracking board, visible only by ED staff, lists patients with their chief complaints, isolation status, and length of stay in the ED, as well as other useful patient information.

On one particular evening, the ED attending physician noted on the electronic ED tracking board the arrival of a patient with the chief complaint of 'sudden loss of vision, right eye.' The physician, looking at the patient locating system floor plan of the ED noted this particular patient was in the ED waiting room. The physician immediately walked out to the waiting room, questioned the patient further, and swiftly brought the patient back to the ED for triage, care, treatment, and services. The physician performed an eye exam and identified a 'central retinal artery occlusion,' a true emergency situation where the patient could go blind in that eye without immediate attention. The physician checked the electronic record for patient allergies and entered a medication order in the bedside computer, and the nurse administered the medication and documented it in the electronic medication administration record. The ED staff contacted the ophthalmologist on call. The ophthalmologist was at the hospital within 15 minutes; he removed water from the anterior chamber of the patient's eye, and the patient was able to see light in a matter of minutes."

Navigating the Paper Maze

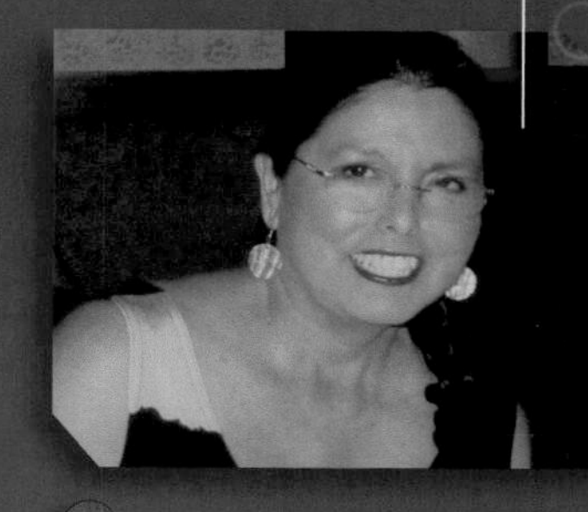

» PROFILE:

Juanita Pahdopony-Mithlo
OKLAHOMA

~ A College Professor and Chronic Disease Patient Struggles to Connect the Details of Her Health History for Electronic Health Records

Juanita Pahdopony-Mithlo began having health problems in 1987, but she was not diagnosed with scleroderma until 2000. Both before and after her diagnosis, Juanita has been the victim of a technologically challenged healthcare system. The inefficiency has only added to her discomfort and prolonged the pain of her condition.

Because her disease is systemic, Juanita has seen multiple doctors and had countless tests performed. She has traveled from doctor to doctor, making her care even more complicated. Juanita has been forced to become a walking file cabinet in order to maintain her volatile health. "I have a big file on myself, and I have to haul medical records from place to place. My doctor from the Indian Hospital has sent me to the rheumatologist. I normally don't see the same rheumatologist from year to year. They've asked me to bring my last few months' charts and copies of my medical records, so I hand-carry them to the rheumatologist." To each new doctor, she brings copies of her extensive medical records, test results, and medication lists, and must retell her entire 20-year ordeal. Most times, a new doctor has no idea what her background is before she walks in the door and plops down her stack of papers and files.

She tells a horror story about seeing a new gastroenterologist for reflux problems associated with her disease. "They did a test on me over and over and over again. And they said, 'We can't understand what's going on ....' I overheard them talking, and I thought they knew what I was there for. They couldn't understand why it wasn't working. I didn't have very much movement in my lower esophagus when I swallowed. Finally, I said, 'I have scleroderma,' and they said, 'Oh! That explains it! Of course.' I thought they should have known why I was there, but apparently they did not have that piece of the puzzle. I had to do that particular test pushing that tube down my throat and into my stomach, at least three times before they figured it out."

Juanita lives in constant fear that the one doctor who knows all about her condition and helps her to coordinate her care will move away. "Since I have my doctor, I feel a lot better knowing that at least one person is somewhat following my case. It scares me to think about what I would do if he left."

"I have a big file on myself, and I have to haul medical records from place to place."

– Juanita Pahdopony-Mithlo

Did You Know?

~ A study by The Commonwealth Fund shows that 63 percent of adults 19 and older do not have a regular doctor for more than five years at a time.

Source: 2004 Commonwealth Fund International Health Policy Survey of Adults' Experiences with Primary Care; www.cmwf.org/surveys/surveys_show.htm?doc_id=245240

Mac vs. PC All Over Again

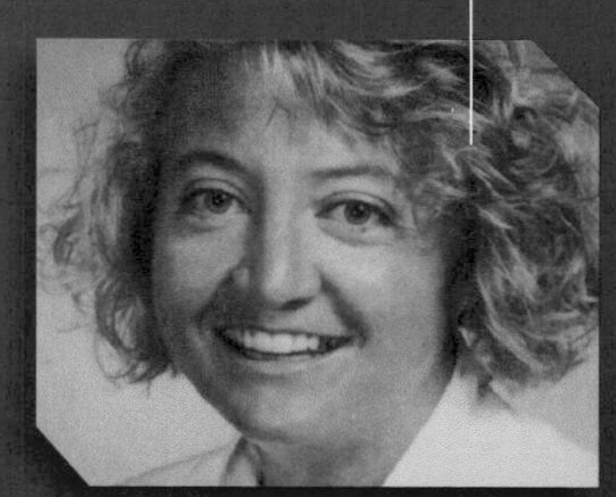

» PROFILE:

Maureen Mays, M.D.
WISCONSIN

~ A Cardiologist with a New EMR System Discovers That Access Without Interoperability Can Be Meaningless

Dr. Maureen Mays looks forward to the day when she will have all her patients' information right in front of her during an appointment. Unfortunately, that day is not today for many reasons. Dr. Mays has discovered that even having an electronic medical record (EMR) system sometimes isn't enough. Interoperability—being able to have her computer system share information with the computer systems of other hospitals, labs, and doctors—sometimes means the difference between a healthy patient and a sick one.

Dr. Mays' HMO started implementing an EMR system a short time ago, and she expects it will still be another year or two until it is fully working. But she is very optimistic about the benefits of the system once it is completed. "Our HMO has four stand-alone clinics, plus the hospital, and then we have satellite clinics. It's a huge area, and it will be amazing when we don't have to have charts sent to us from remote locations, and we will be able to instantly access information when a patient comes in."

One of the problems she has run into early on with the new system is a lack of interoperability. Even though she has EMRs for most of her patients, Dr. Mays orders some very complex labs for some of her patients from labs all across the country. When she sends samples out, most labs cannot send the test results back to her in a format that can be put into the EMR. The result: any doctor that looks at that patient's medical records will not see the whole picture. They will have to go "clicking around" to find lab results that were scanned into the computer and won't see them next to all the other lab results.

"It's funny ... it's sort of like back in the 80s with PCs versus Macintoshes. There was no way they linked. Over the last 20 years that's been resolved. I hope this doesn't take 20 years."

– Maureen Mays, M.D.

One thing Dr. Mays is not concerned about is the security of electronic records. After working with paper records for so long, she knows firsthand just how unsafe they really are. "First of all, they're traveling around in cars. Second of all, charts are exploding all the time! You're walking down the hall and a chart will break open and papers go flying everywhere. And third, even when I'm walking down the hall in the clinic, somebody could look down and look at the name on the side of the chart. So I don't know ... I'm not well-versed in Internet security or in electronic record security, but I don't think it should be a big concern."

Well on the Way

"The laws that inhibit this [interoperability] need to be changed."

– Peter Gross, M.D.

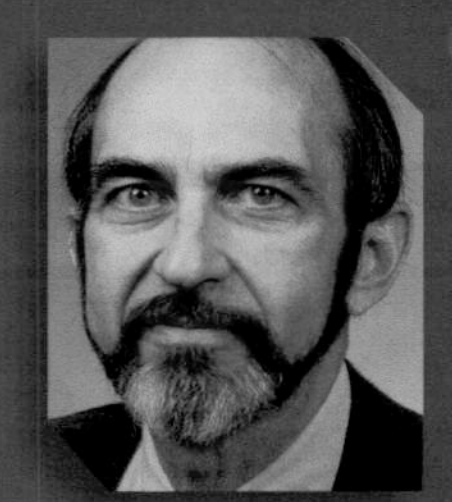

» PROFILE:

Peter Gross, M.D.

NEW JERSEY

~ Changes to HIPAA and Stark Are Needed to Make Interoperability a Reality

Dr. Peter Gross is well-versed in the challenges and benefits of having health information technology (IT) in hospitals and doctors' offices across the country. He teaches medical students about the nuances of such systems and has worked with his own hospital and other organizations to help doctors and nurses get over the initial hump of starting to use these systems in their day-to-day practice. Dr. Gross believes that, with the right legal reforms, health IT can finally give providers the tools they need to practice better, safer medicine.

"I think that the laws that inhibit this [interoperability] need to be changed. There are [Stark] laws that prohibit doctors from cooperating with hospitals and other organizations because it's viewed as collusion. That has to be dealt with. The HIPAA laws have to be dealt with, too, so that they don't impair having a nationwide free exchange of information."

"There are a number of companies out there that are helping us get into e-prescribing. With these systems, if a patient is ready to leave the hospital, I could write all the prescriptions on the computer and send them off to the patient's pharmacy, wherever it is. When a patient is admitted to another hospital in our area—or eventually anywhere in the country—I could go onto the computer, enter the patient's name, birth date, and whatever other identifiers are necessary, and call up all of the current medications the patient is taking. When a patient comes into the hospital and they say, 'I'm on this blue pill for hypertension and this red pill for heart failure,' that doesn't help me. Having a nationwide system where we could find out what medications the patient is on would be very helpful."

Dr. Gross emphasizes that when using these computerized systems to record information about a patient's visit, the most important things to document are not billing codes, but vital information about a patient's health conditions. "When patients go to two or more different doctors, the doctors could enter a brief summary note about what they did during the visit. That summary note should include only critical information that the physician thinks is important to put there, otherwise you'll have so much verbiage that it will be worthless. What goes there should

A system that works best for everyone will be built with allegiance to no particular method, program, or model, but with flexibility for the choices and needs of patients, doctors, nurses, and other healthcare providers.

The convenience of connecting

- **Allows doctors and other healthcare providers to share medical history, lab results, and other pertinent information.** The ability to share information makes consultations easier and permits the consulting physician to review the complete picture of a patient's healthcare as needed. Patients can follow up on the meaning of lab results; record comments about their diet, exercise, and other lifestyle choices; and address questions to their doctors without having to schedule an appointment or a phone call.

- **Easier to secure vaccination records for camp and school enrollment and provide records to other doctors.** Schools and camps usually require confirmation of vaccinations. An interoperable system means the necessary records are available to any authorized person. Treatment while away from home or after a move no longer requires the physical transportation of records, just authorization by the patient for a new healthcare provider to access health information.

- **Better support for adults caring for aging parents.** Adults caring for their aging parents—especially those doing so from far away—can more easily review material made available by their parent's doctor, discuss medical choices, monitor the parent's compliance with a course of treatment, check to see that prescriptions are filled, and stay in contact with on-site caregivers and nurses.

- **Easier to work with doctors after diagnosis and treatment.** An interoperable system allows patients to more easily contact their doctors to confirm adherence to a treatment plan, to ask questions, and to learn more about their condition.

“Information technology is a pivotal part of transforming our healthcare system. We are at a critical juncture. Working in close collaboration, the Federal government and private sector can drive changes that will lead to fewer medical errors, lower costs, less hassle, and better care.”

Mike Leavitt, Secretary, Department of Health and Human Services

Confidentiality is easier to preserve

- **Easier to limit unauthorized access.** Connected systems provide more consistent and measurable security than paper-based systems. Instead of filing cabinets, locks, and guards, electronic records are kept behind log-ins or biometric sensors.

- **Easier to track who views your medical information.** Anyone who attempts to log-in to the system and review private healthcare information will have to provide authorization. Unlike paper records, which can be misplaced or copied, electronic records can be constantly monitored and their access tracked. Patients concerned about the unauthorized release of personal information will realize a level of security that is, in healthcare, thus far unknown—because even those who attempt unauthorized access will have left their electronic "fingerprints" in the system.

Easier and more secure access

- **Records are always available with instant access.** Interoperable electronic health information systems provide constant access to data for authorized users. If a doctor or patient needs a medical history, lab results, or radiological images at any time, the information can be reviewed instantaneously.

- **Records less likely to be lost.** Electronic healthcare information stored on an interoperable system will be preserved in backup copies, so it is highly unlikely that records would be lost.

Improved quality of care

- **Notes, prescriptions, and data are always readable.** Paper records are written at least partly by hand, but electronic records are stored as digitized text, visual image files, and matrices of standard options. There will never be any doubt about text recorded in the electronic information.

- **Patients with chronic conditions can take better care of themselves.** Those with chronic conditions such as diabetes can benefit from improved interaction with their healthcare providers and increased access to healthcare

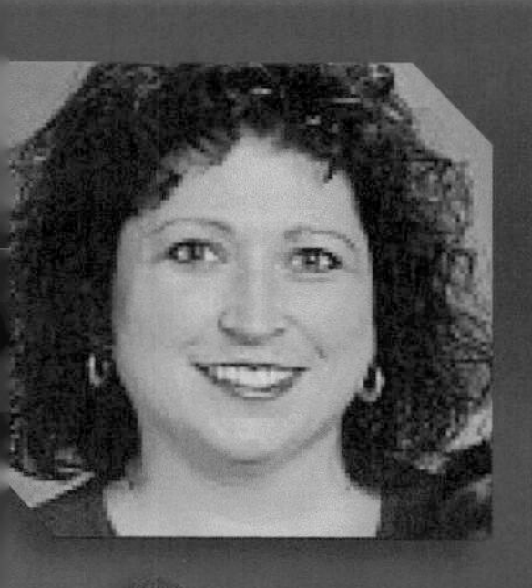

» PROFILE:

Jeanie Stahl, RPh
SOUTH DAKOTA

~ A Pharmacist in Rural South Dakota Says Using Information Systems Should Be Common Sense

Prescription for Efficiency

Jeanie Stahl runs the only pharmacy in a rural county in South Dakota. Jeanie works with all the doctors in the area, but her favorite to work with is Dr. Tad Jacobs, who started using an electronic medical information system about a year and a half ago. She loves it.

When she receives a prescription from his office, either by fax or e-mail, the patient's information and the name and dosage of the drug are all complete and readable, saving her hours of phone calls back and forth to clarify information. "That part of it alone has really improved patient care. In the past, they would call in a prescription, and if you didn't quickly think to ask them all the information you might possibly need, then you had to call them back again and get the birth date to figure out which patient it was. There was a lot of time wasted."

"With the two other doctors I work with, I'm used to reading their handwriting, but there are some days when the only way I can figure out what the prescription is to fax it back to the clinic it came from and say, 'What is this supposed to be, because I can't read anything?' It's very scary."

"My electronic system is also able to check drug interactions for all my customers. Every time I add a prescription to a particular person's profile, it automatically screens through everything. Then it gives me the option, depending on the level of severity, to hit a button and it faxes that right over to Dr. Jacobs, and it tells him that there is an interaction with something else they're on. It's very handy, especially because you do have people going to different doctors and specialists, and they are not always good about saying, 'I have this, and I'm taking this from another doctor.'"

With countless new drugs coming into the market all the time, Jeanie sees the use of information technology as a vital part of practicing healthcare nowadays. "It is not humanly possible for the doctor or the pharmacist to catch all the possible complications. With so many new drugs available, the people at the drug companies coming up with new names are not thinking about how similar the names are to each other. Throw in bad handwriting, and you're asking for a mistake. It's very scary to think that poor handwriting can easily result in a very grave outcome for a patient."

"It's very scary to think that poor handwriting can easily result in a very grave outcome for a patient."

– Jeanie Stahl, RPh

Did You Know?

~ According to the Institute for the Study of Healthcare Organizations and Transactions, over 150 million phone calls requesting clarification from pharmacists to physicians are made annually due to the physician's handwriting being illegible.

Source: John F. Kihlstrom, PhD, Copyright (c) 2000 Institute for the Study of Healthcare Organizations & Transactions, Bad Penmanship Can Lead to Medical Errors; www.institute-shot.com

"Patients deserve the same quality of care in rural areas that they can get anywhere else. In order to do this, I have to be able to have a free flow of information between the tertiary facility and my primary care facility."

– Tad Jacobs, DO

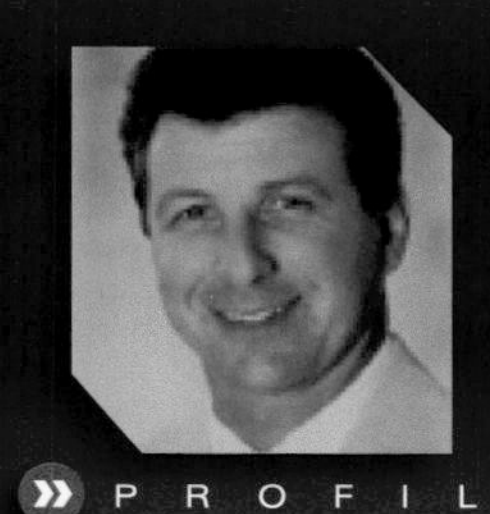

PROFILE:

Tad Jacobs, DO

SOUTH DAKOTA

~ Physician in Rural South Dakota Uses an E-Prescribing System to Ensure His Patients Get the Available Care

The E-Prescribing Difference

Dr. Tad Jacobs' small office in rural South Dakota has been using an e-prescribing system for two years now, and he is already sold. "I went through a lot of frustrations trying to learn the ins and outs of the process, but now that I've gotten used to the system, I probably write 80 to 90 percent of my prescriptions using e-prescribing."

Dr. Jacobs and the other doctor in his practice became part of an e-prescribing pilot program through a larger hospital system about 45 miles away. Dr. Jacobs loves what the new system helps him to do, even though he admits its imperfections. He is able to put prescriptions into the computer, and they are automatically faxed to his patient's pharmacy.

He is also able to keep a record of all the medications a patient is taking, their insurance information, and their allergies. If he tries to prescribe them something they are allergic to, or that might interact with another drug they're taking, the computer alerts him, and he is able to save that patient a possible trip to the emergency room. "One of the biggest frustrations that we have as physicians is knowing at any one time what medicines patients are on—especially when they are seeing multiple doctors. Electronic medical records will eliminate that as a problem."

But the system is not yet perfect, and Dr. Jacobs looks forward with excitement to the day when his system is truly interoperable. "We transfer a lot of patients to our tertiary care center in Sioux Falls. It's frustrated me at times trying to get all the information that we have available on patients down there. You would think that communication between physicians would be a very easy thing, but it's not. We have all the information about the patient on these charts, but the charts can't always go down with them. To have information immediately available if I transfer someone down there would be a huge plus. I see just an incredible waste of dollars from labs and x-rays being duplicated that were already done in rural settings just because they're not available in front of the doc who is seeing the patient at the time."

FACT

~ Sixty-one percent of patients fear being given the wrong medication.

Source: Buckley, Melissa. Improving Drug Prescribing Practices in the Outpatient Setting: A Market Analysis: California HealthCare Foundation, 2002.

information. With an interoperable system, those patients will be able to more easily contact their healthcare providers, allowing those patients to more effectively manage issues of day-to-day care. When healthcare providers establish on-line links to articles and information about various conditions, their patients gain tools for maintaining their health.

- **Notification of recalls can be carried out faster.** When the Federal Drug Administration, a manufacturer, or other authorized party issues recalls or advisories about medical devices and prescription drugs, an interoperable system can help identify and notify doctors and patients far more quickly than an individual search through medical files by healthcare providers.

- **Connectivity makes powerful public-health tools possible.** With an interoperable system, authorized groups can conduct advanced biosurveillance—the acquisition and study of anonymously sourced data for trends, the appearance and movement of disease by geography and demography, the efficacy of treatment, early warnings of epidemic disease outbreak such as West Nile or avian influenza—and ascertain whether trends in data suggest the possibility of biological or chemical attack.

Paving the Way to Interoperability

An interoperable medication record for every American

Having an electronic medication record for every American is a critical step toward achieving true interoperability in healthcare, giving treating physicians the information they need when they need it, allowing more effective care for their patients. It will bring all the medications an individual is currently taking to the doctor's attention at the time important decisions about new prescriptions are being made. With tens of millions of Americans relying on so many different medications to manage everything from elevated blood pressure to high cholesterol, a physician needs a patient's accurate and up-to-date medication list to prescribe the right medication at the right time for an individual's specific health concern, while avoiding the potentially harmful effects of a negative drug interaction.

Consider the following example of how one physician's practice might benefit from a patient's medication record.

2005: A portrait of today's state-of-the-art electronic medical record system

No interoperability

Dr. Vivian Schilling wants to provide her patients with important information about their health. She also wants to have access to information that can help her be a better doctor. She uses an electronic medical record system in her office that allows her to access patient information from her desktop computer, tablet personal computer, handheld computer, or from home. Dr. Schilling is one of the 10 to 30 percent[17] of more than 871,000 practicing physicians in the United States[18] who currently use a full version of an electronic medical record system.

A unique user name and password securely connects Dr. Schilling to a patient's electronic "chart" right in her office, during a visit. While she talks to her patient, she enters information directly into the electronic medical record, documenting every detail of the case as the patient describes symptoms and concerns. She can do so without the potential problem of illegible handwriting because, depending on the device she uses, she can speak, type, or have her writing converted to digitized text.

---

[17] *Advanced Studies in Medicine* 4, no. 8 (2004): 439.

[18] American Medical Association. *Physician Characteristics and Distribution in the U.S., 2005 Edition* and prior editions. < http://www.ama-assn.org/ama/pub/category/12912.html>

Each time Dr. Schilling sees a patient, she reviews and updates the information in the electronic medical record. She also uses the system to view the results of imaging studies and laboratory tests she has ordered to help guide her treatment decisions. And as she determines the best course of care for her patient, the system provides another layer of safety by automatically presenting a series of alerts—potential concerns for a patient that the physician might wish to consider—based on the patient's age, sex, health condition, and medication.

When Dr. Schilling chooses medication, she uses the system's pharmaceutical database, which contains thorough information about each of the drugs she could prescribe. With this tool, she can determine the appropriate prescription and avoid allergic reactions, unnecessary side effects, and potentially harmful interactions between drugs.

The electronic medical record system also gives Dr. Schilling the ability to review all the patients she treats as a single group, so whenever new medication information is released, she can quickly identify all the individuals taking a given medication and quickly provide them with important information that could impact their health. For example, when the U.S. Food and Drug Administration issued a public health advisory about the withdrawal of Vioxx® from the American market, each of Dr. Schilling's patients who were taking Vioxx® were identified through the system and notified within 24 hours to stop taking the medication.

Dr. Schilling understands that patients who feel connected to her as their physician, and who are educated about their own individual health concerns, are more likely to be actively involved in maintaining their health over time. They make better lifestyle choices, tend to eat better, watch their weight, and avoid significant health risks by getting enough exercise and not smoking.

For example, when patient Betsy Clemmons arrives for her first office visit, Dr. Schilling invites her to enroll in a personalized on-line service that provides tools for health management. Describing the system as an "on-line connection to her own electronic medical record," Dr. Schilling tells Betsy about the things she will be able to do, such as viewing information the doctor has entered in the electronic medical record about Betsy's health issues; reviewing information from past appointments, including any patient instructions the doctor recorded; receiving the results of tests almost as soon as they are released; requesting new appointments and prescription renewals; and receiving reminders about when her next health screening or tetanus shot is due—and all this will be available from any Internet connection, any time, day or night.

Perhaps most important, the tool contains links that provide Betsy with reliable information about the issues that matter most to her. For example, Betsy has a history of diabetes in her family. As Dr. Schilling is ordering a blood glucose screening at this first appointment, when Betsy gets home and logs in to the on-line tool, she can click on links to read in detail about diabetes, better understand how she might avoid it, and see how others manage the disease. Of course, Betsy's personal information is encrypted and secure. No one but Betsy, Dr. Schilling, and the nursing and office staff directly involved in Betsy's care can access it.

Although the system significantly improves Dr. Schilling's ability to provide superior medical care, its effectiveness is limited because the information in it is limited to Dr. Schilling's practice. Ideally, a patient's vital medical information should be accessible to any physician treating that patient, no matter where the patient may be when care is needed. Still, Dr. Schilling's system is an important first step toward an interoperable medication record.

2006: Smart personal medication record

Stage 1: Limited interoperability

In 2006, Betsy becomes interested in having her own personal medication record. She wants to include prescriptions from all her physicians, along with over-the-counter medicines she takes on her own—not just prescriptions from Dr. Schilling.

Betsy finds a secure, password-protected on-line service that allows her to enter her medication history and access it at any time. She enters the medications she is currently taking, along with her known allergies, history of drug interactions, and other health conditions. All information will be entered manually by Betsy, but if she enters the Federal Drug Administration's medication product code found on the label of her prescription bottles, official and complete drug information will be automatically linked to Betsy's record. With this, she can be alerted automatically if any of the drugs she is taking are recalled, no matter who prescribed them.

Betsy can grant access to her medication record to anyone she chooses, including physicians and family members. She can print out her medication history when going to a new physician or print out a copy to keep in her wallet in case of an emergency.

The ability for consumers to have a personal medication record is a vital step toward an interoperable medication record. In this stage, anyone who has access to the Web will be able to access their own record 24 hours a day.

2008: Electronic dispensing record

Stage 2: Increased interoperability

In 2008, the medication record becomes more connected to other physicians and information. When Betsy buys medication, the dispensing information is forwarded by the claims adjudicator or pharmacy to a secure clearinghouse. Betsy (and any provider she authorizes) can access this aggregate record of medications via a secure Web site. This automated electronic dispensing record replaces the smart personal medication record of 2006, described in the previous section.

Medicines are now recorded automatically in the record. Betsy doesn't have to remember to do it. All of her providers automatically see what each of them has prescribed. Whenever a medicine is dispensed, it is checked for interactions with Betsy's allergies and with her other medicines. Full information about each medication—including dosing, side effects, interactions, lab conflicts, allergy alerts, disease contraindications, pricing, and drug image identification—is only a click away with this electronic dispensing record. Notification about medication recalls is immediate and automatic.

Betsy and each of her providers will be able to quickly and easily access all drug information in a single, aggregated record. However, the record is still not connected to practice-based e-prescribing systems. Dr. Schilling and any other healthcare provider must open a second display to manually check the aggregated record. During the prescribing process, automatic alerts are still limited to medications prescribed by that practice.

"The only limit to our realization of tomorrow will be our doubts of today."

Franklin D. Roosevelt

2010 and beyond: Interoperable medication record

Stage 3: Complete interoperability

In 2010, Dr. Schilling's office will have a fully interoperable medication record. The electronic medical record of 2005 has been retrofitted to use the standard drug names recognized by all systems. Over the last five years, all of Betsy's other providers have adopted standards-based e-prescribing systems. Providers and pharmacies instantly update each other on every change in medication information and prescriptions in real time. Finally, e-prescribing and dispensing are connected.

Dr. Schilling now has all the advantages of interoperability while maintaining the user-friendly electronic medical record interface of 2005. She can access patient records from home or in the office, allowing her to provide care for patients at any time. For example, when Betsy is admitted to the emergency room, Dr. Schilling, as her primary care physician, is able to connect to Betsy's information from her home. She sees both her outpatient medications and the intravenous solutions being used in the emergency room, and she gives a well-informed opinion of the treatment that should be taken.

Dr. Schilling's electronic medical record allows her to select medications from a drug information database that is updated automatically, at least daily. It includes direct links to all information in the electronic drug label.

With full interoperability now in place, Dr. Schilling can prescribe medications and treat her patients using evidence-based guidelines, concise and easy-to-use clinical care guidelines based on the most updated and accurate medical information available.

For instance, Dr. Schilling often will use evidence-based guidelines in treating pneumonia, asthma, or sinusitis. Having this information available gives Dr. Schilling the information needed to achieve a diagnosis, estimate a prognosis, choose the best therapy, determine potential harm, and provide the highest quality of care in a timely and efficient manner. Information is automatically tailored to avoid drug interactions and comply with the formulary (i.e., the list of medicines qualified for coverage) from the patient's insurer. With an interoperable medication record, the check for interactions is repeated at dispensing to catch changes in the patient's medication list since the prescription was first written.

By 2014, with Betsy's permission, de-identified (i.e., anonymous) abstracts of her medication record, lab tests, and diagnoses are reported to a prescription reporting database for automated postmarket surveillance. Bioinformatics algorithms check regularly for unexpected patterns to help identify safety concerns that might be missed by premarketing trials. These trials often exclude patients who may be at greater risk of certain adverse effects but will likely receive a drug when it is on the market. Premarketing trials that assess safety or efficacy also do not always detect relatively rare adverse events. Through interoperable electronic prescription reporting, the public has the best available tools for storing and analyzing safety reports and possible adverse drug events.

In 2010 and beyond, the benefits of a full interoperable medication record are realized. The building blocks of interoperability that were utilized in 2006, 2008, and 2010 provided the interface, framework, and content for the interoperable medication record. Dr. Schilling and Betsy can now have a better doctor-patient relationship by using all available information technology tools in an interoperable framework.

Timeline to an Interoperable Medication Record for Every American

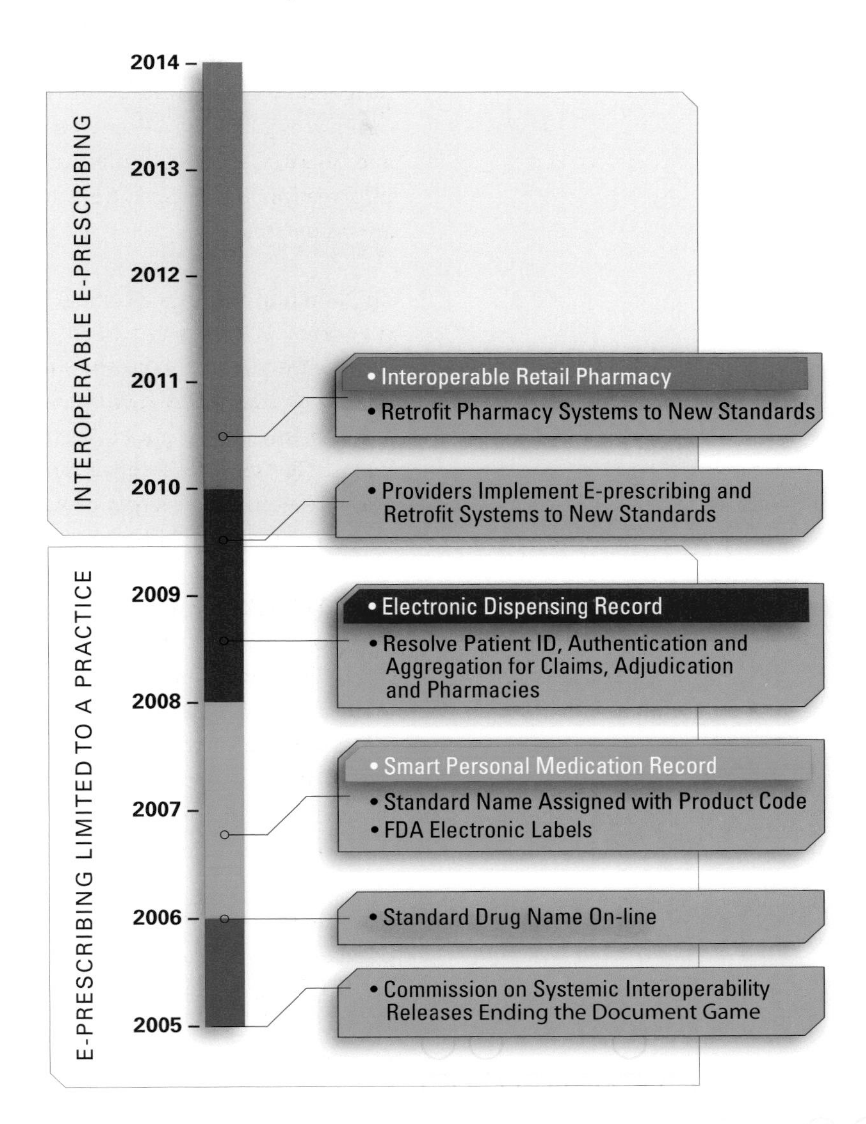

Interoperability—Why Now?

"By computerizing health records, we can avoid dangerous medical mistakes, reduce costs, and improve care."

President George W. Bush

People are dying

In 2000, the Institute of Medicine released a landmark report estimating that 44,000 to 98,000 people die each year from medical errors in this country,[19] many of which can be caused by missing or incorrect information and delays in access. In a more recent study released by Health Grades, Inc. (a healthcare ratings, information, and advisory services company) the number was estimated to be 195,000 people killed by medical error annually.[20] There should be a widespread demand for a connected system, but neither the public nor the healthcare industry is calling for it. This is because many healthcare providers and even more members of the public are not aware that such a system is possible. Put simply, interoperability will save lives.

The government is supporting this initiative right now

For the first time, the President has formally made a high priority of creating a national system of interoperable healthcare records.[21] To support this goal, the Medicare Modernization Act included authorization for the Commission on Systemic Interoperability and a mandate for this report, which is a survey of interoperability and a guide to achieving it. In addition, the Office of the National Coordinator for Health Information Technology has been established to implement the President's vision for widespread adoption of interoperable electronic health records within 10 years.

[19] L. Kohn, J. Corrigan, and M. Donaldson. *To Err Is Human: Building a Safer Health System.* Committee of Health Care in America, Institute of Medicine. 2000.

[20] Ibid.

[21] United States White House, Office of the Press Secretary. *President Discusses Health Care Information Technology Benefits.* January 27, 2005. <http://www.whitehouse.gov/news/releases/2005/01/20050127-7.html>

The technology now exists and is continuously becoming easier to use

Interoperability relies on technologies that already exist: broadband, personal computers, wireless systems, e-prescribing platforms, biometric security devices, electronic imaging software and hardware, touch-sensitive screen input devices, advanced database programming and querying techniques, increased memory and data storage capacity, and simplified network administration software.[22]

Success stories show the system works

Successful implementations cited in this report include efforts in:

- CareGroup, a six-hospital integrated system in Massachusetts;
- Cummings, Georgia, clinics associated with Dr. James Morrow;
- McLeod Regional Hospital, South Carolina;
- Miami, Florida, pediatric cardiology practice of Dr. Evan Zahn;
- New England Health EDI Network;
- Sonoma County, California;
- The Veterans Administration; and
- Wishard Memorial Hospital in Indianapolis, Indiana.

Additionally, more than 300 other efforts and initiatives are identified in the chapter, "Existing Efforts: Connecting the Country."

[22] Kenneth Adler. "Why It's Time to Purchase an Electronic Health Record System." *American Academy of Family Physicians: News & Publications.* November/December 2004. <http://www.aafp.org/fpm/20041100/43whyi.html>

People want interoperability

When people learn about connected systems and their benefits, more than 70 percent of the public say they would use one or more features of a personal health record. In particular:

- Seventy-five percent say they would e-mail their doctor;
- Sixty-nine percent would track immunizations;
- Sixty-nine percent would monitor their record for mistakes;
- Sixty-five percent would transfer information to new doctors; and
- Sixty-three percent would look up and track their own test results.[23]

The technology is ready, and the evidence for the value of connectivity is clear. For the last 27 years, both government and private industry have studied the problem and made hundreds of recommendations.[24] There is still no system in place. It is time to end this aimless trek and implement an interoperable system of healthcare information. Healthcare without connectivity is extracting a price in resources, quality of life, and lost lives too high to continue to pay.

It is time for healthcare providers to receive the tools they have been missing and for consumers to claim the benefits they need and deserve.

[23] Connecting for Health Collaborative. *The Personal Health Working Group: Final Report.* Markle Foundation. July 1, 2003.
[24] See Appendix C for a complete list of past recommendations.

Instant Access, Rapid Results

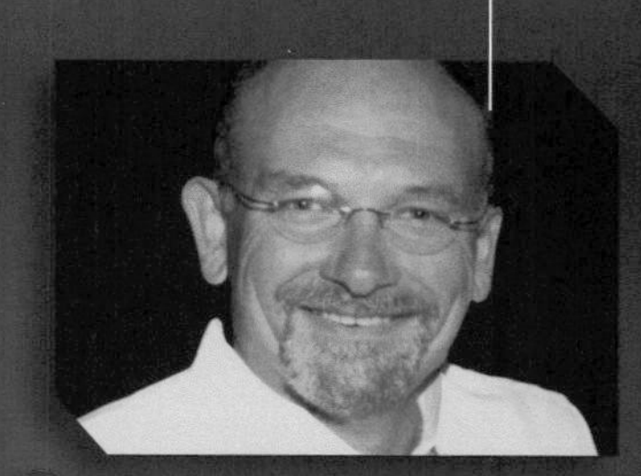

» PROFILE:

James Morrow, M.D.
GEORGIA

~ Significant Improvements in Quality of Care and Efficiency After Implementing an EMR

Dr. James Morrow knows the difficulty of financing a medical practice. However, he has discovered an electronic tool to assist in reducing costs while also providing his patients and staff with tools needed to better manage patient care.

In 1998, Dr. Morrow implemented an electronic medical record (EMR) system at his practice in Cumming, Georgia and costs were immediately cut to both practice and patients. Before the system was in place, a patient visit tracked on paper records cost the practice $112.47. The new EMR system has reduced that cost to just under $80 and has enabled the practice to see three times the number of patients.

More patients require more doctors, and the savings from the EMR enabled his practice to double the number of doctors on staff and to hire additional physician's assistants and registered nurses.

While reducing costs and increasing staff is important to Dr. Morrow, he states, "The big thing is we can practice better medicine." The staff at his office now alert patients when medications are recalled, receive reports in a secure electronic fashion, track tests and procedure results, and communicate more efficiently internally. For patients with chronic diseases, it is possible to track their visits and know when they have missed a visit that could be vital to their care.

The effectiveness and accuracy of electronic records allows Dr. Morrow and fellow doctors in the practice to better utilize resources, see more patients, and provide personalized care. According to Dr. Morrow, "The return on investment for my office is measured in real dollars, in quality, job satisfaction, a sense of accomplishment, and success in today's changing world."

"Everything is about access. Patients need to message us securely and quickly, and they can. They look at lab results, ask for medication refills, and request referrals. It helps them manage their care better."

– James Morrow, M.D.

FACT

~ Physicians spend 38 percent of their time writing up charts. For nurses, this figure is 50 percent. The average office spends $10 per visit to track the paper file.

Source: http://ruralhealth.hrsa.gov/RHC/March16Transcript.htm

Realizing the Importance of Accurate Records

"As we get older, issues come up and you need to know what your medical history is, and even your family medical history."

– Sandy Silins

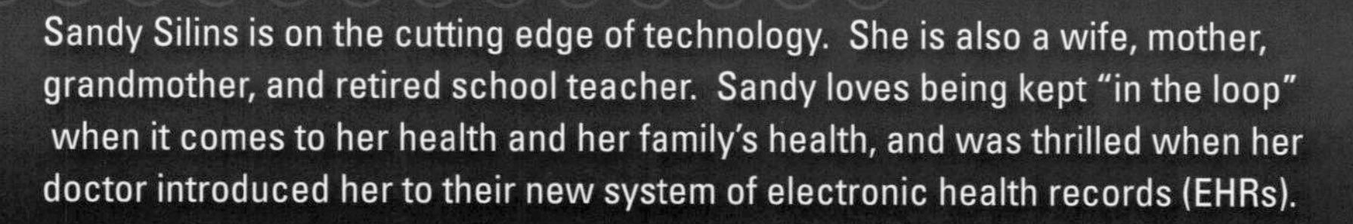

Sandy Silins is on the cutting edge of technology. She is also a wife, mother, grandmother, and retired school teacher. Sandy loves being kept "in the loop" when it comes to her health and her family's health, and was thrilled when her doctor introduced her to their new system of electronic health records (EHRs).

"I am on the computer a lot, so for me it was a very seamless switch to being involved with my doctor. I use it to keep in touch with my doctor, track all my health records, make appointments, get test results, refill medications; all without having to be involved in telephone calls with office staff and so forth. I find it to be tremendously efficient, time-saving, and accurate."

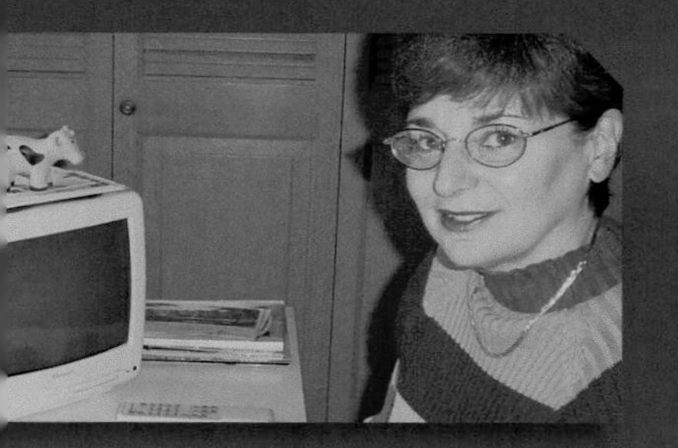

» PROFILE:

Sandy Silins

ILLINOIS

~ Retired School Teacher and Grandmother Knows the Value of Accurate Medical Records to Her Family's Health

Sandy was the first in her family to start using the EHR, and within just a few months she had the rest of her family—including her daughter, Lisa Tumpowsky—sold on the system. Having access to her health information brings her peace of mind and reassurance and makes switching doctors easy. When her mother-in-law moved to Illinois from Florida, Sandy made sure that the doctor she chose had an EHR so that she could be involved in health decisions. Sandy is also comforted that she can reach her mother-in-law's doctor anytime she has a question.

Sandy first became interested in electronic health records after she lost her own mother a number of years ago. "I spent enormous amounts of time in the hospital with her, talking to doctors. If I had this it would have made my life so much easier."

"When my mother-in-law became chronically ill, I spent half my life trying to reach doctors and get answers. The other issue was accuracy. She was in the hospital a lot, and every time we went into the hospital, there was the whole issue of having to have her whole history repeated again, and there were mistakes made because they didn't have accurate records. I used to carry a book with me with all of her information because it was so long. I became very concerned about medical records after that."

Now, Sandy has the peace of mind that she is in control of her health and her family's health. Going to the doctor is no longer guesswork.

Did You Know?

- Caregivers of people over the age of 50 spend an average of 17.9 hours per week providing care. Twenty percent (4.5 million out of 22.4 million) of those caring for family or friends aged 50 and older spend over 40 hours per week providing care, with some providing constant care.

Source: Family Caregiver Alliance. "Selected Caregiver Statistics." August 5, 2005. http://www.caregiver.org

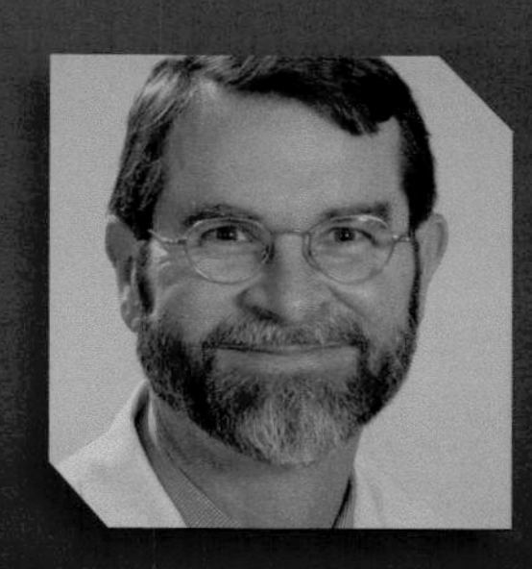

» PROFILE:

John Cole, M.D.
LOUISIANA

~ The Downfalls of an EMR System That Isn't Interoperable

"We have patients who come back and forth from other hospitals and research centers—and we spend a lot of time assembling information or waiting for information from those different places. If you could automatically send that in an electronic fashion, the amount of time spent would be greatly decreased, and the accuracy and completeness would be enhanced."

– John Cole, M.D.

Plays Well with Others

Dr. John Cole treats many patients with rare and deadly forms of cancer. He also likes to stay on the cutting edge of medical discoveries and is in constant contact with a major cancer research institute. He e-mails with doctors there, and gets feedback about his patients and information about clinical trials. Many of his patients move back and forth between cancer research centers, and they will often go for second opinions and specialized treatment. Altogether, this amounts to numerous doctors he must be able to communicate with in an efficient and effective way every day.

The hospital where Dr. Cole practices recently started using an electronic medical record system with amazing capabilities ... within their own system. The downfall, he says, is that he has no way to quickly send information or his patients' medical records to their other doctors or research centers hundreds of miles away.

While he believes that the ability to quickly and accurately share information is vital to his patients' health, his main concern is that he may "accidentally" violate HIPAA, a law recently enacted to protect patient privacy. "I think that is a barrier for some people, because they would like to be helpful. If they are not sure where to send the information, it can get misdirected, which is not always in their control. I think most people would like some sort of protection against that from a HIPAA standpoint. I think people are so scared that somehow they're going to get dinged for unintentional violation of HIPAA regulations that when medical records start being transferred it's going to be a concern."

Did You Know?

- Eight percent of patients are referred to another physician.

Source: CDC/NCHS, 2002 National Ambulatory Medical Care Survey.

Consumers
Table of Contents

Consumers

"A patient-centered system absolutely demands an electronic health record. To empower wired consumers with information, choice, and control, we need to harness the explosive power of information technology."

Senate Majority Leader Bill Frist

Introduction

A personal story of "The Document Game"

Ashley Shaff was born with a chromosomal abnormality that has caused lifelong problems with her eyes, ears, and heart, and contributed to developmental delays, sleep apnea, lung disease, and a host of other conditions. Peggy Frank, Ashley's mother, has had to take personal charge of Ashley's medical records to ensure that complete and timely information reaches doctors and providers caring for Ashley. The sustained effort has been wrenching. Below is an excerpt from Peggy's testimony before the Commission.

> [My daughter] Ashley has been seen by one dozen medical facilities, spanning 3,000 miles—literally coast-to-coast. She has had approximately 35 hospitalizations. She has been seen by [at least 36 medical specialists and therapists].... I have had to be ... a "connector," literally running interference between the various physicians and health care facilities to ensure that Ashley's medical records physically get from place to place ... in a timely manner, often under extreme emotional conditions.
>
> Trust me, playing "the document game" is disturbing, especially at times of considerable duress.
>
> The same holds true for ... asking endless medical history questions [that have been asked and recorded by others many times before, but rarely shared with other doctors]. They ask everything that has happened during her entire life and seek great detail on absolutely every single medical procedure, hospitalization, etc., that has occurred over the span of Ashley's life.
>
> I cannot tell you how many times I was reduced to tears.

I remember in Northern California sitting at Ashley's post-operative bedside, crying as I was trying to provide the medical history. I was just told, not minutes before, that she was terminally ill and had about five months to five years to live. This is wrong. It is unkind, and perhaps even a medical mistake waiting to happen. What if I make a mistake, an error or an omission, that has a grave impact on her care, then or in the future?

There is a lot of talk about reducing medical costs by increasing patient safety. Where does having a medical record, easily accessible, fit into this picture?

I believe it to be pivotal.[1]

You deserve constant access to your personal health information

Your personal medical information helps guide your medical treatment, but sometimes your complete information is hard to come by.

Parts of the data may be easy to get, usually because you are standing in the office of the doctor who stores that record in the first place, or you are seeing a doctor who works in the same medical practice. Other parts of the information may be much less readily available, because separate information is stored in different doctors' offices, hospitals, and labs. This lack of connection—lack of "interoperability"—among people and among sources of information can result in bad diagnoses, duplicate testing, conflicts in prescriptions, wasted time for doctors and patients, diminished quality of care, needless expense, unnecessary worry, and even the loss of lives.

Problems that arise from a lack of information do not have to happen.

The most basic information about your health—medicines you take, tests you've had, doctors you've seen, conditions you've had—ought to be available to any doctor you choose at any time.

Once a patient has granted permission, healthcare providers should be able to access personal healthcare information when and where they need it, so they can provide the best care possible, whether the patient has a scheduled visit … or has just fallen off a ladder.

The Parallel to Cell Phone Technology

No one knew the extent of what could be done with cell phone technology until the market got hold of it, and gave us the cell phone-address book combination, the camera phone, the Internet-ready phone, and more. We still do not know what new uses will be developed for cell phone technology. The same holds true for a connected system of medical information.

[1] Peggy Frank. Testimony before the Commission on Systemic Interoperability. March 15, 2005.

You have three seconds to remember every doctor you've ever seen, every procedure you've ever undergone and every medicine you've ever taken.
You could do just that if your medical history was altogether, safe and sound and in one place. That's why online medical records are such a great idea. They mean you can get to your medical information instantly. That could be a real life saver in the event of an accident or sudden illness.

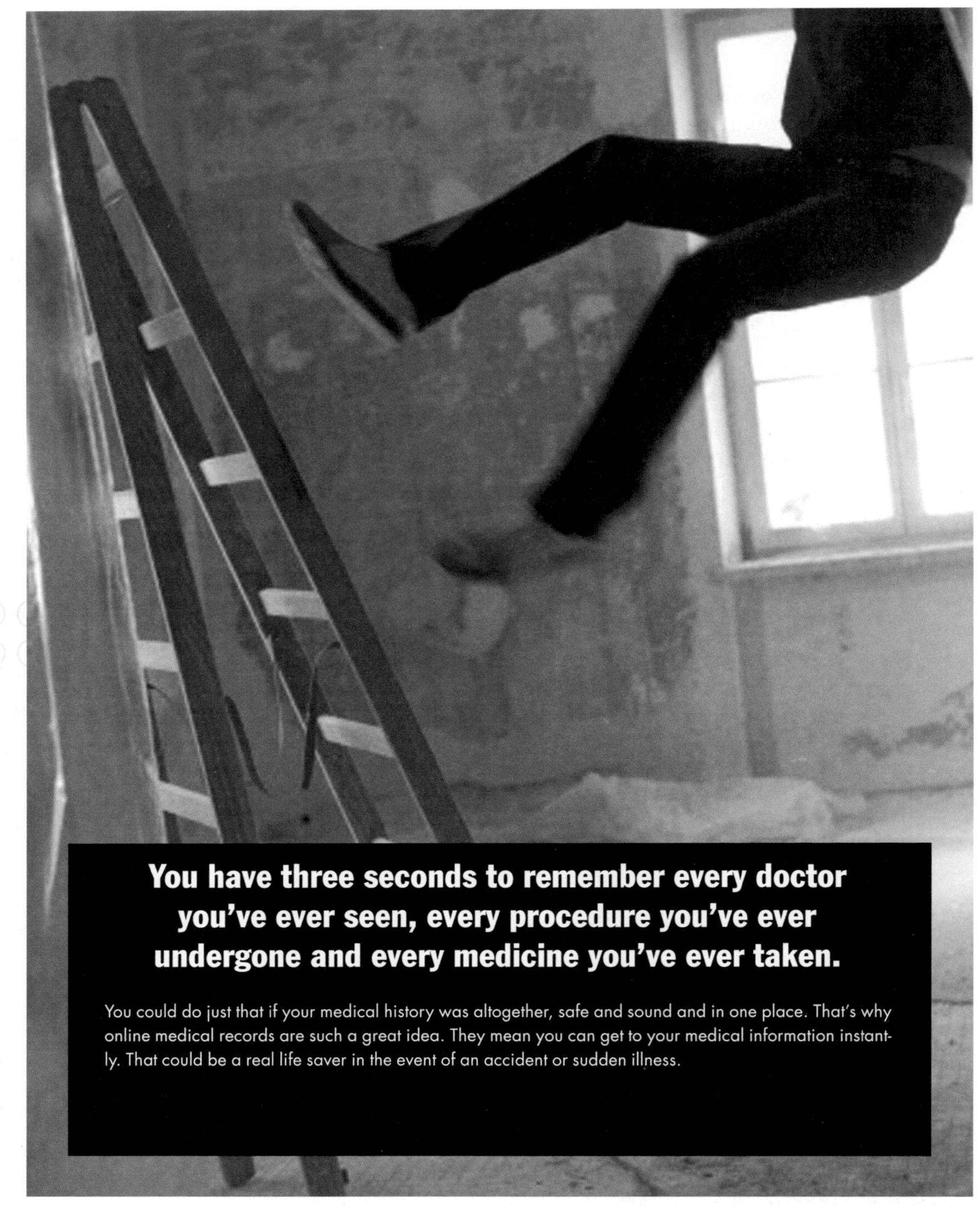

This document was provided by **the Markle Foundation.**

A Culture of Safety

» PROFILE:

Jandel Allen-Davis, M.D.
COLORADO

~ HMO Physician Supports Electronic Records for Quality Patient Care

Dr. Jandel Allen-Davis puts the safety of her patients at the top of her priority list every day. With a system of electronic medical records (EMRs) and e-prescribing, Dr. Allen-Davis has the information needed to provide the best care possible.

While the integrated healthcare delivery system she works with is almost completely integrated inside its own walls, its systems cannot communicate with the systems of other hospitals. Still, for the average patient, Dr. Allen-Davis and others are able to help their patients find better and safer treatment options and be more involved in their overall health. "One of the biggest bangs for the safety buck is when I order medications. When I enter a certain disease into the computer, it automatically gives me all the possible treatments and the correct dosage for my patients. This is a tremendous tool, especially when I have patients with diseases I'm not as familiar with."

"Instead of sending them to another doctor or calling someone to get their opinion about what medicine would work best, all the most recent and accurate information about all of these drugs is right there, in the medical record. In a given department or with a clinical situation, we look at what would be the best way to use the system to keep patients safe, to alert doctors to anything new that might be going on or new warnings for medications. Many of our patients, especially our older patients, are on multiple medications, and there's always the potential to harm somebody by not being aware of drug interactions."

"Many of our atients, especially ur older patients, are on multiple medications, and here's always the otential to harm somebody by not being aware of rug interactions."

– Jandel Allen-Davis, M.D.

But safety is not the only benefit. Dr. Allen-Davis frequently uses the system to help connect her patients with other doctors and the treatment they need, especially for those with chronic diseases. "Last week I had a patient whose labs came back and showed that her blood sugar was elevated. I was able to call her, let her know that based on the information, it looks like she's developed diabetes. I then ordered the appropriate follow-up lab work and told her to 'make sure you call your primary doctor.' But with the EMR, I was also able to say, 'I'm going to send a copy of this note to your primary doctor, so that she can be involved in your care right away.' Her primary doctor called her to make sure she came in, and we got her connected into the right programs of diabetic counseling and nutrition teaching. I think those little nudges begin to change the culture of safety for patients."

FACT

~ Chronic conditions make up 29.6 percent of the reasons people visit their primary care specialists.

Source: CDC/NCHS, 2002 National Ambulatory Medical Care Survey
http://www.cdc.gov/nchs/about/major/ahcd/officevisitcharts.h

Electronic Access Equals Peace of Mind

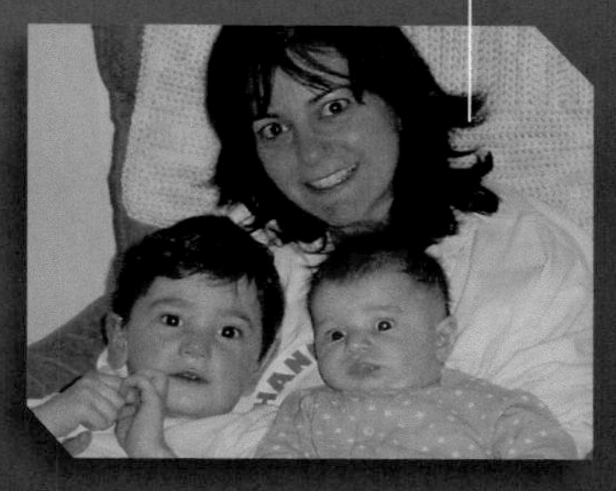

» PROFILE:

Lisa Tumpowsky

ILLINOIS

~ Busy Working Mother of Two Young Boys Wishes Her Sons Could Have Access to Electronic Records

"You don't always remember, 'What was the name of that drug I was allergic to?' 'When was the last tetanus shot I had?' It just simplies life a lot."

– Lisa Tumpowsky

Lisa Tumpowsky was diagnosed with a thyroid condition called Graves' Disease in April of 2004. At almost the same time, her doctor started using a system of electronic health records—a change that revolutionized the way Lisa thought about her health and her children's health.

This electronic system helped her when she changed to a new endocrinologist. Lisa had discovered she was allergic to a particular thyroid drug, but when she went to the new doctor, she couldn't remember the medicine's name. The new doctor simply went to her computer, looked up the information, and prescribed a different medicine. Lisa's pharmacy is also connected to all her doctors, who are able to send prescriptions directly to her local pharmacy, saving her the hassle of carrying around the paper with the prescription scribbled on it.

Lisa's dealings with her doctor were not always this efficient. Until last year, she was—like so many others—at the mercy of her doctor's office staff to get her health information. She is still at their mercy when it comes to her children's health. "I still have issues with my children's doctors, who are not on any sort of system whatsoever."

But the lack of access for Lisa's children's doctors is more than just inconvenient. It is dangerous. Lisa never knows which doctor of the four in the practice she will see, or whether they have all of her sons information available to them. Not long ago, her one-year-old son was given a chickenpox vaccine, and a short time later he came down with a virus. The doctor she saw at the time was unaware of the recent vaccine and prescribed a steroid treatment that would have reacted with the vaccine. Lisa caught this as she was reading the label on the prescription bottle, which said: "Do not administer if the child has been exposed to the chickenpox vaccine." In today's world of technological marvels and instant access, this is more than ridiculous, it is an outrage.

For Lisa, convenience—as well as safety—is the key. "If my children's doctors were on a system like this, every single time I sign my son up for school or for summer camp, I wouldn't have to fill out a manual form, go to the doctor, wait in line, wait for the receptionist to fill in the information, you know, allow human error to intervene. I would just be able to push a button and send my child's health records, or proof of immunizations, directly to the school."

Lost in the Mail

"We don't know whether the mail lost my records or whether they got lost at the clinic. We just don't know."

– Mary Blades

Mary has suffered from scleroderma—a potentially life-threatening condition—for nearly nine years. When she was first diagnosed, the doctors in her hometown of Springfield felt that she would be better served by going to a clinic.

So Mary packed her bags—and copied her medical records to hand-carry the numerous papers and files to her new doctor. "I had gone to my doctors that I'd been to and got copies of all their information that they had on me. And for some reason, I made copies before I mailed them, which turned out to be a very good thing, because when I mailed them ... we don't know whether the mail lost my records, or whether they got lost at the clinic. We just don't know."

Now, copies of Mary's health information have been "misplaced," leaving her with concerns about her privacy and the security of the records her doctors are keeping about her condition.

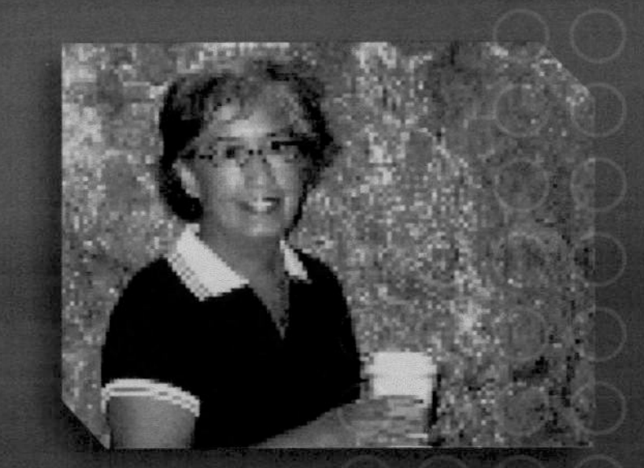

PROFILE:

Mary Blades
MISSOURI

~ 63-Year-Old Woman Longs for Efficient, Secure Communication with Doctors

Transforming Dentistry with IT

"Having an electronic health record system makes sure the right people know the right information at the right time."

– Jung-Wei Chen, DDS

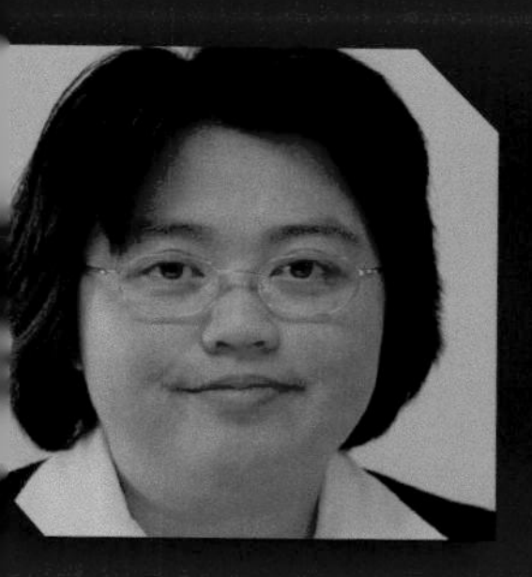

PROFILE:

Jung-Wei Chen

DDS
TEXAS

~ A Pediatric Dentist Turns to Health Information Technology

Pediatric dentistry and health informatics are not two fields that would normally be considered a common pair, but for Dr. Jung-Wei Chen, the combination makes perfect sense. At the university where she teaches, Dr. Chen supervises the undergraduate and post-graduate dentistry clinic and serves on a committee that is evaluating electronic dental records systems for patient care and teaching purposes.

The electronic record currently in use at the dental/medical school does not allow all forms of medical and dental information to be stored. Patient radiographs cannot be entered, and much of the information cannot even be exchanged. "Sometimes we have to ask the patient to fill out the same information over and over, and then go to a referral doctor and fill out all the information again. Those things can be limited if all the information can be transferred or can be united."

According to Dr. Chen, electronic health information in dentistry, like that in medicine, can do a multitude of good, from tracking oral hygiene to tracking the medical actions and the learning progress of a dental student while giving clinical care to patients. While many electronic tools have not yet been developed, currently chronic illnesses can be tracked. Rural health systems benefit greatly from having access to tools and doctors. "If you have diabetic patients, electronic records keep track of their hemoglobin A1C levels, or it helps keep track of drug allergies or drug interactions. And it is very helpful for rural areas. For example, you're the only dentist in a small town, but you see a big lesion in the patient's mouth, you're thinking, should I send this patient 500 miles away to a big medical center to do the cancer screening, or should I just give the patient a Tylenol?"

With the added tools that an electronic health information system can provide, the rural clinician would not have to send a patient hundreds of miles away to an oral pathology or cancer specialist for consultation on a possible benign mouth sore. Any doctor could track the history and disease pattern of a chronically ill patient and exchange this information electronically with the specialist for consultation. Dental students would be exposed to a new way to treat patients. There are as many possibilities for health informatics in the dental profession as in the medical profession.

A Healthier System Means Healthier Kids

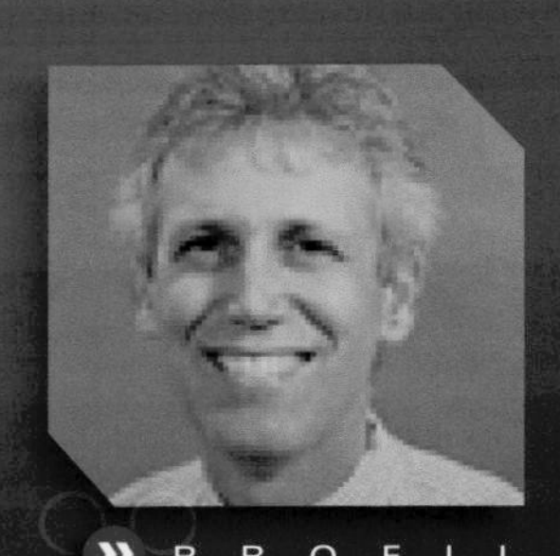

» PROFILE:

Stephen Borowitz

M.D.
VIRGINIA

~ A Pediatric Gastroenterologist Praises Progress and the Use of Technology

"I think that one of the problems with healthcare is the lack of trust of other people's data, so we tend to duplicate. Anybody who has ever gone into a doctor's office knows that you fill out your history form for every new doctor you go to see."

– Stephen Borowitz, M.D.

Dr. Stephen Borowitz can see infinite benefits to using electronic medical information systems in medical practice, especially when working with so many growing children. But he also sees many things that need to change with the current system to truly improve patient care.

Dr. Borowitz sees electronic tools as a key that could unlock many medical mysteries—for patients and for doctors—in real time. "I think it's a tremendous opportunity for just-in-time education, not only for the patient, but for the practitioner, since all adults are problem-oriented learners. If I have a patient in front of me with a problem I don't understand and I can deliver educational content in the context of that encounter, I'm going to get much more out of it, because it's real to me, rather than going to a lecture three weeks later that may or may not be pertinent to a particular patient."

He also sees that simply having access to patient data could make a huge difference in caring for children. "One of the major focuses of taking care of children is immunizations. To have access to immunization data, so that we know what immunizations the child has or has not gotten across the continuum of care, enables us to at least do somewhat of a better job of catching that child up, or making sure that they're up-to-date on their shots."

"One of the struggles that I had with this whole process is that a lot of people when they move to an electronic medical record simply automate what we've previously done on paper, instead of stepping back and saying, 'What information do I really need to take care of this patient, and how might I codify it in a way that enables me to look at the information in a different way?' A lot of people continue to rely on dictation, transcription, and free text, which I think is the only way we could do it in the near term. However, if we codified it, we could do all sorts of creative things."

The U.S. healthcare system needs a connected electronic system of personal health information that allows doctors to share information and find critical data instantly. Systems that make the most of shared data and interaction are all around us: in banks, over the Internet, in libraries. Such a system for healthcare is possible. The technology exists and can be implemented—and no one can predict all the possible benefits that will arise from making it part of our lives.

"In health there is freedom. Health is the first of all liberties."

Henri-Frederic Amiel,
Poet and Philosopher (1828 – 1881)

Helps healthy people stay healthy

Healthcare is episodic, but health is daily. You make decisions about your health every day, and the overall task of staying healthy is in your own hands. Healthy people stay healthy longer when they closely monitor their own health and seek out current information on how to stay well. Armed with information and knowledge, a patient not only gains new perspective on his or her choices, but also learns what the range of choices is. You choose what kinds of foods to eat, how much to eat, how much to exercise, whether or not to take vitamins, and a host of other things. Those living with chronic conditions usually monitor and maintain their health on a daily basis by, for instance, measuring blood sugar and blood pressure, or receiving outpatient therapy.

A system of electronically connected medical information will help create a more active partnership between patients and healthcare providers and promote healthier lifestyles. Doctors will be able to more easily and frequently monitor the progress of their patients, and patients will be able to more easily contact their doctors—or access a doctor's expertise through recommended articles and other material—to better follow a course of treatment.

Seven "Rights"

According to Andy von Eschenbach, Director of the National Cancer Institute, there are seven "rights" to a high-quality system of healthcare:

1. The **right** patient
2. Receives the **right** treatment
3. At the **right** time
4. For the **right** reason
5. In the **right** location
6. With the **right** outcome in real time
7. At the **right** price.[2]

Problems with the paper-based system

The paper-based system of maintaining health information has critical shortcomings. There is no consistent and complete access, only limited control over access, no record of who has accessed the healthcare information, a risk of mistakes in care resulting from illegible handwriting and missing information, wasted time on tasks that could be streamlined, and no agreed-upon "language" for recording medical data.

[2] Andrew C. von Eschenbach. "Director's Update: Clinical Trial System of Future." *NCI Cancer Bulletin* (October 26, 2004): 2.

Seven Ways to Know If Your Healthcare Provider Uses an Interoperable System of Healthcare Information

1. The patient and the healthcare provider can always see the information in the record of the patient's healthcare.
2. Neither the patient nor the healthcare provider ever has to reenter information that has not changed.
3. The patient and the doctor can always obtain access through the system to all health studies, whether they were done in hospitals, clinics, laboratories, radiology facilities, rehabilitation centers, or nursing homes.
4. The patient can grant access to his or her entire health record to a healthcare provider in any part of the United States. This is especially important in the case of emergencies during travel.
5. The portions of the computer-based health record necessary for business processes (e.g., payments, insurance reimbursements) can be automatically and simply provided to appropriate parties.
6. The portions of the record that are relevant to quality of care studies can be readily provided.
7. The patient, doctor, and participating healthcare entities are protected from improper access to private medical records by any third party under severe penalty of Federal law.

Electronic medical records, interoperability, and the difference between the two

An electronic medical record is your current medical information and your patient history. It may include anything found in a typical paper-based file, including electronic imaging reports.

While electronic medical records have the capacity to be interoperable, they are not naturally so. That is why most existing electronic medical records cannot be used in multiple clinical care environments.

When interoperability exists, distant systems can exchange information. For instance, if you were on a trip to Los Angeles and ended up in the hospital, an interoperable system would allow your doctor there to view your entire medical history as recorded by your doctor back home, as well as any other information from any other time you had an encounter with the U.S. healthcare system.

If paper has so many drawbacks, what is the alternative?

The better answer is connected health information—interoperability. Part of this connected information for each patient is a personal medical history, maintained on a computer: an electronic "safe" where medical history is stored. Instead of having information written on sheets of paper in filing cabinets, medical records are accessible instantly by any healthcare provider who has received permission from the patient.

What is in the interoperable electronic health record? The same things that are in a paper record: your x-rays, MRIs, prescriptions, treatment history, lab and other test results, physician's notes, and anything else you or your doctors deem important to your health.

Electronic medical information that is accessible by computer is easy for doctors to find in an emergency, because they can pull it up from wherever they are—there is no waiting for someone to rifle through a filing cabinet to find the needed information.

Benefits: Moral, intellectual, and practical

The possible benefits of interoperability in healthcare fall into three categories:

- **The moral benefit.** In 2000, the Institute of Medicine estimated that 44,000 to 98,000 Americans are killed by preventable medical errors each year.[3] Since that time, follow-up studies have indicated that the number of preventable deaths is even higher. For example, Health Grades, Inc. reported in 2004 that as many as 195,000 Americans were killed in 2000, 2001, and 2002 by medical mistakes in hospitals nationwide.[4]

- **The intellectual benefit.** In the 21st century, Americans should expect more from the healthcare system, a critical field that has less connectivity than many other parts of life: Kids are on-line in school, families care for grandparents through on-line services, and on-line shopping includes everything from shoes to stocks and bonds. The technology and skill exist but have yet to be purposefully applied.

- **The practical benefit.** An end to the document game—the problems that result from delays and inefficiencies inherent in a paper-based system of records. It is time to eliminate the shuffling of papers and the wait for critical medical information to be sent to the right person or place via phone calls, faxes, or "snail mail." An electronic system that connects caregivers and patients with information anytime and anywhere will:

    - Eliminate the need for repetitive, difficult, and often inaccurate retelling of medical history each time a patient sees a new caregiver;

    - Eliminate the one-size-fits-all approach that the lack of personal information forces on doctors and nurses as they diagnose and treat patients; and

    - Eliminate the problem of personal health information being scattered far and wide with no way to bring it together for basic healthcare, let alone emergency treatment.

---

[3] L. Kohn, J. Corrigan, and M. Donaldson. *To Err Is Human: Building a Safer Health System.* Committee of Health Care in America, Institute of Medicine. 2000.

[4] HealthGrades. *In-Hospital Deaths from Medical Errors at 195,000 per Year, HealthGrades' Study Finds.* July 27, 2004. <http://www.healthgrades.com/aboutus/index.cfm?fuseaction=mod&modtype=content&modact=Media_PressRelease_Detail&&press_id=135>

Convenience

"Never before in history has innovation offered promise of so much to so many in so short a time."

Bill Gates

You can have constant access to your own information

With an interoperable healthcare system, you will be able to review your personal medical information in private, at your leisure. You will also be able to add information as you see fit, such as family history, over-the-counter medicines you take, self-monitored data for blood sugar or blood pressure, and exercise history.

High-touch and low-touch

With some services, you want human interaction. Other times, you just want to get what you came for and go.

At the gas station, you want to get in and out. The trend toward self-service began when the price of gas got so high that few stations could afford to pay someone to pump the gas and still maintain a competitive price. Once people began pumping their own gas, they did not want to be bothered with having to go inside to pay, and "pay at the pump" systems emerged. In 2004, more than half the transactions at gas stations happened at the pump.[5] It has become a "low-touch" industry.

But when you go to a nice restaurant on a special occasion, you expect personal service—"high-touch" attention. It is the same with any place where people want service tailored to their own needs. Hair salons, high-end clothing stores, auto repair shops—when people walk in, they want reassurance, handholding, and attention.

In the healthcare world, high-touch attention is more than something nice to have. It is what most patients truly want, need, and expect.

[5] Jeff Lenard. Commission on Systemic Interoperability staff interview. May 2005.

Healthcare is a hybrid—a high-touch activity that can benefit from low-touch support. It is easier to order prescriptions, make appointments, and keep up with medical records using an automated system—a low-touch approach. But when a person goes the doctor, it should be a high-attention, detail-oriented experience—a high-touch experience. However, according to the Health Resources and Services Administration, under the current system, physicians spend 38 percent of their time writing up charts.[6] For nurses, that figure is 50 percent.[7]

Less time filling out forms

With connectivity, the first round of filling out forms can be the last round. Since all healthcare providers can share data, patients do not have to fill out a medical history or insurance form more than once. Wherever authorized providers are located (whether the patient has visited that provider before or not) the information will be readily available.

Easier contact with your doctor means improved personal and family care

Interaction with the healthcare system is most often episodic. With an interoperable system in place, you can refer to your physician's information network and find information you need to make a doctor's appointment go more efficiently or reduce the number of follow-up visits you might have to make.

Sometimes you need to ask your doctors detailed questions in person. At other times, e-mail would be a better medium. For many questions, doctors will be able to direct you to on-line resources such as MedlinePlus.[8] Such a system could take into account the details of your medical condition and guide you to informative articles.

Avoid the Redundancy and Possible Error of Retelling Medical History

Nearly everyone has had the experience of going to a new doctor or hospital and having to fill out a huge pile of forms. Those forms usually include a request for medical history, something most people will have given to other healthcare providers several times before. When recounting that history, there is always the risk of forgetting something. People with many health problems cannot be expected to remember all the details of their treatment.

Even the healthiest person can have a lengthy record, and the dates and details can be impossible to remember. In an emergency, a reliable recounting is even less likely and even more critical. For patients with chronic conditions, retelling a medical history is often quite emotional and painful and omissions can be deadly.

An interoperable healthcare system will eliminate the need for retelling medical history by making that history available to every provider authorized by the patient and by allowing doctors and others to add to the history as treatment progresses. The system will minimize and ultimately eliminate the need to transmit medical records by phone, fax, courier, or mail.

---

[6] Bill Finerfrock. "Presentation on Electronic Medical Records in Rural Health Clinics" (teleconference transcript). *Health Resources and Services Administration*. 2005. <http://ruralhealth.hrsa.gov/RHC/March16Transcript.htm>

[7] Ibid.

[8] URL: www.medlineplus.gov. MedlinePlus allows consumers to conduct free searches for up-to-date medical information, including extensive information about drugs, an illustrated medical encyclopedia, interactive patient tutorials, and the latest health news. MedlinePlus also provides access to medical journal articles.

A connected system makes it easier for parents to obtain copies of vaccination and other medical records for camp and school. It eases the task of caring for aging parents. It also provides a way for patients to get the information they need to ease their own health concerns.

Millions of Adults Monitor Healthcare of a Loved One from a Distance

According to a survey conducted by the Family Caregiver Alliance,[9] over seven million Americans are managing care for a loved one over age 55 who lives at least an hour away. Caring for an aging parent is hard enough, and distance only increases the difficulty.

According to the same survey, the average long-distance caregiver lives 450 miles away from the loved one he or she is caring for. Those polled reported spending an average of $392 a month for out-of-pocket expenses and travel, not counting missed job time and income.

On-line Support: One Patient's Experience

In 2003, Pat McGinley of Cleveland, Ohio, registered for an on-line program created to help patients monitor their health. She signed up at the request of her physician, but it never crossed her mind that she would actually use it. "I am not a real techie person," she said. "I did it to appease my doctor." A few weeks later, following routine blood work, the doctor's nurse called to inform her that she had both high cholesterol and high triglyceride levels. Pat was upset at the news and resigned herself to living with her worries and unanswered questions until the follow-up visit in two weeks.

Then something happened that Pat did not expect: She received an e-mail telling her that she should log on to her on-line healthcare program to review new information. She went from being worried to being relieved when the program directed her to comprehensive, easy-to-understand information about her test results and likely condition. She could compare her results with normal levels and click on embedded links for additional material. Pat began to feel more at ease, and at her next appointment she was prepared with important, informed questions for her doctor about her health and what she needed to change.

The system "really empowered me to think about what was going on. It made me feel like I was part of the decision-making process," she told President Bush at a public event at the Cleveland Clinic in January 2005.

With the help of an interoperable healthcare system, Pat and her doctor were able to work together to make critical lifestyle changes. As a patient, Pat understood her medical situation better than she ever had before, and she credits that to her access to private, personalized information delivered electronically. "I went from feeling helpless to feeling completely in control of the situation," she said.[10]

[9] Michael Hill. "Moving Creates Boom in Long Distance Care," *Washington Post*. March 17, 2005.
[10] White House Office of the Press Secretary. *President Discusses Health Care Information Technology* Benefits. Press release. January 27, 2005.
<http://www.whitehouse.gov/news/releases/2005/01/20050127-7.html>

'Dentistry is just one part of the uman body, and e same principles apply there as other medical are. It's such an integral part of he total health of the patient. It's ot separate from medicine."

– Joseph Chasteen, DDS

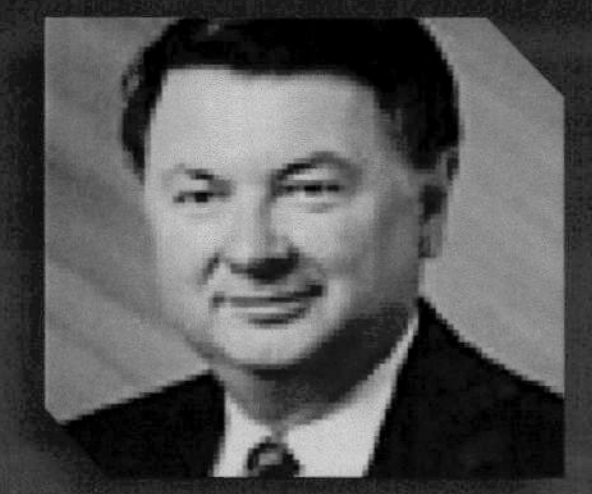

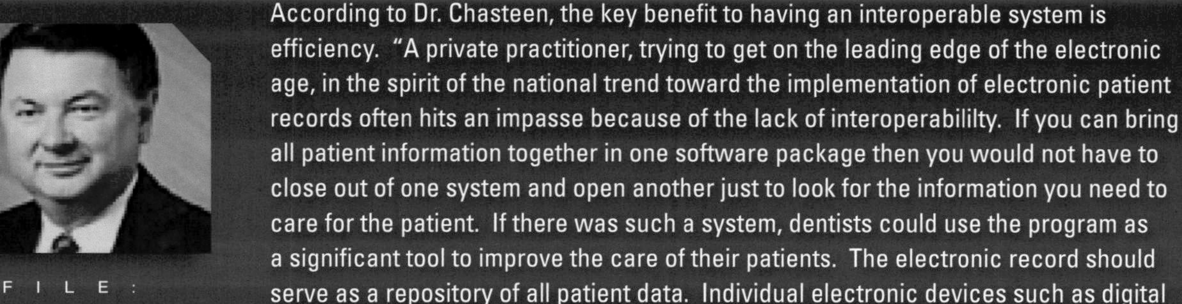

» PROFILE:

Joseph Chasteen
DDS
WASHINGTON

~ A Dentist Pleads for Dentistry To Be Included in New Health Technologies

Seeing the Big Picture

Dr. Joseph Chasteen is frustrated that some sectors of the medical community continue to see dentistry as something apart from medicine in terms of patient care. Dr. Chasteen is the Director of the Office of Educational and Information Technology at a university in the state of Washington and he knows firsthand the benefits and barriers to using information technology effectively in a dental practice.

Dentists have recently seen a boom in new, high-tech devices to help them in the diagnosis and treatment of their patients. But as remarkable as these devices are, they can be more of a hassle than helpful because each individual device is designed to store information in its own software program. When the information cannot be transferred or shared with a universal, electronic patient record system, it prevents dentists from being able to see the complete picture of their patient's oral health status in one information system.

According to Dr. Chasteen, the key benefit to having an interoperable system is efficiency. "A private practitioner, trying to get on the leading edge of the electronic age, in the spirit of the national trend toward the implementation of electronic patient records often hits an impasse because of the lack of interoperabililty. If you can bring all patient information together in one software package then you would not have to close out of one system and open another just to look for the information you need to care for the patient. If there was such a system, dentists could use the program as a significant tool to improve the care of their patients. The electronic record should serve as a repository of all patient data. Individual electronic devices such as digital radiographic equipment and periodontal charting devices should be designed to work with the electronic patient record using established standards."

A major advantage of an electronic patient record for both dentists and patients is the ability to see the whole picture of the patient's health. "If a patient has a history of hypertension, I want to know that so I can avoid using incompatible medications and anesthetics during treatment. A standardized electronic patient health history could be integrated with a drug interaction program to automatically prompt warnings of any potential incompatibility of current patient medications with planned treatment. Such innovations would be welcome tools in a contemporary dental practice."

Did You Know?

~ There are 176,063 professionally active dentists in the United States.

Source: American Dental Association, Information Line.

Views from the Floor - The Nurse Perspective

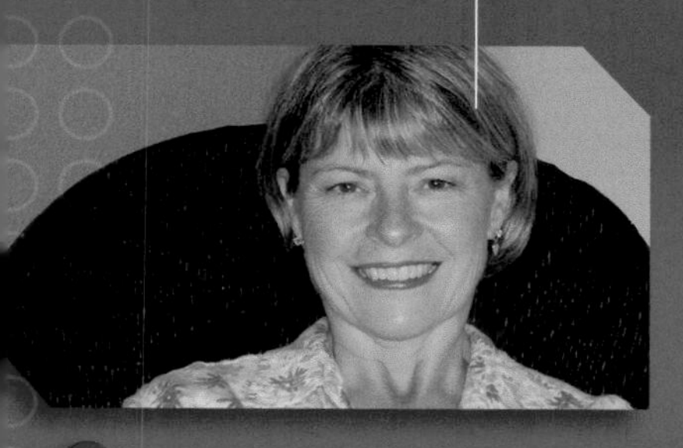

PROFILE:

Roz Willis
RNC
WASHINGTON

~ Treats Children at a Child Protection Center and a Juvenile Detention Center

"A 14-year-old female was brought in to be seen by the medical staff of a shelter due to neglect at home. The only history we got was that she had school phobia, was hiding in closets, and had bladder control problems. The only concern she initially reported was having problems with bed-wetting. An exam showed that she was pregnant and had a bladder infection; further cultures revealed she also had a sexually transmitted disease. She was not sure who her primary care physician was or when she was last seen. She was not aware of any allergies and gave us limited medical information. We needed to initiate treatment for her and get her established with an Ob-Gyn specialist. Having an electronic system in place to check allergies, immunizations, and other medical history would have been helpful in providing safe and effective care, especially when prescribing antibiotics. We had to contact the new doctor and send records, culture results, and treatment plans in order for them to continue with treatment and ensure proper follow-up. Having a system in place where we could check medical information and treatment would be helpful so we don't overtreat or give insufficient care to our clients.

I also worked with a young teen who was removed from his home due to substance abuse. I had to provide care for him at the Juvenile Detention Center (JDC) because he was a frequent runaway. He was diagnosed with hepatitis C and needed follow-up. He returned several times to the JDC after ingesting large amounts of drugs. While investigating follow-up situations, it was discovered that he was seen and treated several times at a downtown emergency room (ER) and had given an alias. One time a friend dropped him off at the ER close to death, and he had to be resuscitated. Unfortunately, he left with an unknown person before anyone could be called. He had also been seen and treated at other ERs in the city at which drug testing wasn't performed because they didn't know his history. My involvement continued with him in order to get immunizations information and lab data, which were needed in order to schedule him for a liver biopsy. There was no one person who had all the information, since he was shuffled between treatment centers. It is frustrating trying to provide services for him and trying to get the medical follow-up that is necessary and that could have a major impact on his life."

Views from the Floor - The Nurse Perspective

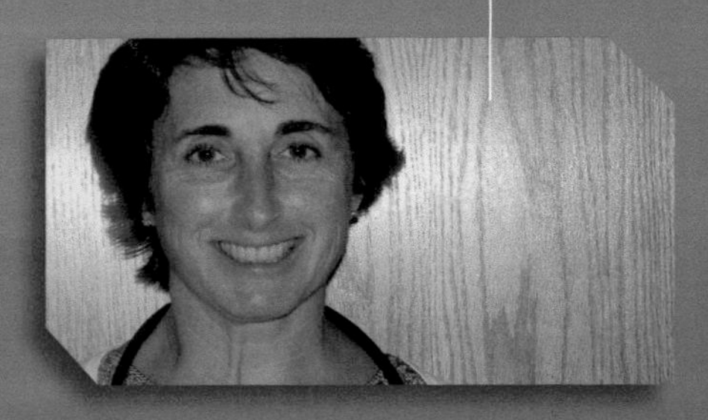

PROFILE:

Deborah Bretl
RN, MSN, APNP
WISCONSIN

~ Acute Care Nurse Providing Care at the Bedside Sees a Need for Electronic Information

"Some of the history for the admission paperwork is available from previous visits, so I can start my admit paperwork before the patient arrives on our floor. Patients get frustrated having to give their history, medication lists, etc., to the emergency room staff and then repeat it for the floor staff. Those patients that have frequent admissions would benefit from on-line information facilitating the admission process.

The ability to document at the bedside in real time would eliminate the scramble to document just before a shift change. This would also improve the accuracy of documentation. Recently, I spent 10 minutes looking for a chart, time I could have spent on patient care. One of the doctors had taken it down the hall and left it there. On-line documentation and information would greatly enhance patient care by ensuring accurate documentation, legible orders, fewer errors, and available information for those who are providing the care."

PROFILE:

Alex Vassserman
RN, CPHIMS
FLORIDA

~ Critical care at the bedside needs clinical decision support

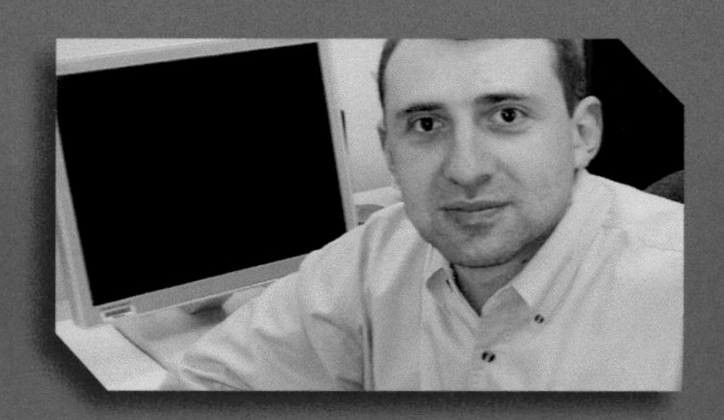

"I often find myself at a patient's bedside desperately looking for meaningful data to support my clinical decision-making. With real-time information, evidence-based nursing practice becomes the everyday routine."

"I have to travel to make a living, and everytime I get on a plane, I put myself at extreme health risk. I've got to make sure I'm awake long enough to give whatever medical professional who is going to be treating me the appropriate information so that they don't kill me!"

– Amye Leong

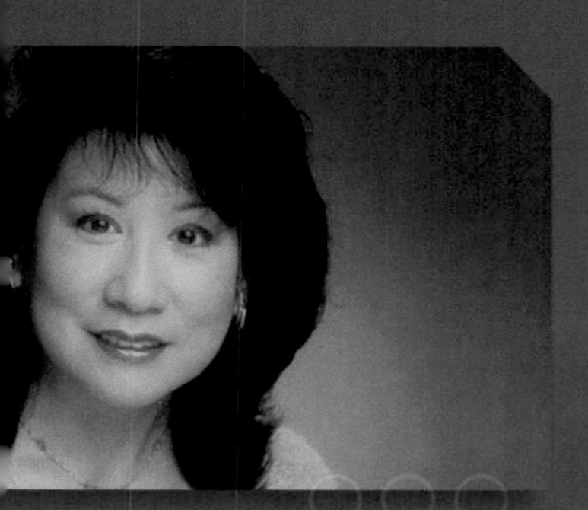

» PROFILE:

Amye Leong
PENNSYLVANIA

~ A California Native Copes with the Complications of Constant Travel with a Chronic Disease

Living with a Chronic Condition

Traveling today is dangerous enough, but traveling with a chronic disease can be life-threatening. Amye Leong tells her story of one particular incident where the lack of medical information could have abruptly ended her life. "I've had rheumatoid arthritis (RA) for 26 years, since I was 18 years old. I've had to focus more energy on it than anything else I can remember."

"Two years ago I was based in Paris but happened to be in Washington, D.C., for a conference. I awoke one morning at the hotel vomiting and in such physical pain. I know arthritis pain but this was very different. I called the hotel concierge and the conference organizers, who all suggested that I get to an emergency room right away. I was scheduled to take my flight back to Paris but I was going into shock and was beginning to feel like I was going to pass out. Unfamiliar with the medial terrain of D.C., I had the conference organizer call a friend a National Institutes of Health. If they got me to a certain hospital, a physician friend would be waiting for me.

"I got into a cab at my hotel with another person from the conference. I was doubled over in extreme pain, throwing up and having a hard time focusing. We told the cab driver which hospital to take me to. He did not take us there, but of course, I didn't know that. I didn't know one hospital from another I was so out of it. I didn't even have my eyes open. He took us to the closest hospital because he thought I was going to die in the cab."

"We got to the ER and told them our doctor was waiting for us and they said, 'What are you talking about? You have to fill out these forms.' I was passing out. They threw me into a wheelchair and said to the woman with me, 'You have to fill out these forms if she can't.' So my conference organizer, who knows nothing about my medical background, and only knew that I had RA, had to keep me awake long enough so I could give her the information to fill out the form."

"Finally, she just started screaming and said, 'Can't you see this woman's in distress? She needs help!' She started screaming so loud that the triage nurse came out to find out what was going on. And she took one look at me and said, 'Get her in here right away.' So it was a health professional that finally usurped the clerk who wanted me to fill out forms. She immediately got me into medical care. They instantly put me through tests and hospitalized me for a kidney stone that lodged itself in the worst possible spot."

Continued

"Then we found out we were in the wrong hospital all along. It was too late to be transferred, so we had to go through all kinds of, 'What's her medical history? What kinds of drugs is she taking?' I passed out cold at that time. Someone who only knew me as a speaker at a conference—did not know my medical history, did not know the drugs I was taking, only had a phone number of my mother who was not home—was responsible for telling them all this vital information. They had to wait until I was awake long enough, and they hoped by treating me they weren't going to do something to me that would be counter-indicated for the medications I was already on."

"When I woke up, I was in a hospital room with three doctors standing over me. They told me I had a kidney stone and needed surgery as soon as possible, and then I passed out cold again. The only thing I remember after that is someone saying, 'Stat, stat, get her into surgery.' When I woke up, it was a day and a half later. I had gone through surgery, which would normally have taken only an hour and a half, but because my blood levels were so low and my condition was unstable, I was in recovery for seven hours."

"When I finally got out of surgery, my friends who live in Washington were at the hospital. They are not my blood relatives so the hospital would not let them in to see me. We convinced the hospital that my friends who were there to help me were not necessarily blood family, but they were the closest thing to me at that time. My friends were the ones who knew my medical condition and treatments. I ended up spending 12 days in the hospital, most of it waiting for treatment because the doctors didn't have the information they needed."

"I can tell you the importance of having some kind of electronic record as someone with a chronic disease who faces all kinds of problems. I go through airports all the time and set off all kinds of alarms, because I've been through 16 surgeries. Twelve of those were joint replacements. I've been hospitalized for 298 days in my lifetime so far. But that has not stopped me from being a productive member of society."

"Chronic disease, unfortunately, is more mainstream than not. We are a highly mobile society. For people with chronic diseases who are trying to lead active lives, who travel as I do, we put our lives on the line every time we leave home. What do we do when we're not at home in our neighborhood medical care system? I have to travel to make a living, and every time I get on a plane, I put myself at extreme health risk. I've got to make sure I'm awake long enough to give whatever medical professional who is going to be treating me the appropriate information so that they don't kill me!"

FACT

~ Nearly half of the U.S. population, more than 125 million Americans, suffers from some sort of chronic medical condition.

Source: www.gingrichgroup.com/Transforming_Examples/Transforming_Examples_Resource_Center/139.cfm

Empowering Patients and Improving Care

"Health IT can enable transformation of healthcare by allowing a better way to care—consumer by consumer, physician by physician, disease by disease, and region by region."

David Brailer, M.D., Ph.D., National Coordinator for Health Information Technology

Continuity of care

With accessible personal health information, each new caregiver a patient sees can have access to that patient's history as the patient sees fit. Doctors no longer have to worry that the medications and the course of treatment they prescribe may be in conflict with those prescribed by other providers. In short, an interoperable system of electronic health information allows not only doctors but also hospitals, pharmacies, insurance providers, labs, diagnostic centers, nursing facilities, assisted living centers, and hospices to see the big picture—to know and understand the courses of treatment in progress, the intentions and goals of other healthcare providers, and the details and general trends of a patient's health and courses of treatment.

In addition to helping patients who see multiple doctors, the system will help ensure continuity of care for people who have moved from one place to another, an important benefit in a mobile society. How frequently does this issue come up for people? A study by the Commonwealth Fund, a private foundation supporting research on medically underserved communities, shows that nearly two-thirds of adults change doctors at least once every five years.[11]

Fewer errors and less wasted time

Since patients can give any provider access to their medical records any time, anywhere, they will no longer have to recount their medical histories every time they see a new doctor. That means that everyone saves time and there is no risk of forgetting a critical detail of treatment or condition.

[11] Harris Interactive. *2004 Commonwealth Fund International Health Policy Survey of Adults' Experiences with Primary Care,* Commonwealth Fund. 2004 <http://www.cmwf.org/surveys/surveys_show.htm?doc_id=245240>

An Increasingly Mobile Society

Americans are refusing to stay put and today's technology reflects that more and more. People travel greater distances frequently, whether for business or pleasure.

Visiting family, moving around the country to find work, traveling on business... all of these realities create huge demand for new technologies and devices to accommodate busy lives and constant motion. Personal digital assistants, cell phones, laptop computers, wireless Internet access, portable DVD and MP3 players, and Global Positioning Systems are just some of the gadgets that are available to the average consumer.

Amazingly, though, our cars benefit from more connectivity than our bodies do. If your car breaks down, you can take it to almost any dealership service department where the mechanic can access a history of the work that has been performed on that car and make an appropriate decision on what to do next.

Healthcare should be no different. In today's economy and travel culture, even healthcare professionals are more mobile than they were just a few decades ago. Healthcare information should be mobile and available wherever patients and professionals happen to be. Your health information should be designed to travel with you, not limit your travel.

“All of a sudden, the more educated you become, the more comfortable you become, not only about figuring out what's wrong, but, more importantly, figuring out how to cure the problem.”

President George W. Bush
(on patient-accessible electronic medical records)

Both doctors and patients are better informed

Healthcare providers will also be able to monitor compliance to find out if patients are getting their prescriptions filled, following up with referred physicians, and getting tests as ordered. Patients will be able to access the details of their treatment on the network and read as much or as little about their condition as they like. When health information is made available by doctors for patient review, the patients will be more informed, better prepared to ask questions, and better able to find peace of mind.

Better management of chronic conditions

Diabetes and other chronic conditions require frequent monitoring. Seven out of every 10 deaths in the United States each year are attributed to chronic diseases such as cancer, arthritis, muscular dystrophy, diabetes, and cardiovascular disease.[12] These often are prolonged illnesses that decrease quality of life and cause critical physical limitations, and they affect 90 million Americans.[13] When patients follow the treatments doctors prescribe and make lifestyle changes, such as getting more exercise, they can better manage chronic diseases.

Communication between doctors and patients can improve the management of chronic diseases, because patients will have a better understanding of their condition, how to manage pain, and how to deal with personal limitations. Chronic diseases often manifest themselves in ways that appear minor but are in fact significant indicators of serious problems. With better communication, patients can learn to recognize these symptoms so they can properly manage their healthcare.

Electronic prescribing (e-prescribing)

With an electronic healthcare system in place, doctors' prescriptions will instantly be sent to a pharmacy for patients to pick up. The prescription will be signed with an electronic signature that is readable at the pharmacy, so the notoriously illegible handwriting of doctors will no longer be an issue. There will be no paper

[12] National Center for Chronic Disease Prevention and Health Promotion. <http://www.cdc.gov/nccdphp/>
[13] Ibid.

prescriptions to lose or to drop off at the pharmacy, so patients will save time, trips to the doctor, and phone calls. E-prescribing systems will be able to check for harmful drug interactions as the doctor writes the prescription, long before the patient picks it up at the pharmacy.

Improved care for expectant mothers and their unborn babies

Obstetrics is an ideal place to introduce patients to connected healthcare information. On average, a pregnant patient will visit her provider's office 14 times during the pregnancy,[14] more than any other time in her life. Since prenatal exams may occur at many different locations, and different practitioners in a group may examine the same patient, interoperable records promote continuity of prenatal care. Expectant mothers may go into labor at unexpected times or places; accessible health information ensures that the mother's history is always available, wherever and whenever the delivery takes place.

Makes personalized care possible as future medical advances warrant

Medical advances such as DNA research might reveal that medicines will have different effects on people depending on their genetic makeup. Today a doctor may adjust a dosage on the basis of a patient's weight. In the future, a doctor will be able to order medications with specific characteristics, probably down to the molecular level, depending on the genetic makeup of a patient.

To take full advantage of these precise, customized medications, physicians will need access to voluminous and complex genetic information about a patient. These details will not be as simple as dates of treatment and names of conditions; that is, they cannot be memorized or easily carried around. These details will be stored in secure computer data files. For patients to benefit from new medicines, authorized healthcare providers will need to be able to review personal health information through an interoperable healthcare system.

[14] Donald Miller. "Prenatal Care: A Strategic First Step Toward EMR Acceptance." *Journal of Healthcare Information Management* 17, no. 2 (2003): 47–50.

Confidentiality, Privacy, and Security

"We want to know that the record is secure and that it remains confidential. But information technology actually works perfectly to document that. If you left a medical record on paper in a room, how will you know who saw it? You can't know. When it's in electronic form, when anyone logs on to the system, we know. We know who they are, we know where they are, we know what they were looking at, and we can keep logs of all that information so that we can confirm for our patients that their information is secure."

Dr. C. Martin Harris, Cleveland Clinic

Common Electronic Transactions

ATMs. 371,000 ATMs processed 10.8 billion transactions in 2003 in the United States. That is about 80 transactions a day or about 29,000 each year per ATM.[15]

Buying movie tickets on-line. Nearly one in four moviegoers has purchased tickets on-line.[16]

Travel. 39 million people booked travel on-line in 2002, an increase of 25 percent over 2001.[17]

Banking. The 29.6 million U.S. households banking on-line in 2003 is forecast to increase to 56 million by 2008.[18]

Income taxes. Over half of all income tax forms in the 2005 tax season were filed on-line.[19]

The power of technology to create trust

When it comes to using technology—actually making it a part of day-to-day life—attitudes have changed dramatically in a short period of time. Not so long ago, many people were intimidated by and distrustful of computers, but now most people welcome them and wonder how life went on without them:

- Most people enjoy 24/7 access to cash through ATMs;
- Fewer checks are used because of debit and credit card readers in stores;
- Computers in your car tell you when you are due for maintenance, how much gas is left in the tank, how many miles you have traveled and how many you have to go, and even the temperature outside. Global Positioning Systems tell you exactly where you are, and how to get where you are going;

[15] Miller, Donald. "Prenatal Care: A Strategic First Step Toward EMR Acceptance." *Journal of Healthcare Information Management* 17.2 (2003): 47-50.
[16] "This Summer's Blockbuster Hit: The Internet." *Freelance Writing.* July 2004. <http://www.freelancewriting.com/survey-072004-01.html>
[17] Mintel International Group Ltd. "Internet Travel: Abstract." September 1, 2003. <http://www.marketresearch.com/product/print/default.asp?g=1&productid=931785>
[18] Kim Komando. *Online Banking's Best Lure: Online Bill Paying.* Microsoft: Small Business Center. 2005. <http://www.microsoft.com/smallbusiness/resources/technology/business_software/online_bankings_best_lure_online_bill_paying.mspx>
[19] Internal Revenue Service. *2005 Tax Filing Season Sets Records.* July 2005. <http://www.irs.gov/newsroom/article/0,,id=138112,00.html>

- Cell phones are small, specialized computers. You can make calls wherever you are, and you are not limited by wires and cords. Some cell phones compete with desktop computers in their ability to accommodate e-mail, Internet access, word processing, and even photographs and video.

Why Americans (and the world) have so readily adopted technology

Your most personal and important information is entrusted to secure electronic systems. That security is one key to quick and widespread acceptance of connected healthcare systems.

It was not just convenience and fun that earned technology mainstream acceptance. A critical concern was first addressed: Would personal information such as tax returns and bank accounts be kept private? Had technology been introduced to the U.S. culture through government efforts, legislators could have simply mandated the use of interoperable systems, then improved the system after they were in place.

But private investors in technology could take no such risks. Privacy and security issues had to be anticipated and resolved by the businesses creating the systems. The public had to accept a system's security, then make their opinion known by using the system—or by turning it into a very expensive white elephant.

For the ATM network, on-line banking, bill paying, and e-commerce to succeed, the system had to thoroughly protect privacy. And the public had to believe—correctly—that the system was reliable as advertised. This confidence in technology was acquired incrementally. The benefits were great enough for Americans to assume a relatively minor risk.

“Information technology has radically changed business and so many other aspects of American life. It is time we use the power of the information age to improve health care. If we do, we can dramatically improve the quality of care, safety, efficiency and patient control over their health care decisions.”

Statement by Senate Majority Leader Bill Frist and Senator Hillary Rodham Clinton

People are growing more comfortable with using technology for healthcare

Trust in technology's ability to protect privacy is beginning to spread to its use for medical information:

- Eight in 10 Internet users—about 95 million Americans over the age of 18—have looked on-line for health information.[20] They are especially interested in diet, fitness, drugs, health insurance, experimental treatments, and particular information about doctors and hospitals.[21]
- Fifty-nine percent of women who go on-line have read up on nutrition.[22]
- Thirty-eight percent of parents on-line have checked for health insurance information.[23]
- Forty-one percent of Internet users with broadband connection at home have looked up a doctor or hospital.[24]

This is an encouraging start, but the level of American confidence needs to be much higher for an interoperable healthcare system to be accepted. Over 70 percent of people want to see technology used to improve the quality of healthcare, but nearly as many (67 percent) are concerned about privacy.[25]

Trusting Technology at the Gas Pump

How often do you take a receipt after filling up your gas tank and paying with a card? When you do take the receipt, do you usually throw it away after looking at it? When the bill comes at the end of the month, do you just assume it is correct, or do you go through a stack of paper receipts to reconcile it?

Most people discard the receipt if they take a look at it at all, and when the bill comes in they glance at the total to make sure the bill is in the normal price range.

This example of trusting technology to consistently get important details right is a good indicator that people will eventually trust technology with other critical information—such as personal healthcare records.

[20] Susannah Fox. "Eight in Ten Internet Users Have Looked for Health Information Online, with Increased Interest in Diet, Fitness, Drugs, Health Insurance, Experimental Treatments, and Particular Doctors and Hospitals." *Health Information Online.* May 17, 2005. <www.pewinternet.org/PPF/r/95/report_display.asp>

[21] Ibid.

[22] Pew Internet. *More Internet Users Do 'Health Homework' Online.* Press release. May 17, 2005. <http://www.pewinternet.org/press_release.asp?r=106>

[23] Susannah Fox. "Eight in Ten Internet Users Have Looked for Health Information Online, with Increased Interest in Diet, Fitness, Drugs, Health Insurance, Experimental Treatments, and Particular Doctors and Hospitals." *Health Information Online.* May 17, 2005. <http://www.pewinternet.org/PPF/r/95/report_display.asp>

[24] Ibid.

[25] Harris Interactive. "Many Nationwide Believe in the Potential Benefits of Electronic Medical Records and Are Interested in Online Communications with Physicians." August 2005. <http://www.harrisinteractive.com/news/allnewsbydate.asp?NewsID=895>

The good news: Prevention and confidentiality are attainable goals

No system can be perfect, but you can expect much higher quality outcomes from an electronic healthcare system than you receive from the current paper-based system. After all, most electronic information systems perform flawlessly every day. If they didn't, bank accounts would be wrecked and bills would be inaccurate every month.

That is not to pretend there are no problems in the world of electronic data exchange. But those problems are the exception, not the rule. For every incident of lost data, billions of transactions occur without incident every day. Still, recent events involving data loss deserve consideration. The following information was published by the *Wall Street Journal* in May 2005:[27]

> In February 2005, consumer-data compiler ChoicePoint announced the theft of data on about 145,000 consumers. Within two weeks of that incident, Bank of America announced the loss of up to 1.2 million credit card numbers belonging to the Federal government. In March, retailer DSW Shoe Warehouse announced the discovery of theft of data potentially affecting over a million people. In June, CardSystems Solutions Inc., a payment processing company, was infiltrated by hackers, exposing more than 40 million credit card and debit card accounts to potential fraud. Similar events followed at Lexis-Nexis, Boston College, Polo Ralph Lauren, Ameritrade, and Time-Warner.

In some cases, fraud against consumers was discovered quickly. In other cases, customers were advised to closely check their credit card statements for several months to make certain fraudulent charges did not appear. In a few cases, the problem was not data theft but the loss of backup data media, such as reels of computer tape during shipping; this would have led to fraud only if the tapes had been found, identified, and translated.

The Living Will Registry: An Application of Electronic Connections in Healthcare

More and more Americans are writing "living wills"—instructions for medical care in the event that they become too incapacitated to communicate with their doctors. It's a good idea, but the problem with a living will is that healthcare providers do not always know that their patient has one.

That is why, in 1996, Joseph Barmakian, MD, created the U.S. Living Will Registry.[26] The registry is a way to provide instant access to physicians nationwide for patients who maintain a living will. In fact, healthcare providers are required by Federal law to check for a patient's advance directive and place a copy of the will in the patient's medical record. Access to the registry is password-protected, and a patient's information is shared with no one other than his or her healthcare provider. This service is provided free to the public.

---

[26] United States Living Will Registry. "Living Will—Health Care Proxy." July 2005. <http://www.uslivingwillregistry.com/info-english.shtm>

[27] E. Perez and R. Brooks. "File Sharing: For Big Vendor of Personal Data, A Theft Lays Bare the Downside." *Wall Street Journal.* May 3, 2005.

While all data loss is potentially serious, these events are notable for their real-life impact relative to the number of records lost or stolen:

- At ChoicePoint, only 750 cases of fraud appeared out of the records of 145,000 consumers—about one-half of one percent.
- At Lexis-Nexis, only 59 incidents have been reported out of stolen information on 310,000 consumers—0.019 percent, or less than two-hundredths of one percent.

The Limits of Security: An Important Note

While a system of interoperable health information can be designed to carefully monitor the access and use of information, it's not possible to ensure that there are absolutely no "prying eyes." The limits of safeguards will be determined primarily by the state of technology. Today, unauthorized use is minimized by log-ins and passwords for authentication that limit access to medical information. In time, the system will be strengthened with biometrics. Improvements will also be made in encrypting data during storage and transfer. But even the most basic system of connected health information will provide more consistent security and improved tracking of access than any paper system can.

The organizational responses to these incidents are promising. In each case, the organization modified the way it handled consumer information to improve the systems of protection:

- Bank of America is moving away from backup tapes to computer-to-computer data transfers. In instances where backup tapes cannot be eliminated, encryption is being considered.
- Since the thieves posed as legitimate customers, ChoicePoint no longer sells sensitive personal data to clients outside government and accredited corporate entities.
- Lexis-Nexis reduced access to personal data.[28]

All the companies worked with Federal authorities to find the culprits and to improve procedures for security.

Public confidence in these companies has remained strong, as measured by the value of the companies' stock and their sales. While stock prices for some of the companies took an immediate dip when the breaches were publicized, almost every firm has rebounded. Polo Ralph Lauren's stock price dropped 55 cents (1.4 percent) the day it confirmed data theft;[29] however, quotes bounced back to near 52-week highs in late June. DSW Shoe Warehouse's sales actually saw a considerable increase; revenues grew more than 60 million dollars (not adjusted for inflation) for the first five months of 2005 compared with 2004.[30] Other

[28] Lucas Mearian. "Data Snafus Spur IT Action: Bank Mishap Prompts Call for Network Backup." *COMPUTERWORLD*. March 7, 2005. <http://www.computerworld.com/?source=nav_tab>
[29] Associated Press. "Update 5: Polo Ralph Lauren Customers' Data Stolen." *Forbes*. June 2005. <http://www.forbes.com/business/feeds/ap/2005/04/14/ap1947570.html>
[30] J. McGrady. "May Sales Report." Retail Ventures (June 2005). <http://www.retailventuresinc.com/index.jsp>

companies, such as Time-Warner and Bank of America, showed no significant fluctuation in stock prices.

If consumer confidence was shaken, that confidence seemed to return quickly.

Individuals want access to and control of their own records

Dr. Alan Westin is a retired professor at Columbia University and a widely recognized advocate for privacy rights. He has examined the task of winning public support for a system of electronic health records.

Dr. Westin conducted a survey to see if people believe that the expected benefits of a system—whatever they think those benefits might be—outweigh the potential risks to privacy.[31] In his survey, Dr. Westin asked whether consumers think it is important to be able to track their own information and "exercise privacy rights." The result was no surprise: More than 80 percent of the respondents rated availability of their medical records as important.[32]

As a connected electronic healthcare system is integrated into the practice of healthcare, the system must be transparent—each element of an interoperable system must be fully known to the public, its function clearly understood, and its mechanisms available for inspection. Explanations to the public must use straightforward language to create confidence and must acknowledge—not dismiss—doubt. In particular, the system should allow individuals:

- To access personal clinical data;
- To make additions to the record; and
- To review the audit trail of who accessed the records, what was viewed, when, and for how long.

[31] Alan Westin. *How the Public Views Health Privacy: Survey Findings from 1978 to 2005.* PrivacyExchange. February 23,2005. <http://privacyexchange.org/>
[32] Ibid.

There is no more direct way for people to check the accuracy of their records than to simply review the information themselves.

At the launch of the interoperable healthcare system, any particular piece of information will almost certainly be maintained at its source (e.g., lab reports at the lab or at the office of the requesting physician, treatment records at the doctor's office, hospital records at the hospital). This may change as new technologies emerge and are implemented, but security, confidentiality, and transparency to patients must remain top priorities in deciding how and where data are stored.

Confidentiality: The core of the doctor-patient relationship

The core of healthcare is the relationship between the patient and the provider. That relationship is built on trust—not an abstract notion of confidentiality or security, but a personal belief that what a patient tells a doctor or nurse remains confidential.

In a healthcare relationship, individuals disclose highly confidential—sometimes embarrassing and definitely private—information about themselves, information they may not tell anyone else.

Doctors need to know this information to better understand a patient's problem and to better prescribe treatment. There is no other way to deliver the right care.

Technology cannot be allowed to disrupt this relationship. Rather, technology must fit seamlessly into the existing "psychology of trust" found in the healthcare world. The trust a patient holds in a healthcare provider helps build trust in new elements added to the healthcare system, leading to an attitude of, "If my doctor trusts this new system, then I do, too." Doctors will need concrete facts to tell their patients about the security and privacy of the system. Companies that provide systems will need to support physicians and hospitals in efforts to educate patients.

Better Health ... Anytime, Anywhere

"I really feel kind of comforted that I can get access almost immediately to my doctor, my records, and everything else just by stopping at an Internet café anywhere along the line."

– Keith Belcher

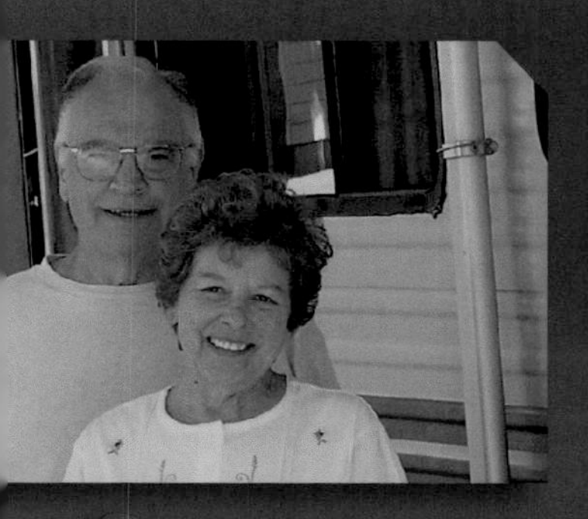

» PROFILE:

Keith and Margy Belcher
OREGON

~ On-the-Go Couple Managing Chronic Diseases While Traveling

Seventy-year-old Keith Belcher and his wife, Margy, feel right at home almost anywhere. They've spent the last several years of their retirement traveling the western United States in their RV—despite the fact that both Keith and Margy have chronic health conditions that require regular contact with their many doctors. They have been able to live their dream of traveling because of their doctors' commitments to making their patients' health information electronically available to them—and to their other doctors—anytime, anywhere.

Keith and Margy decided to move from northern California to Sweet Home, Oregon, in 2002. Originally, they had planned to find a new primary care doctor after the move, but they found it difficult to find someone who was taking new patients in the small rural town. They eventually decided to keep their doctor in Palo Alto, partly because they planned to go back to visit family at least three times a year. It would be easy for them to come in for annual checkups, but mostly because they could stay in regular contact with her via a Web portal and e-mail.

Keith has struggled with diabetes for years and more recently learned he had heart problems and underwent triple-bypass surgery. "When I was down there for an annual checkup, having absolutely no clue as to anything being wrong, I went in and had my normal checkup, and she put me on a treadmill test, which I failed. And I failed my echogram, and I failed the angiogram, and ended up about 10 days later having a three-way bypass." Although it was a scary situation for both Keith and Margy, they feel much better knowing that they are able to contact their doctor anytime with any questions or concerns.

Now Keith is managing both his heart condition and his diabetes no matter where he is. Keith's doctors order tests and treatments for him while he is in Oregon, and they check on his status and test results almost immediately, even though they are hundreds of miles away. "Because all the treatment I get here, whether it be therapy or anything else, all of that is initiated through the prescriptions from my doctor in Palo Alto." Margy also manages her arthritis on the road, and she is able to e-mail her doctor about any changes in her treatment or unusual symptoms or side effects. Her doctor orders tests for her that she can have done near home as well.

Continued

For the Belchers, their newfound freedom means more than just convenience. They can rest with the knowledge that wherever they are, their health information is accessible. "When we're in eastern Oregon, or we're thinking about possibly going to Lake Powell, I really feel kind of comforted in that I can get access almost immediately to my doctor, and my records, and everything else just by stopping at an Internet café anywhere along the line. If I were ever on the road and I needed to go to another hospital, I could just log on and wherever I was my medical professionals could be on the same page."

FACT

~ One in five Americans live in rural areas and only one in 10 physicians practice in rural areas.

Source: Rural Emergency Response - the Safety and Health Safety Net;
www.cdc.gov/nasd/docs/d001701-d001800/d001781/d001781.pdf

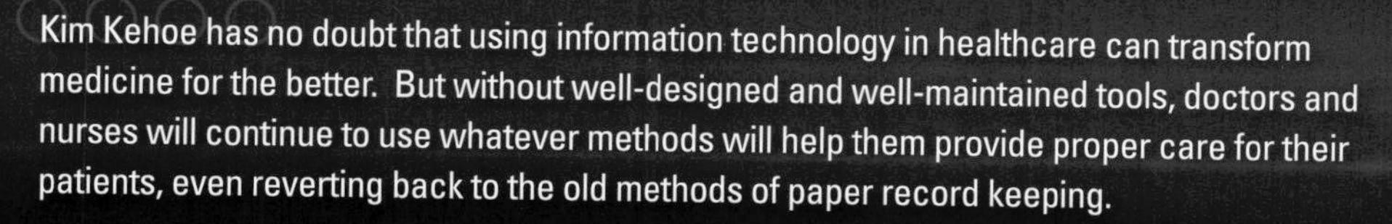

Free is Not Always Best

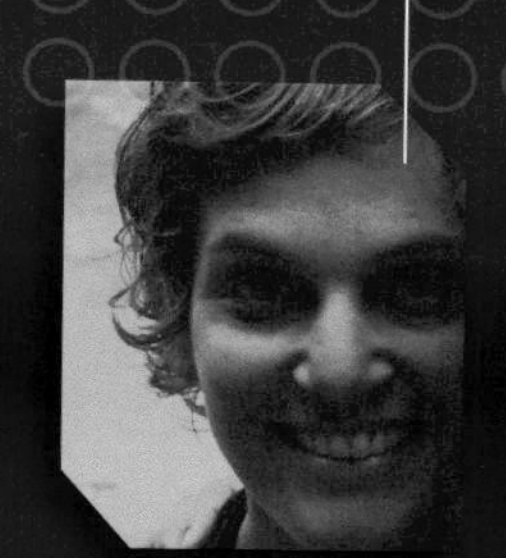

PROFILE:

Kim Kehoe

HAWAII

~ Nurse Practitioner Urges Health IT Advocates to Consider Providers' Needs

"It's got to work for the providers. Already we're dealing with a system that doesn't make it very easy to practice good medicine. So if it doesn't make our lives easier, it's not going to work."

– Kim Kehoe

Kim Kehoe has no doubt that using information technology in healthcare can transform medicine for the better. But without well-designed and well-maintained tools, doctors and nurses will continue to use whatever methods will help them provide proper care for their patients, even reverting back to the old methods of paper record keeping.

Kim works as a nurse practitioner for a community health center in Hawaii. The center recently was given a government-funded electronic health records system and used the system for a six-month period. However, the small office with only three doctors and two nurses found the system to be more of a hindrance than a help. "Part of the problem was that we're a small community health center and we don't have tech support. Our tech support was basically an out-of-town computer consultant whom we called anytime we had computer problems." After six months, they went back to using paper.

"The whole idea of electronic medical records from a provider's perspective is that it's supposed to make the visit and the billing more efficient, so we could see a patient and click everything on the electronic medical records, and by the time the patient left the room, it was immediately transmitted to billing. The problem was we couldn't really customize the electronic system for our purposes. We've heard of other products that might be more user-friendly, but ours wasn't working in that way."

"It was taking a long time to complete the record in the room with the patients. There was also an issue with interviewing patients. You couldn't look them in the eye because you were looking at a computer screen clicking buttons. It was sometimes very difficult to find buttons that fit every person, so you ended up free-texting a lot. It ended up taking a lot longer. It was not saving us time, at least from the providers' point of view."

"We definitely see the benefit of it, mostly around issues like medication lists and chronic health problems. If you came into the clinic and we changed your medication, it would change it on your master list. If you were hospitalized for some reason, the ambulance would have instant access to that medication list, or your list of allergies to medications or chronic health problems. We see the benefit of every provider having access to that information, but in terms of the patient encounter with a provider, you're limited. Most patient visits are 15 minutes. So if the system isn't making you more efficient, it makes your job more complicated and less personal."

In Need of a Lifesaving Tool

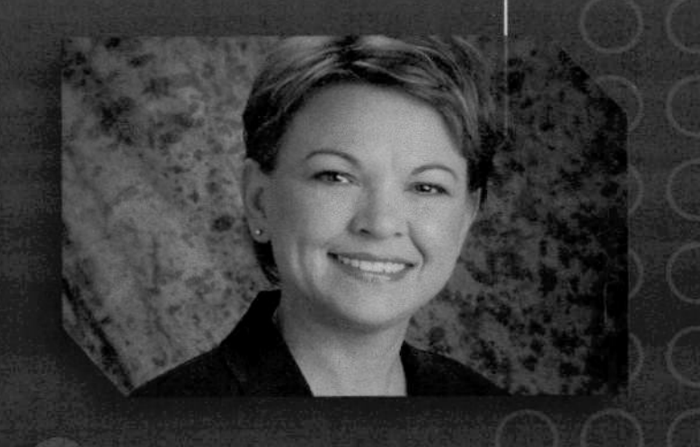

» PROFILE:

Lisa Amiotte, M.D.
SOUTH DAKOTA

~ A Psychiatrist in South Dakota Struggles with an Antiquated Information System

"Doctors are spread pretty thin. Information is scattered throughout the various clinics and doctors, which makes it very complex to navigate."

– Lisa Amiotte, M.D.

Dr. Lisa Amiotte knows firsthand the difference in care that a patient receives with—or without—information available to their doctors and nurses. She tells one horror story of a young patient who was brought to her hospital last winter. The young man had been found wandering around a reservation in western South Dakota in freezing cold conditions. When he finally arrived at the hospital, he was severely frostbitten and unable or unwilling to speak. Rather than being able to pull up his information on a computer and find out why he was not speaking, Dr. Amiotte, along with countless other doctors, nurses, and social workers, began the painstaking process of trying to scrape together any information that would help them properly treat the sick young man.

Days later, and after hours of searching for information and medical guesswork, they were finally able to contact his primary care doctor miles away. At that point, they learned that the young man had paranoid schizophrenia, and also had severe problems with substance abuse. Dr. Amiotte sees this incident as an example of how lack of information can severely hurt patients.

But even on a day-to-day basis, Dr. Amiotte knows that having a reliable system of accessible electronic medical records could revolutionize the way she treats her patients. "From the standpoint of just being able to get collateral information from another clinician, not just having the information from the patient's standpoint, but having the information from another clinician's standpoint, you'd be able to avoid a lot of pitfalls (like what other medications the patient is on, their history, etc.). A lot of times it's trial and error until you get the actual release of information and paperwork back from that other physician's office. You have to just go on your own good judgment and clinical experience, and on what the patient has given you. My patients don't always have an accurate recollection."

Dr. Amiotte sees many possible benefits to healthcare providers in rural areas, like her. "Doctors are spread pretty thin. Information is scattered throughout the various clinics and doctors, which makes it very complex to navigate."

"I was told I ask too many questions about Tommy's health ... but what the doctor says is not always clear to the patient. It is my right to know."

– Gay Quick

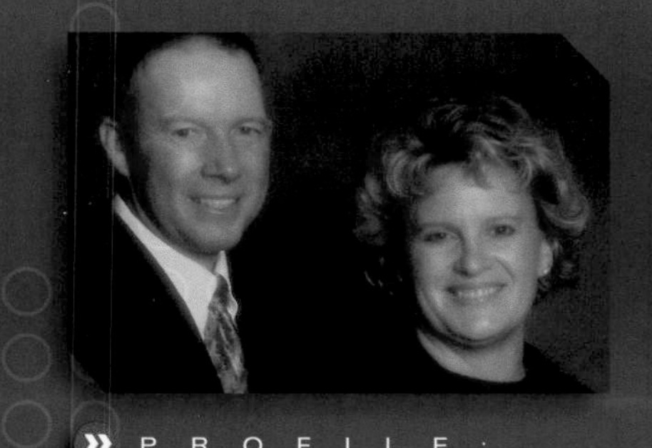

» PROFILE:

Gayetta and Tommy Quick
MISSOURI

~ Dedicated Wife Acted as a Walking Medical Record for her Husband Dying of Cancer

The Waiting Game

Beginning in April of 1985, Tommy Quick's family was introduced to "the waiting game." He was diagnosed with a brain tumor and had his first brain surgery in Minnesota in 1986. This was to be the first of Tommy's 19-year battle against cancer. Next came a string of over 100 magnetic resonance images (MRIs), multiple rounds of chemotherapy and radiation, and more than three brain surgeries in four hospitals nationwide. During this time, Tommy would not have been able to accurately recite his medical history without the help of his wife, Gayetta (Gay).

Managing Tommy's medical record became Gay's full-time job. His life depended on real-time information in order to receive quick and accurate treatment. In 1985, his doctors in Missouri and Minnesota told Tommy he had only two to three years to live. The Quicks lived on a farm 100 miles away from his nearest doctor, and his battle against cancer took place between Kansas City, Minneapolis, and San Francisco.

Gay understood the importance of accurate and quick medical information. By setting aside a few days to schedule his medical needs, Gay learned to schedule Tommy's blood work, MRI, and doctor appointments on the same day. To speed up his appointments, Gay says, "I finally wrote down everything, so when he went to the doctor, I would take my satchel ... Tommy's life was in my satchel." This included a list of significant dates, descriptions of seizures, doctor visit details, medications, insurance information, and even a collaboration of all of Tommy's MRIs that doctors would not otherwise have.

In 1996, when his tumor began to grow more rapidly, communication between San Francisco and Kansas City became vital. MRIs traced the tumor growth and because San Francisco made many treatment decisions, including two major brain surgeries, MRIs needed to be sent from Kansas City to San Francisco quickly. Gay took the responsibility when the hospital informed her that it could take up to a few weeks to mail the MRIs. Gay called every day to ensure that Tommy's doctors in San Francisco received the MRIs that were overnight mailed at about $20.00 each. Tommy's condition called for routine blood work and a MRI every six months beginning in 1996. Following each test or appointment, the Quick family began a new round of the waiting game—waiting for an update on Tommy's battle against cancer—afraid to leave home and miss a call from San Francisco or Kansas City.

Continued

Gay's efforts to manage Tommy's medical records were especially vital when he lost the ability to speak and to use much of the right side of his body. Gay went above and beyond to maximize Tommy's quality of care. Tommy passed away in September 2004 following his long fight against cancer.

"The waiting game was the hardest game to learn to play."

– Gay Quick

Did You Know?

- The National Cancer Institute estimates that approximately 8.9 million Americans with a history of cancer were alive in 1997.

Source: American Cancer Society. Cancer Facts and Figures, 2002.

Health Issues for Individual Communities

"Information technology holds the promise of reducing healthcare disparities for those living in rural communities. We can measure our success in building an IT infrastructure by the provision of quality of care in these communities challenged by long distances and scarce medical resources."

Senator Chuck Grassley

Access for everyone, including the poor and indigent

The need for healthcare is universal and critical, and a system of accessible and accurate interoperable records can extend benefits to everyone. It would not merely equalize healthcare opportunities; it could raise the quality of healthcare for everyone. This is especially important for the indigent and the working poor populations, who often have the most challenging healthcare issues and the least continuity of care.

Connecting Migrant Workers

The health problems of migrant workers are often compounded by constant travel, along with language and cultural barriers. But a new system in Sonoma County, California, is changing that. This interoperable healthcare network allows migrant workers and their families to enroll in a program that stores their health history, conditions, and treatments as an electronic health record. The records can be accessed by healthcare providers from clinics anywhere in the United States and Mexico.[33]

Better care in community health centers

Thirty-six million Americans lack access to a regular source of healthcare—that is nearly one out of every eight people.[34] Twenty-six percent of all health center visits are for chronic diseases, including asthma, diabetes, hypertension, HIV/AIDS, mental health issues, and substance abuse.[35] These centers serve:

- One in eight uninsured Americans;
- One in five low-income uninsured Americans;
- One in nine Medicaid beneficiaries;
- One in seven members of minority groups;

[33] "Internet Medical Records for Migrant Workers." *Local Frontiers–Sonoma Medicine* 55, no. 2 (Spring 2004). <http://www.vwsvia.org/>
[34] National Association of Community Health Centers. *A Nation's Health at Risk.* 2004.
[35] Ibid.

- One in ten Americans living in rural areas; and
- One in five low-income children.[36]

The following are among the benefits of an interoperable system to individuals who rely on these centers:

- Preventing abuse by checking all medications taken and supplying only appropriate medications;
- Providing accurate records of immunizations for children; and
- Preventing chronic disease with more effective primary care for patients through monitoring of conditions and adherence to treatment.[37]

Issues in rural areas

Four-fifths of the United States is rural,[38] and in 29 states at least one-third of the population is classified as rural. Rural residents face serious healthcare issues not only in terms of illness but also in terms of lack of easily accessible services. For instance:

- One in five Americans live in rural areas but only one in 10 physicians practice in rural areas;[39]
- Forty percent of the rural population lives in a medically underserved area;[40]
- Fire departments are the primary provider of medical services in rural areas;[41]

[36] Ibid.
[37] Ibid.
[38] For practical purposes, "rural" can be considered areas of relatively low population outside cities and suburbs. "Urban" can be considered the cities and suburbs themselves. For purposes of analyzing statistics, consider the U.S. Census Bureau definitions: "urban" is "[a]ll territory, population and housing units in urban areas, which include urbanized areas and urban clusters. An urban area generally consists of a large central place and adjacent densely settled census blocks that together have a total population of at least 2,500 for urban clusters, or at least 50,000 for urbanized areas. Urban classification cuts across other hierarchies and can be in metropolitan or non-metropolitan areas." "Rural" is "[t]erritory, population and housing units not classified as urban ... and can be in metropolitan or non-metropolitan areas." Source: U.S. Census Bureau. "Urban and Rural Definitions." October 1995.
[39] Gary Erisman. "Rural Emergency Response–The Safety and Health Safety Net." National Ag Safety Database. 2001. <http://www.cdc.gov/nasd/docs/d001701-d001800/d001781/d001781.pdf >
[40] Ibid.
[41] Bruce Evans. "Rural Health Care's Missing Link." *Fire Chief.* June 2002.

- For motor vehicle accidents, the average response time of emergency medical services in rural areas is 18 minutes.[42] This is eight minutes longer than the response time in urban areas.[43] (The average response time from the point of injury to the arrival of medical assistance for transport during the Vietnam War was eight to 10 minutes);[44]

- Compared with patients in urban areas, patients in rural areas tend to be older, have higher rates of chronic illness, and exhibit poorer health behaviors such as smoking and obesity;[45] and

- Rural residents often have to travel great distances to reach medical care.[46]

With access to care an average of 30 miles away,[47] rural areas have much to gain from the ability to access healthcare information at a distance. In an emergency, interaction with a doctor may be limited to phone advice. For routine care, increased communication with healthcare providers will increase patients' quality of life because they can better follow treatment guidelines and more easily receive feedback from healthcare providers. This is especially valuable for the many rural areas that offer few preventive services.

The American Indian and Alaskan Native populations most often live in rural areas, and their healthcare problems mirror many of those of the rural population. Like the rural population, these individuals tend to have more serious and more frequent health problems than the general population, and they enjoy less access to the healthcare system. As a result, they tend to use health services less often than other groups.

[42] National Rural Health Association. *What's Different About Rural Health Care?* July 2005. <http://www.nrharural.org/about/sub/different.html>
[43] Ibid.
[44] Gary Erisman. "Rural Emergency Response—The Safety and Health Safety Net." National Ag Safety Database. 2001. <http://www.cdc.gov/nasd/docs/d001701-d001800/d001781/d001781.pdf >
[45] American Society of Health-System Pharmacists. "IOM Sets Strategy for Improving Rural Health Care Quality." December 15, 2004. <http://www.ashp.org/news/showArticle.cfm?cfid=19987294&CFToken=93416380&&id=8935>
[46] National Rural Health Association. "What's Different About Rural Health Care?" July 2005. <http://www.nrharural.org/about/sub/different.html>
[47] Bruce Evans. "Rural Health Care's Missing Link." *Fire Chief.* June 2002.

An Institute of Medicine committee has recommended that the government develop a strategy for transitioning rural health clinics (along with community health centers, critical access hospitals, and other rural providers) from paper to electronic health records.[48]

Tracking disease and nationwide medical concerns

A connected system of healthcare would allow the U.S. government to monitor health concerns such as vaccination rates, disease outbreaks, and disease trends nationwide. This kind of bio-surveillance would mean that West Nile virus, avian influenza, environmental health concerns, disease outbreaks from flooding due to hurricanes, such as Hurricane Katrina, and numerous other issues could be better targeted and monitored, allowing containment efforts to be established with more precision and efficiency.

"You won't find a solution by saying there is no problem."

William Rotsler, Author (1926 – 1997)

Military

The U.S. military service branches do not have an efficient way to transmit medical information in critical, time-sensitive situations. For soldiers extracted from the battlefield, injury notes, medical history, test results, and surgical history are not always communicated from one doctor to the next. This forces service-men to undergo duplicate tests and surgeries, and to settle for less than the most efficient treatment.

Veterans

The U. S. Department of Veterans Affairs (VA) currently provides medical care for over five million veterans.[49] The VA maintains electronic copies of all patient information—including information from doctor's appointments, medications, and laboratory and imaging data—constituting a closed interoperable network of healthcare information for this specific population. Any of this information can be stored and transmitted among doctors within the VA medical system. The success of this system suggests that a nationwide system of connected health information is possible.

[48] American Society of Health-System Pharmacists. "IOM Sets Strategy for Improving Rural Health Care Quality." December 15, 2004. <http://www.ashp.org/news/showArticle.cfm?cfid=19987294&CFToken=93416380&&id=8935>

[49] United States Department of Veterans Affairs. *Facts About the Department of Veterans Affairs.* June 2005. <http://www1.va.gov/opa/fact/vafacts.html >

Improving Health Through Online Access

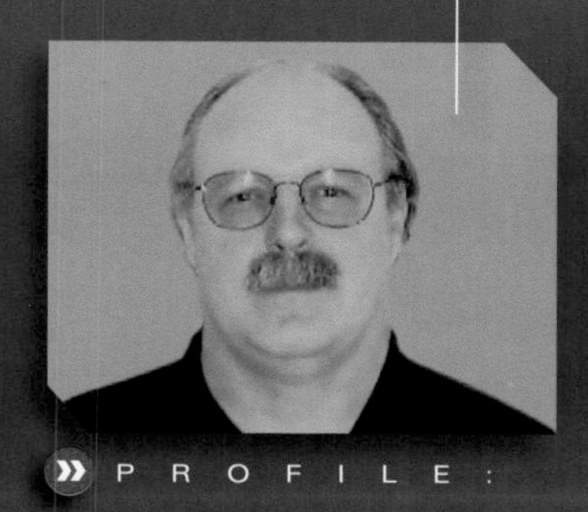

» PROFILE:

Ron Brimmer

MARYLAND

~ 50-Year-Old Veteran and Frequent User of My HealtheVet, an Electronic, Interactive Medical Record

"Going to the doctor is no longer guesswork."

– Ron Brimmer

Ron Brimmer's health is a lot better these days because of My HealtheVet. The Department of Veterans Affairs (VA) began the interactive electronic medical records program in 2003 at VA hospitals to better connect doctors with patients and to provide both of them with critical medical information whenever they need it. Ron was one of the first veterans to test this new electronic patient records system, and he is now one of its biggest advocates.

Nearly 30 years ago, Ron injured his back, knee, and both shoulders. He is mobile only with crutches or using his electric scooter. Maintaining mobility is an ongoing process, which includes physical therapy and visits with three to five doctors on a regular basis. But My HealtheVet makes managing his care a lot easier. It enables him to access his VA medical records at home; review his prescriptions, blood test results, and notes from the doctor; and even add information or update his record.

With My HealtheVet, Ron is healthier because his visits to a VA doctor are now more focused, and his care is more personally directed. Ron is better informed about his treatment and as his health has improved, his visits to the doctor have actually decreased. When he sees a doctor outside of the VA system, he can print his VA medical records and take them along—that's a real time and trouble saver for Ron, who lives 35 miles from the hospital and would otherwise have to drive in and request his records in person. In addition, My HealtheVet allows him to e-mail his doctor at any time with questions. Electronic records at the VA have even kept Ron from taking medications that would interact with each other.

Did You Know?

~ Of the 25 million veterans currently alive, nearly three of every four served during a war or an official period of hostility. About a quarter of the Nation's population—approximately 70 million people—are potentially eligible for VA benefits and services because they are veterans, family members, or survivors of veterans.

Source: www.va.gov/about_va/

A Medical Battlefield

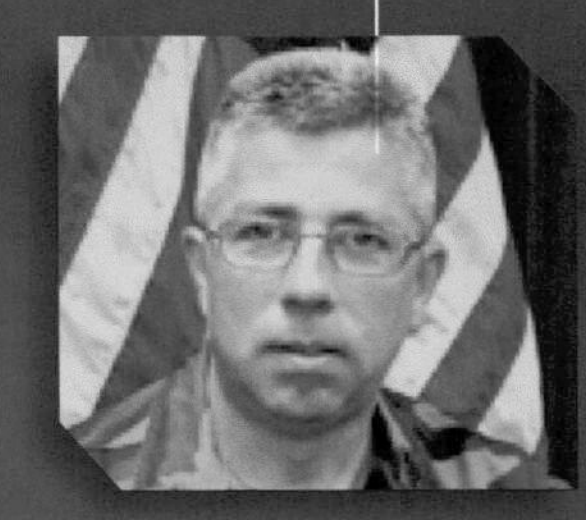

» PROFILE:

Colonel John Holcomb
TEXAS

~ Challenge of Adding an EMR on the Battlefield Without the Internet Available

We have hospitals in fghanistan and Iraq, d many of the soldiers vould arrive without records in Germany, vith no record of the CAT scans or what happened in surgery in Afghanistan or aq. The clinicians in ermany would have to operate on the patient, ould have to redo all eir x-ray evaluations, CAT scans, etc ....”

– Colonel John Holcomb

Most American citizens do not see Black Hawk helicopters and falling mortars as daily scenery, but the American soldier on tour in Iraq or Afghanistan does. Receiving medical treatment on a battlefield is dramatically different than in a hospital stateside, but today interoperable information holds the power to change military medicine.

Colonel Holcomb is a researcher and clinician in the Army. He testifies to the importance and need for interoperable electronic health information in the military, especially in a war zone. “Without an electronic medical record (EMR), we're relying on pieces of paper that are inadequately filled out or if they are filled out, they get lost as soldiers move from a small little surgical site to a larger site by helicopters or ground, and then get transported on a cargo plane to Germany. Then another cargo plane transports them to the United States, and pieces of paper get lost in the shuffle.” When pieces of paper holding medical information get lost in the military, soldiers pay the price as their doctors try to put the puzzle pieces of medical information together. However, a soldier's health can hold the key for how daily operations are carried out for fellow soldiers on the battlefield.

Colonel Holcomb works with the Joint Theater Trauma Registry, which is a database that allows injury patterns and outcomes to be tracked. “It's an extraordinary research opportunity to help find out what was going on at each level, and how patients did, and what their outcomes were, but the Joint Theater Trauma Registry is really hampered by not having electronic data at every site that is compatible from one site to the next, and transferable from one site to the next. It is limited in its scope, quality, and timeliness.”

“If we had that timeliness factor we could respond with injury patterns, changing tactics, and techniques and procedures of the enemy, and we would recognize injury patterns.” However, military hospitals in the United States do not have the tools needed to track injuries and relay preventative information to those in command in a timely fashion.

FACT

~ Tricare, the largest military health plan, has nearly nine million beneficiaries.

Source: Weiner, Tim. "A New Call to Arms: Military Health Care" New York Times. April 14, 2005.

Coping With Chaos

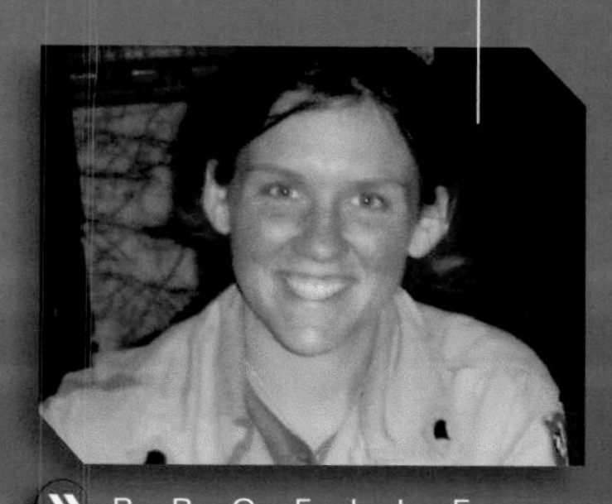

PROFILE:

Abbie Pickett
WISCONSIN

~ An Army National Guard Specialist Injured in Iraq Tells Her Own Personal Health Horror Story

"Out in the field, there's no reliable record keeping system to verify what happens to soldiers."

– Abbie Pickett

Abbie Pickett's life was forever changed by her experience in Iraq. As a specialist for the Army National Guard, Abbie found herself in the middle of a mortar attack on a base recreational facility in October of 2003. While she was physically injured in the attack, Abbie found that much deeper and more painful wounds would show up later on.

Abbie's eardrum was punctured in the attack, but she heroically helped care for her fellow soldiers who were more seriously wounded during and after the attack. Abbie and two other soldiers who were involved were seen by a physician's assistant after the incident. The man filled out all the paperwork documenting the attack and their wounds and informed them that he had also put in for them to receive Purple Hearts. But that paperwork was lost. It is now almost two years after the incident and Abbie has yet to find an effective course of treatment for her Post Traumatic Stress Disorder (PTSD).

Shortly after the attack, Abbie began developing symptoms of PTSD, but because her injury could not be "verified," her diagnosis was delayed. She was bounced around from caregiver to caregiver for almost two years. Instead of being treated appropriately, Abbie has been given numerous drugs for everything from depression to insomnia, and has to recount her trauma again and again with each new provider. "Out in the field my care was shifted from person to person so that every time I went to get help or get my medications refilled, I had to start at square one."

"Because mental health has such a bad stigma in the military, they try to keep it as hush-hush as they can. They tell you that as soon as you leave their office, they'll destroy your records and they'll never exist. The problem is, when you come back, you have to prove that you've been in a traumatic event or that your depression was a result of being over there, but those records have been destroyed. There are a ton of soldiers coming home trying to get help, but the waits are so long that unfortunately, in that time, there are car accidents, suicides, and they're abusing alcohol and drugs trying to self-medicate."

Continued

Abbie also had a horrible time trying to claim promised benefits because she could never "prove" that she was injured in combat. "It took me a little over a year from when I got home to get my compensation. Out in the field, there's no reliable record keeping system to verify what happens to soldiers. I'm over the bitter state. Right now, I'm just struggling to get by and deal with my symptoms." To top it all off, she will never receive a Purple Heart or a Bronze Star for the wounds she sustained or the heroism she displayed in Iraq, all because of an archaic and horribly flawed system of medical record keeping.

Did You Know?

- There are nearly 11,600 wounded from the war in Iraq and Afghanistan.

Source: PBS OnLine News Hour, April 26, 2005.; "Coping With U.S. Combat Injuries"; http://www.pbs.org/newshour/bb/middle_east/iraq/postwar/mfacts_casualty.html

Reducing Medical Errors While Saving Patients' Time and Money

"Today in America, thousands of patients are having unnecessary tests, undergoing surgeries they do not need, and taking harmful drugs due to our paper-based health care system, and the consequences are deadly and costly. Because of this, sadly, hundreds of patients will die today and thousands more will be put at risk. And all of this can be prevented. Simply put, paper kills."

Congressman Tim Murphy

The bottom line

Medical errors are killing more people each year than breast cancer, AIDS, or motor vehicle accidents.[50]

The scope of the problem: by the numbers

- One of every seven primary care visits is affected by missing medical information, leading to duplication of, or delays in, care and testing, along with unnecessary costs to the patient.[51]

- According to the Center for Information Technology Leadership, approximately one-fifth of medical errors are due to inadequate availability of patient information.[52]

- In an article published in the July/August 2004 issue of *Annals of Family Medicine*,[53] medical errors were studied as a chain of events rather than isolated incidents. Two-thirds of all errors in treatment and diagnosis were found to begin with errors in communication. These included missed communication among physicians, misinformation in medical records, mishandling of patient requests and messages, inaccessible records, mislabeled specimens, misfiled or missing charts, and inadequate reminder systems.

[50] Institute of Medicine, Centers for Disease Control and Prevention; National Center for Health Statistics: Preliminary Data for 1998 and 1999. 2000.
[51] Peter Smith. "Missing Clinical Information During Primary Care Visits," *Journal of the American Medical Association*. 2005.
[52] Global Technology Centre. *Reactive to Adaptive: Transforming Hospitals with Digital Technology*. 2005.
[53] Woolf, Steven H. *A String of Mistakes: The Importance of Cascade Analysis in Describing, Counting, and Preventing Medical Errors*. Annals of Family Medicine 2:317-326 (2004). <http://annalsfm.highwire.org/cgi/content/abstract/2/4/317>

- According to a survey by Research America, 41 percent of Americans have been or know someone who has been the victim of a medical error.[54]

- According to the Institute of Medicine, over a half million people are injured each year because of adverse drug events, many of which could be avoided if healthcare providers had complete information about which drugs their patients were taking and why.[55]

Relative risk of healthcare

Of activities seen as potentially risky, travel by rail in Europe and commercial air travel are actually among the safest activities, with fewer than one in 100,000 fatalities per personal encounter or trip. Driving is far more dangerous: about 42,000 people die each year in automobile accidents. It is no surprise that, statistically, mountain climbing and bungee jumping are among the most dangerous activities. But the biggest surprise of all is there are more deaths per encounter with the healthcare system than for any of these other activities.[56]

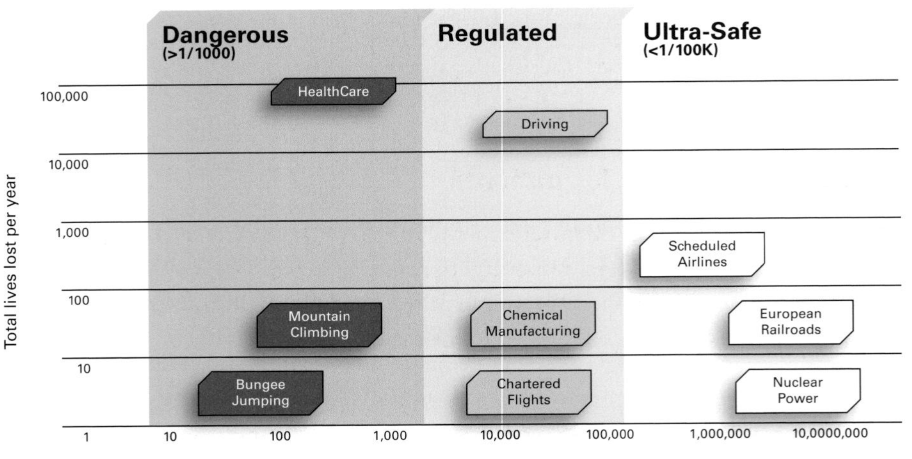

[54] Wooley, Mary. *Research for Health: The Power of Advocacy.* January 14 2005. Research!America. PowerPoint. January 14, 2005. <http://www.nlm.nih.gov/csi/research_america_011405.pdf

[55] Agency for Healthcare Research and Quality. "Reducing and Preventing Adverse Drug Events to Decrease Hospital Costs." *Research in Action: Issue 1.* March 2001.

[56] Scott Young. *The Role of Health IT in Reducing Medical Errors and Improving Healthcare Quality & Patient Safety.* PowerPoint. Agency for Healthcare Research and Quality. August 2005. <http://www.ehealthinitiative.org/assets/documents/Capitol_Hill_Briefings/Young9-22-04.PPT>

The financial costs

Total national costs (lost income, lost household production, disability, and healthcare costs) of preventable adverse events (medical errors resulting in injury) are estimated to be between $17 billion and $29 billion, of which healthcare costs represent over one-half.[57] According to a Markle Foundation report, the U.S. healthcare system spends $30 billion to as much as $293 billion annually on unnecessary paperwork.[58]

Severity of Injury in Preventable Adverse Drug Events

Source: Bates, David J. Cullen, Nan Laird, et al. "Incidence of Adverse Drug Events and Potential Adverse Drug Events: Implications for Prevention." *JAMA* 274(1): 29-34 (1995).

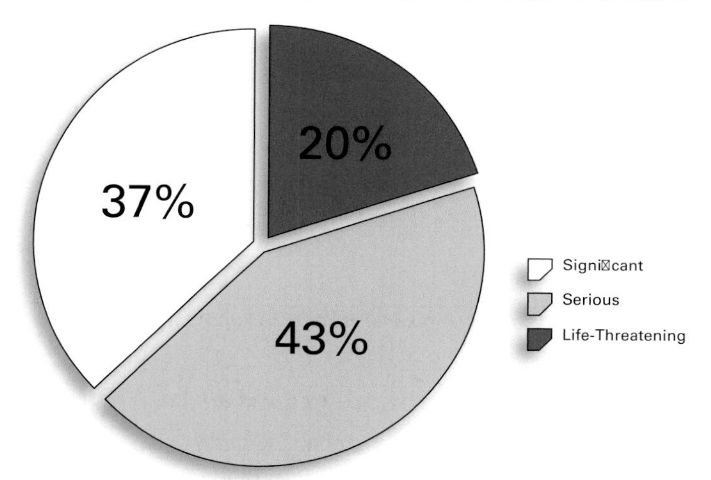

Financial advantages for patients

Because 90 percent of the financial benefits from health information technology goes to payers and purchasers,[59] financial benefits to consumers will be indirect. In particular, patients will spend less time at the doctor's office and miss fewer days at work while enjoying increased quality of care.

[57] L. Kohn, J. Corrigan, and M. Donaldson. *To Err Is Human: Building a Safer Health System.* Committee of Health Care in America, Institute of Medicine. 2000.

[58] MedStar eHealth Initiative, Verizon. "At a Tipping Point: Transforming Medicine with Health Information Technology, A Guide for Consumers." MedStar eHealth Initiative, Verizon. April 1, 2005. <http://ccbh.ehealthinitiative.org/communities/community.aspx?Section=100&Category=211&Document=621>

[59] N. Menachemi and R. Brooks. *Exploring the Return on Investment Associated with Health Information Technologies,* p. 36. Florida State University College of Medicine. February 2005.

Some savings can be realized by giving providers updated and cost-effective information during the prescribing process. One e-prescribing system now in use alerts doctors to the most cost-effective treatments for patients, including generic medications, less expensive alternatives to medications in the same therapeutic class, and more appropriate drug utilization.[61] The Center for Information Technology Leadership says this type of technology, which supports the ordering of medications, would save Americans about $27 billion annually in medication spending.[62]

Families Feeling the Pinch

In 2003, 43 million people reported financial problems related to paying medical bills.[60]

Reduce duplication of tests

Medical tests can be painful, and sometimes they involve great risk. In addition, tests can cost a lot of time and expense: up to $500 billion is spent on unneeded or duplicative care, which is nearly a third of our annual healthcare spending.[63] But under a system of connected medical data, a doctor can avoid unnecessary tests by accessing a patient's record to see if another doctor has already completed the test.

Reducing Fraud and Abuse

In 2003, Florida Medicaid implemented a voluntary medication management and e-prescribing program for physicians caring for Medicaid patients. Since its implementation, this program has saved Florida taxpayers an average of $700 per doctor each month. But there has been more than financial benefits: there has been a four percent drop in significant drug interactions since the program began.[64]

Dramatically reduce drug interactions

Patients will benefit from an extra layer of protection against drugs being prescribed that, when taken together, have adverse effects. This extra protection will come from the personal health information that is provided to physicians, nurse practitioners, and others who prescribe medicine. Today, providers have no way of knowing what other healthcare providers have prescribed for a patient.

[60] U.S. Department of Health and Human Services, Office of the Assistant Secretary for Planning and Evaluation. *Effects of Health Care Spending on the U.S. Economy 2005.* August 2005. <http://aspe.hhs.gov/health/costgrowth/report.pdf>

[61] Cap Gemini Ernst & Young. *TouchScript Medication Management System: Financial Impact Analysis on Pharmacy Risk Pools.* October 2000.

[62] Center for Information Technology Leadership. *The Value of Computerized Provider Order Entry in Ambulatory Settings.* March 2003.

[63] Statement of Mike Leavitt, Secretary of Department of Health and Human Services, before the Committee on the Budget, United States Senate, July 20, 2005.

[64] Florida State. Agency for Health Care Administration. Florida Medicaid Nominated for National Award. Press release, August 3, 2004. <http://www.fdhc.state.fl.us/Executive/Communications/Press_Releases/archive/2004/08_03_2004.shtml>

A High-Stakes Puzzle

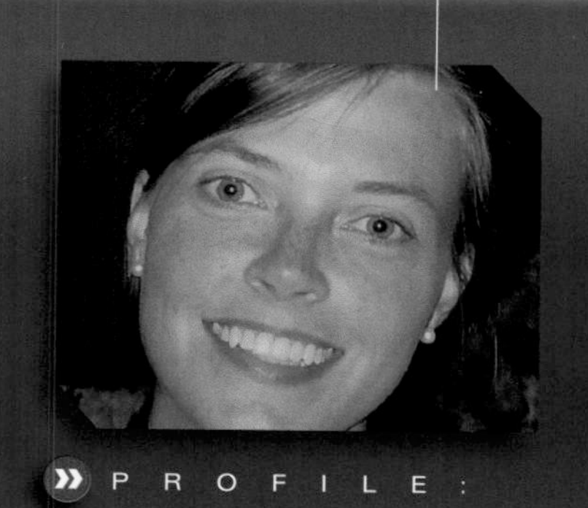

» PROFILE:

Anne Henegar

GEORGIA

~ Woman Struggles with a Chronic Disease, Multiple Doctors Across the Country ... and a Life of Uncertainty

For Anne Henegar, uncertainty has become a way of life. For 10 years she has struggled with a disease without a name, and all the confusion and frustration that has gone along with it. Her husband is a minister, so she has lived in four different cities since she first became sick and has seen numerous doctors and specialists along the way. With each new doctor and city, Anne has accumulated piles of paper: test results, x-rays, and forms. She has been forced to carry her extensive medical records to each new physician, always fearful she is missing a critical piece of information.

Anne is most concerned that a missing piece of paper could hold the key to unlock her mystery condition. "For me, my condition is very systemic. I have to have somebody that's constantly thinking of me as a whole, because one thing affects the other. Each part of the puzzle is very important, and I'm the one having to remember that." But even more than that, Anne wants to be more in control of her health, to be able to work with her doctors and look for patterns in her condition that could allow her more days of feeling good.

"Being able to access my records is important because it's my life and my health. I mean, it's who I am. All these details and the time and money that I've put into having these tests and going to see doctors, I need to have access to my records because I want to be able to analyze them and interpret them myself. I'm as much a major contributor to this investigation and discovery as they are, but I'm not privy to that information. I'm the one that lives with this body 24/7, and I think I'm one of the most important people to have the information. I feel like there's got to be some kind of pattern I've gone through with this illness, but I'm the only person who could probably see that, because no doctor has my vantage point."

"Each part of the puzzle is crucial, and I'm the one having to remember each piece."

– Anne Henegar

The scattered information means more than just inconvenience for Anne and her family. It also means countless dollars lost due to duplicated tests and repeated procedures. "A lot of repeat tests have been done. Every time new doctors see me, they want to run their own tests. I feel like the conductor of a really bad orchestra; like I'm trying to make sense of all these incongruent parts."

More than anything, Anne wishes that her many doctors could have the same information available to them at the same time. She knows that someday, having all the facts could mean more than a convenient trip to the doctor—it could mean finally having the answers she has searched for and the peace of mind she craves.

"The time spent responding to all the paperwork collectively took more time than it took the surgeon to remove my tumor!"

– Tracey Ryan

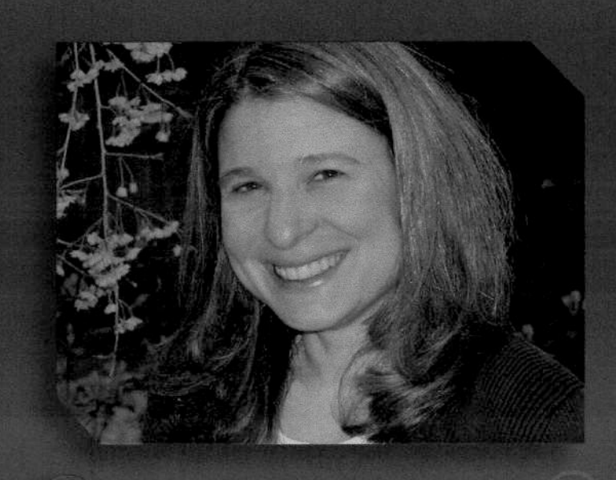

» PROFILE:

Tracey Ryan
CONNECTICUT

~ A Psychologist and Cancer Survivor Says the Stress of Endless Paperwork was Worse Than the Cancer Itself

Surviving a Mountain of Medical Forms

Tracey Ryan went through a terrible ordeal at the end of 2004. Within just a few months, she discovered she had brain cancer, saw up to 12 different doctors, underwent surgery to remove the tumor, and became cancer free. While the experience of having cancer by itself is more than most people think they can handle, for Tracey, the stress of playing the document game between all her different doctors was much more trying.

"Each specialist, each physician that I saw, each institution that I dealt with had their own set of forms, waivers, and requirements. There was no communication between them except if you requested verbal communication. But even when the doctors talked to each other verbally, you still needed to go back and fill out all the forms again. I spent hours filling out forms."

As a professor of psychology, Tracey is keenly aware of the effects of stress—she had plenty of it due to her doctors' inefficient record keeping. She was able to cope with the stress of having cancer because she knew her options—she knew what she was dealing with. With her medical records, it was another story. She never knew what the doctor knew or didn't know, and she eventually delegated the task of filling out piles of paperwork to her willing husband. "It was the minor hassles that really got to me more than the major ultimate health problem that I had to deal with, which I could deal with because I had the information about it."

"It wasn't a problem going to the doctors. The most stressful aspect was really filling out these forms—the really minor hassles associated with the bigger problem. It was kind of a running joke ... another form, another paper." The scariest part was that even with the information on the forms, many doctors acted surprised when, for example, Tracey told them about a medication she was on, even though she had indicated it on numerous forms.

Tracey found it hard to believe that, with all the other amazing advances in healthcare—such as those that saved her life—doctors were so far behind the times in the way they handled her medical records, most often faxing or mailing them from one place to another and having her repeatedly give the same information that they had on file. "The time spent responding to all the paperwork collectively took more time than it took the surgeon to remove my tumor!"

Views from the Floor - The Nurse Perspective

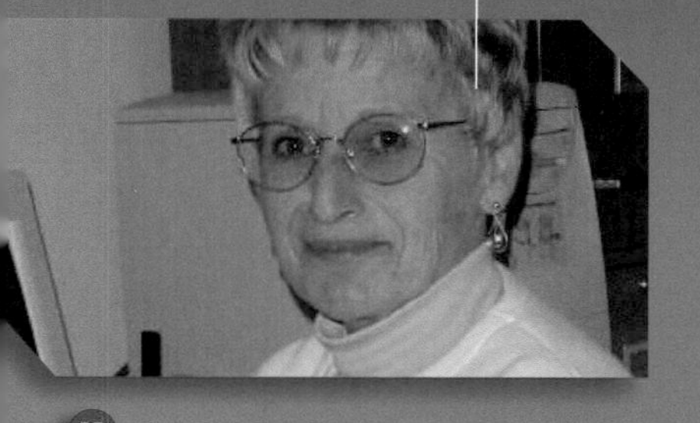

PROFILE:

Sylvia Suszka Hildebrand

RN, MN, ARNP, CCNI
WASHINGTON

~ Empowering Patients by Connecting Care

"I have had the opportunity to instantly access broad clinical practice teams that are geographically isolated using electronic medical records (EMRs), computerized physician order entry (CPOE), and virtual private network (VPN) e-mail. With these systems, the teams are only a few clicks of the mouse away. I am able to offer direct prescriptions and lab orders. As a nurse, I have a wealth of standing orders to implement using the CPOE function. With today's handhelds, I have instant access to pharmacology programs to quickly access drug interactions, side effects, and patient teaching information.

Our patients have the ability to join My Group Health to gain entry to their EMRs to view lab results, write personal e-mails to their providers, reorder medications, and make future appointments. They can also access a wealth of health education topics for assistance in monitoring their chronic health conditions. They have access to our knowledge base on-line to review diseases and symptoms, and often pictures are provided for health conditions from A to Z."

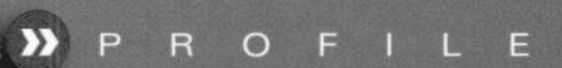

PROFILE:

Amanda Barley

RN, BSN
PENNSYLVANIA

~ MS Candidate in Nursing Wants Access to Data for a Reduction in Medical Errors

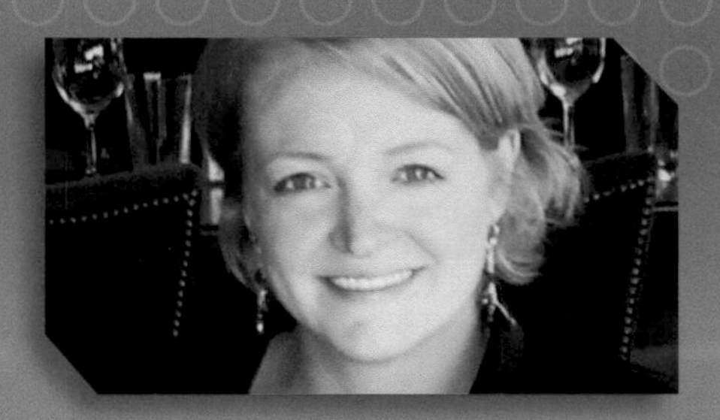

"Clinicians rarely have access to clinical test results ordered by other clinicians on shared patients, causing expensive and sometimes risky tests to be reordered or critical facts to be missed when evaluating a patient's health. Giving clinicians access to data about their patient's care from providers outside their organizations would likely result in fewer medical errors and better continuity of care. Creating an environment that encourages this transformation represents an opportunity that must be seized."

Views from the Floor - The Nurse Perspective

"Linking electronic medical records (EMRs) would be very helpful to public health nurses dealing with a tuberculosis (TB) outbreak in a homeless shelter. There are many steps before treatment is started: identifying the resident who may have TB; taking and interpreting chest x-rays; collecting, processing, and reporting laboratory specimens; clinically evaluating the patient; starting and managing treatment and care; and notifying the health department.

With linkage of EMRs, public health nurses would be able to access lab reports, x-rays, and pharmacy reports earlier and could recognize a TB case earlier. The nurses would then be able to manage the issue in the homeless shelter by quickly screening people at risk for TB (skin testing and chest x-rays); collecting results; coordinating the medical review; and teaching residents, staff, and others who are concerned. Earlier diagnosis, treatment, and management of the issue in the homeless shelter will lead to decreased transmission of the disease."

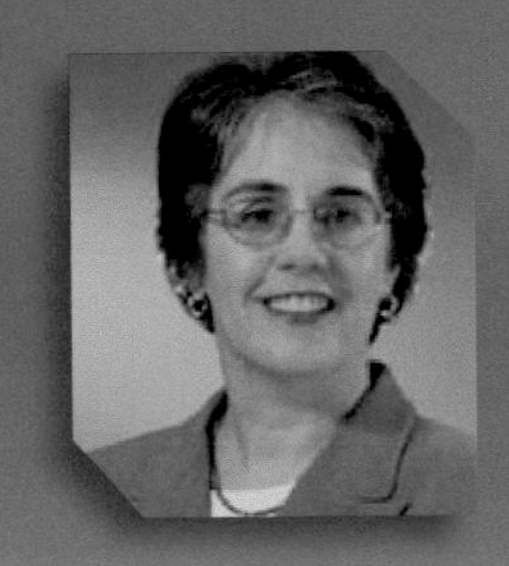

PROFILE:

Derryl Block
PhD, MPH, APRN-BC
WISCONSIN

~ Public Health Nurse/ Nurse Educator Working to Contain Tuberculosis

Deadly Disconnect

The Name of This Person Has Been Changed to Preserve Anonymity

» PROFILE:

Tameka Blackwell

MINNESOTA

~ A Minnesota Woman Struggles to Come to Grips with the Lack of Information That May Have Cost Her Father His Life

"If the lack of information didn't lead to my dad's death, it definitely led to a lot of misery on his part."

– Tameka Blackwell

Tameka Blackwell knows firsthand that being able to access important health information can mean life or death for a patient. Three years ago, Tameka's father was a relatively healthy 70-year-old. He was a smoker and had mild emphysema, but he was not taking any medicines and led a fairly active life. Everything changed when he developed a common cold. At first, he refused to go to a doctor, but when he started having trouble breathing, Tameka took him to an urgent care facility. They did a chest x-ray and told him to go home and take an over-the-counter cold medicine. His condition continued to deteriorate, and three days later Tameka's mother called to say that her father was sitting in his chair unable to breathe and shaking.

When they arrived at the hospital, her father and her mother were both diagnosed with pneumonia, but her father's condition was much worse, and he was immediately admitted and began undergoing tests.

Once Tameka confronted a nurse hanging up a bag of medicine to be given to her father through his IV and asked her what it was. The nurse explained that it was a heart medication. When Tameka asked why her father was taking such a drug when he had absolutely no history of heart problems, the nurse replied by saying that she could not discuss the medications, but to ask a doctor. "Find me a doctor," Tameka quickly responded. She tracked down a resident, who asked her what medication her father was taking for his heart before he came to the hospital. Tameka was flabbergasted. "My father was on no medications when he stepped into this hospital, not even aspirin. I mean, if you look at your records you would know that," she said. A week later, a surgeon explained to Tameka that they did not know who initially prescribed the heart medicine, but that "everything seems to be working so let's just leave it alone."

Multiple surgeries and several months in intensive care later, Tameka's father eventually passed away. But not from cancer or pneumonia. Tameka's father died of sepsis, an infection that developed after one of his last surgeries. "The only thing that I would like is to have information accessible to all the parties who are taking care of a patient. With my father, it seemed at many times they did not have it readily available, or it was too difficult for them to go back and look at. He had many different teams of people taking care of him at separate times, and it seemed like the right hand never knew what the left hand had done. If the lack of information didn't lead to my dad's death, it definitely led to a lot of misery on his part."

Did You Know?

- More than one in five Americans report that they or a family member had experienced a medical or prescription drug error."

Source: The Commonwealth Fund website; www.cmwf.org/publications/publications_show.htm?doc_id=221270

Most people try to do what they can to stay well—exercise and make healthy choices. When you get sick, you go to the doctor. It's an age-old formula. Healthcare providers do what they're supposed to do, patients do what they're supposed to do, and everyone hopes that the outcome will be favorable.

But much more is possible. An interoperable system of healthcare information will allow you to expand the healthcare relationship—to transform yourself from patient to partner. You can be better informed consumers, better able to make healthy choices, and better able to find treatment that reflects all your needs based on complete information, not just the information a single provider might know at any given time.

Opportunities and responsibilities usually appear together; they represent the partnership that drives progress. You as consumers must also become partners in improving your healthcare and creating needed change.

“Without continual growth and progress, such words as improvement, achievement, and success have no meaning.”

Benjamin Franklin,
Inventor and Statesman
(1706 – 1790)

The Healthcare Delivery System
Table of Contents

Digitizing the Healthcare Delivery System

"In a digital healthcare system, providers can have the information they need right at the point of care. Computer algorithms can catch mistakes and prompt to ensure consideration of latest scientific developments. Public health officials can be alerted nearly immediately of unusual patterns that might indicate a natural or bioterror infectious outbreak, or to catch the next Vioxx® before tens of thousands are put at risk. Researchers would have vast new databases to learn more about what works."

Congressman Patrick Kennedy

Information Saves Lives

For patients of Dr. Evan Zahn, immediate access to personal medical records can mean the difference between life and death. That is why, in 1995, he and his colleagues decided to "go digital."

"We make decisions [based on images]," said Dr. Zahn, a pediatric cardiologist in Miami, Florida. "We realized that there was virtually no information-sharing among members of our discipline. We were still running, looking for lab slips, and if I wanted to see an x-ray I had to go find it in its envelope. The kids we deal with are for the most part critically ill—we deal with little babies with very bad heart disease—and we needed detailed information quicker than that. Often when people relay things verbally, the details are left out. We needed a free exchange of information."

Today, Dr. Zahn and his colleagues can instantly share digital images of their patients' hearts and other medical data with other doctors around the state. They use the system before, after, and even during surgery.

"When I want to know something about the inside of the heart that I can't see, and the child's on bypass, and time is critical, the computer is in the operating room and one of the technicians can just punch it up. We've even been working on voice recognition so that ultimately I won't even need a technician. I'll just be able to say, 'Angiogram on John Smith, show frame 16,' and it will do just that."

The system works over any Internet connection. "I can actually put up my laptop tonight when I'm watching the game in my living room and pull up all the same information that I can at work," he said. "I could sit at my computer and go on the Internet anywhere in the world, and I have a database and a log-in and a password. It's encrypted, and it's HIPAA [Health Insurance Portability and Accountability Act] compliant. I can go in and I can work with any of my patients. I get digital images of their operation; I can even view a 30-second delay of their monitor in the intensive care unit, looking at their heart rate, respiration, oxygen saturation, and a number of other things.

"In the bad old days, which still goes on in most places, the doctor performing a procedure would call me—provided I wasn't out of town or unavailable—and I would pick up the phone and try to describe what I saw. We wanted a system where we would have instantaneous access to that type of data.

"Today I was doing a case, and I wanted one of my partners in Orlando, about 250 miles away, to render a second opinion. I just told him to go to the monitor and look at the case I was doing—it was almost in real time—and review with me the images of this little boy so we could make an accurate decision about where to go.

"You only get one chance at it to make this right, and if you do it wrong, it's potentially fatal. If you do it right, you're going to save this baby an open-heart surgery and all the complications from that. This child had a very unusual anatomy, and it didn't look quite right. I wasn't comfortable taking my chances performing the procedure based on the information I had—even though this is all I do, and I've done it a lot for a long time.

"I wanted somebody else's opinion, but the only person I trusted with something like this was 250 miles away. It was as simple as ringing him up on our speakerphone from the lab. He was in his lab in Orlando. We have desktop computers, and we share a common network. My images immediately were uploaded to the network, and all he had to do was click on the patient and look at a few frames, and he basically agreed with where I was going to put it. We put it in and the baby did great.

"But I don't know that I would have proceeded with it without a second opinion. That's one of about a million examples I can give you. We rely on this type of image-sharing and information-sharing all the time. We share data about the patients, and not just images.

"I can look at all those things, including digital images of their operation as it is occurring. For every kid that comes in here, I know exactly who he or she is, exactly what he or she had done, I have pictures of everything, and I can talk to their physician and make a logical decision about what needs to be done. They don't have to rely on me being able to fax a piece of paper, or the parent's recollection. They just go in and they look at the whole hospitalization, everything you can think of—labs, progress notes, admission notes, operative notes, catheterization pictures, echocardiogram pictures—everything you would want to take care of a child with heart disease.

"Take a child with complicated heart disease. I get called to the emergency room to evaluate them. All their heart surgery was done eight miles away at another institution, but I can't get any information from them: nobody knows what I'm talking about; it's 11 o'clock at night. Without the information, their heart is a black box to me. It's a terrible way to treat patients.

"I understand people's fear of this, and the privacy issue. But I think we'll look back on this period in 20 years and not be able to imagine it having been any other way.

"The value that our society and individuals will get from the ability of having their medical information viewed at multiple sites by multiple healthcare providers who are trying to help them is going to so far, far outweigh any problems, that I think it will go down as one of those things that we can't believe we ever lived without."[1]

"I think it will go down as one of those things that we can't believe we ever lived without."

Dr. Evan Zahn, Pediatric Cardiologist

[1] Evan Zahn. Commission on Systemic Interoperability staff interview. July 2005.

Concerned Mother Takes Control

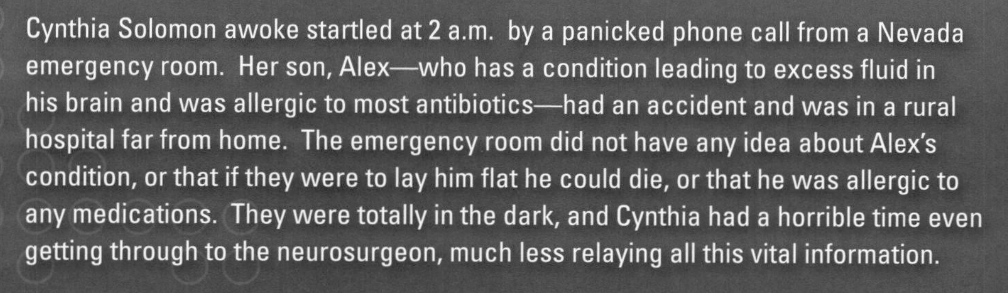

Cynthia Solomon awoke startled at 2 a.m. by a panicked phone call from a Nevada emergency room. Her son, Alex—who has a condition leading to excess fluid in his brain and was allergic to most antibiotics—had an accident and was in a rural hospital far from home. The emergency room did not have any idea about Alex's condition, or that if they were to lay him flat he could die, or that he was allergic to any medications. They were totally in the dark, and Cynthia had a horrible time even getting through to the neurosurgeon, much less relaying all this vital information.

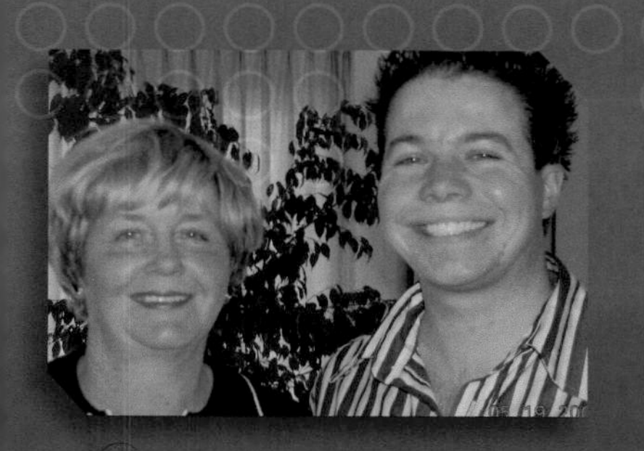

» PROFILE:

Cynthia and Alex Solomon

CALIFORNIA

~ Mother Creates a Personal Health Record Following Son's Medical Emergency

"Medical errors aren't just the fault of doctors or hospitals; it's really the issue of not having the right information at the right time."

– Cynthia Solomon

At that time, all of Alex's medical information—scans, test results, history, surgeries—were stored in numerous boxes and binders at his mother's house in California. Alex came through the ordeal alright, but Cynthia and her son were left shaken.

Cynthia, with the help of some college-age computer whizzes, went on to develop a personal health record (PHR) where she was able to store all of her family's medical information and access it over the Internet—and allow her doctors to do the same. The reasons for creating and using such a record are common sense, she says. "Because doctors and clinics close, and hospitals consolidate, the information that we used to count on being with the local doctor for 20 years of our life is no longer the case."

Today, Cynthia's PHR has expanded into a dynamic business, and she has been able to help hundreds of people from all backgrounds and financial positions become more in control of their health. The most widespread success the system has seen is within the migrant farm worker communities of California. With a modest grant from The California Endowment to local nonprofits, Cynthia's company has been able to connect numerous families to their health information, creating a personalized account complete with e-mail and printable medical history and emergency card.

The biggest challenge Cynthia sees to being able to truly help people become connected to their health is the systems themselves. Once the standards are in place, she says, these systems will no longer be reserved for large hospitals and established doctors, and everyone will be able to communicate freely, which will ultimately save thousands of dollars and lives.

Allowing patients to be in control of their own information will be empowering, and families will be better off.

Electronic Access is a Birthright

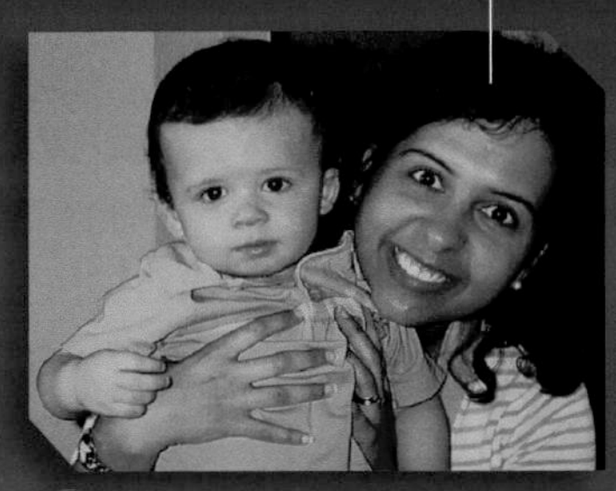

PROFILE:

Jennifer and Jack Edwards

FLORIDA

~ Mother Wants Electronic Access to Her Son's Medical Record

"I believe having access to Jack's health information is a basic right I should have."

– Jennifer Edwards

Jennifer Edwards is the mother of Jack, a healthy 18-month-old baby boy. Fortunately, she has not had to deal with multiple doctors and a sick child, but she is aware of the way technology would help her family's health.

When Jennifer's son was born she had many questions. She was a first-time mother and needed answers quickly to basic questions about Jack's health. These questions led to multiple phone calls and a game of phone tag with Jack's pediatrician's office. Jennifer simply needed to ask the things that a new mother would not know the answers to, such as the results of her son's anemia screening as an infant. Jennifer states, "It would have been helpful to be able to e-mail Jack's doctor questions and receive an answer quickly, and to see basic test results on-line."

Earlier this year, Jack cut his foot on a rusty carpet tack, requiring an after-hours call to the doctor to find out if Jack needed a tetanus shot. This incident, while minor, could have been simplified by an electronic record showing Jennifer the status of Jack's immunizations. Jennifer knows just how valuable having a complete history of Jack's doctor visits, medications, and immunizations would be in providing the best healthcare for her son at her convenience.

Last winter, Jack had several ear infections and was on a variety of antibiotics. Some worked for him, some didn't, and others had side effects. If Jack needs antibiotics again in the future, Jennifer will have to rely on her memory or the pediatrician's notes to know which ones to use. With an electronic record, Jennifer and any healthcare provider Jack visits could easily access an accurate medication history whenever it is needed.

Even providing daycare for her son requires a copy of his up-to-date immunizations, and a lack of this simple piece of information can keep Jack out of daycare. According to Jennifer, "If you've got the [immunization record] on-line, you can always go at your convenience and check it or print it out."

A Win-Win Situation

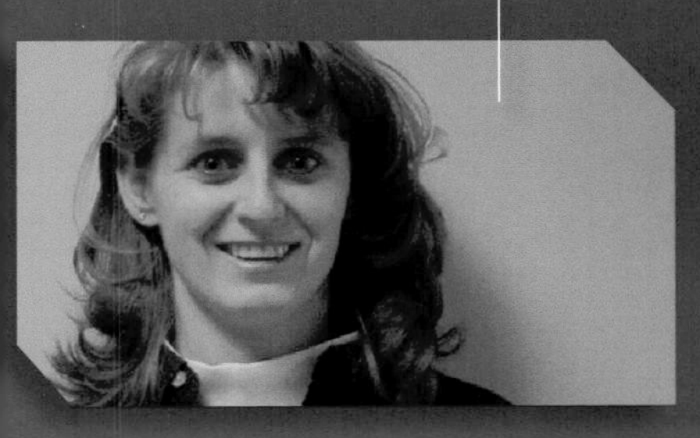

PROFILE:

Sharon Yearous, PNP
IOWA

~ A School Nurse Who Wants Health IT Tools to Provide Better, More Consistent Healthcare for Kids

"With the system we have now, when a kid comes in with asthma or diabetes, we have to fend for ourselves. Most of the time, we don't have any information other than what the child can tell us."

– Sharon Yearous, PNP

"Having access to information is crucial for school nurses. Kids are in school nine months out of the year, five days a week. Who is there that can help provide the healthcare but a school nurse? The school nurse can provide that continuation of care. A child may have seen a healthcare provider earlier in the week or over the weekend, or you may have a child with a chronic illness like diabetes, asthma, seizures, etc. If the nurse has access to an electronic patient record, then she can provide the best care possible because she would have updated, accurate information, up to the last time the child saw a healthcare provider."

So says Sharon Yearous, a high school nurse in Iowa who is also involved in state and national school nursing organizations. She has seen firsthand the challenges school nurses face every day, and she knows that giving nurses access to accurate health information about their students can help them provide better healthcare to millions of children across the country, one school at a time.

"Most school nurses are struggling just to get a computer on their desk. Some of them don't even have e-mail access. I think every school nurse probably knows of the concept of the electronic patient record. Would they like to have it as a school nurse? Absolutely. Do they talk about it? Not really, because they're already feeling like they're struggling just to get one nurse in a building. They know that there are so many kids out there that aren't even served. I think a majority of parents have a misconception that their child is in a school with a school nurse. Nobody realizes that their school nurse may be covering three or four buildings with 1,500 to 2,000 kids. How can we expect to be put on track to get this up-to-date, state-of-the-art electronic patient record? It would be ideal, but it sounds like a pipe dream. Most nurses are just trying to survive day to day with what comes through their door."

"Especially for younger kids, electronic health records would help keep track of things like vaccinations and the routine things that they are supposed to have. Kids move all over, either within town, or out of State, and within school districts, and it's hard to keep track of their health records. We're flying blindly most of the time."

"I've found it impossible to become totally paperless until everything is really interoperable. We still get x-ray reports, lab reports, and consultation letters in the mail. I would have to hire a full-time person to scan all that stuff into a patient's chart, and it's just too costly for me."

– Ernesto Africano, M.D.

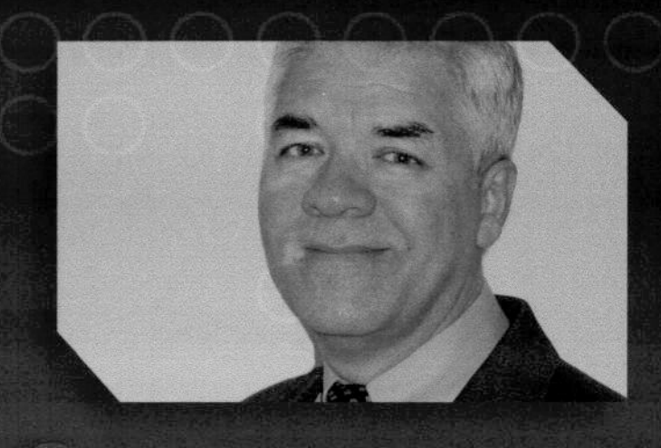

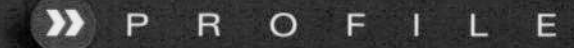

PROFILE:

Ernesto Africano
M.D.
MARYLAND

~ A Specialist in Suburban Maryland Looks Forward to the Day When Medical Records Can Be Easily Shared Among Doctors, Labs, and Pharmacies

Impossible to Achieve Total Interoperability

Dr. Ernesto Africano uses a basic electronic medical record (EMR) in his solo office. While the system doesn't really have any "bells and whistles," it definitely helps him keep track of his patients' progress, saves him time, and ensures that their records are legible and easy to share with his patients' primary care doctors after they come to see him. The biggest benefit he sees is being able to provide better, more efficient healthcare to his patients. But he has been frustrated that more offices and labs are not able to connect to his office. He still has to maintain paper charts because of the volume of information he still receives via fax and "snail mail."

"We get a number of requests for copies of medical records from other physicians and my handwriting is not the most legible, even to myself, so I felt that having very clear and legible records was a definite benefit in organizing my information and patients' charts, and being able to generate reports, letters, and photocopies of reports for other physicians and agencies requesting the medical records, which is almost a daily occurrence." But even while Dr. Africano is able to share his notes and charts with other offices, he still receives all his lab test results, x-rays, and consultation letters on paper. They then either have to be scanned into his EMR or manually entered, which is very time consuming.

Dr. Africano wishes he could connect with other offices, but without interoperability, he is forced to continue sifting through paper charts to find the information he needs. "I would absolutely want to become interoperable with laboratories and pharmacies, so instead of having to print out and sign or fax prescriptions or give them to patients, I would be able to e-mail prescriptions, receive lab reports back, send information electronically to other doctors, or receive existing medical records from my patients when they're referred to me. I think that's where the future is headed."

Benefits to the Healthcare Delivery System

"We have the most advanced medical system in the world, yet patient safety is compromised every day due to medical errors, duplication, and other inefficiencies. Harnessing the potential of information technology will help reduce errors and improve quality in our health system."

Senator Hillary Rodham Clinton

Classes of benefits

The bottom line for healthcare providers is to improve the quality of care for patients. An interoperable system helps achieve that: it reduces time spent on administrative tasks, phone calls, and office business, and provides immediate access to more complete information about patients. That means:

- More complete information available for treatment decisions;
- New and more efficient options for patient interaction;
- Enhanced ability to demonstrate performance consistent with regulations and recognized professional standards;
- Potential for reduced operational costs and more effective use of resources;
- Reduced or streamlined management responsibilities;
- Less paperwork;
- Automation of repetitive tasks; and
- Better efficiency in dealing with other providers and outside parties.

Benefits Appear at All Levels, from Emergencies to Routine Office Visits

The benefits of interoperability will appear everywhere—because secure access will be available from any location that has an Internet connection. This means electronic healthcare information will be available in ambulances, emergency rooms, doctors' offices, hospital rooms, staff rooms, nurses' stations, and clinics.

In fact, benefits to healthcare providers fall into four categories:

- Quality of care;
- Administrative efficiencies;
- Patient communication; and
- Public health and security.

Quality of care

- **Enhanced doctor-to-doctor communication.** With an interoperable system of healthcare, physicians can instantly share test results with other doctors, healthcare providers, labs, pharmacies, and clinics. The system will also allow doctors to highlight particular parts of the record and "point" or "link" that information to other parts of the patient record—in practice, any physician authorized by the patient will be able to look at a patient's chart with another physician who is far away. This will naturally streamline the process of consultation and improve healthcare delivery.

- **Available in any geographic location.** Physicians and other healthcare providers will be able to review the complete medical history of a patient, regardless of the location of either the patient or the provider. An individual on vacation on the West Coast who lives on the East Coast could go to any doctor and have their information available instantly. At each visit, healthcare providers add to the record, so no matter where and when the record is examined, it will be up-to-date.

- **Available in any treatment setting.** Access to medical histories will be available in any treatment environment: in an emergency room, in an exam room, in locations around a hospital, in a doctor's home or office, in public and private clinics—anywhere an Internet connection is available.

"In medicine, seconds can mean the difference between life and death. If you have a heart attack tonight and are rushed to the hospital, your life depends on timely access to accurate and current information. That's why it makes no sense that today's healthcare is not advancing in the Information Age; it's stuck in the Stone Age."

Senate Majority Leader Bill Frist

- **Improved emergency room support.** Doctors in emergency rooms (ERs) often have to work without any patient history at all. Treating an ER patient with no records can be like trying to navigate a country road in the dark with no headlights. However, interoperable tools can be physicians' "high beams" that help them make the best decisions. Since many patients use the ER as their primary care facility, and ongoing and consistent treatment for such patients can be difficult, an interoperable system could reduce suffering and save lives. In addition, the consistency the system provides can help caregivers personalize the experience for the patient. That will help doctors and nurses to encourage patients to form relationships with healthcare practices and clinics, instead of waiting until a problem becomes so severe that it requires emergency treatment.

- **Immediate access to lab results.** A connected, interactive system of healthcare will allow physicians to review test results as soon as they become available—no more waiting for a phone call or fax. Even the most basic system will provide doctors with the ability to "query the database"—to look for patterns that appear only under intense scrutiny and to find patterns and clusters of data that indicate other problems or treatments. By itself, the interconnectivity of lab information with drug information can provide more comprehensive data at the time of care. Today, such information is not available at the time of initial treatment, meaning that more refined treatment has to be postponed until the necessary data have been collected in one place—and that is just what an interoperable system is designed to do.

- **More evidence-based medicine.** Interoperability will promote evidence-based medicine[3] by giving doctors access at any time to databases that offer updated clinical decision support. Interoperable systems will be equipped to provide protocols for various medical situations. Physicians will choose protocols as they see fit, and as outcomes are measured, the data can be used to revise best-practice standards. Interoperable health systems will improve this process in ways never before possible.

A Lack of Information

In healthcare, having the correct information about a patient is crucial, and getting to medical information quickly can save lives. But one Stanford University study showed that 81 percent of the time, physicians lacked the necessary information to make informed medical decisions.[2]

[2] P.C. Tang, D. Fafchaps, and E.H. Shortliffe. "Traditional Hospital Records as a Source of Clinical Data in the Outpatient Setting." *Eighteenth Annual Symposium on Computer Applications in Medical Care.* Washington D.C. (1994): 575–79.

[3] Also known as "best-practice guidelines."

An Example from Emergency Care

When a 40-year-old female arrived at Indianapolis's Wishard Memorial Hospital, all Dr. John T. Finnell knew was she had lost consciousness while waiting to see a doctor in an outpatient clinic.

Dr. Finnell used her driver's license number to pull up an electronic record listing the patient's recent hospital visits. The listing showed the woman had been diagnosed with a seizure disorder, and she had not been taking her prescribed medication. With this information in hand, Dr. Finnell was able to treat the woman appropriately.

If there had been no accessible medical record indicating the most likely cause of her unconsciousness, Dr. Finnell would have administered drugs to stop her breathing, then inserted a breathing tube and ordered tests.

If the file had not been accessible via an electronic network, the delay in securing a paper file—which could have been any number of places—would have taken hours.

"When you're in an emergency and you can't find information about a patient, everybody suffers," said Dr. Finnell.

If Dr. Finnell had not had access to crucial information about the 40-year-old woman who was rushed into his ER, would he still have been able to save her life? Would he have been able to avoid the potential negative effects of his treatment? Would he have been sued if he had not?

Though it cannot be known for certain what would have happened without the electronic record, what happened when the record was available is a matter of fact. Dr. Finnell received the information he needed to come to the aid of an unconscious patient by sparing her redundant testing and risky emergency procedures. Access to her healthcare information helped him to save her life.[4]

In addition, digital systems are much easier to update than medical textbooks, which will speed the adoption of superior science into practice. Under the current system, the delay between new discoveries and their incorporation into common practice is, on average, 17 years.[5] With some 10,000 clinical studies conducted each year, medical knowledge is doubled about every 42 months.[6] But medical studies are often duplicated because one researcher does not know what another is doing, and they may not learn of work similar to their own until a scholarly article is published. This delay in sharing information causes resources to be wasted and ultimately delays the delivery of new and better treatments to patients.

- **Enhanced support for management of chronic disease.** The treatment of chronic conditions often involves multiple physicians and healthcare providers. The proportion of a typical medical practice focused on treatment of chronic conditions is growing every year, as our healthcare system is

[4] Susannah Patton. "Sharing Data, Saving Lives." *CIO Magazine.* 2005.
[5] Ruth Larson. "Medical Advances Can Outpace Doctors: Retraining Not Enforced, Critics Say." *Washington Times*, March 21, 1999.
[6] Ibid.

transformed from a base of infectious to chronic conditions.[8] Already, half the U.S. population lives with chronic disease.[9] A connected healthcare system will make it easier for patients to find information to help them prevent such conditions, since many chronic illnesses are preventable. With patients and doctors in more frequent and casual contact—made possible by interoperability—patients can make better lifestyle choices to avoid chronic disease or improve their management of it.

- **Improved prescription writing and pharmacy interaction through e-prescribing.**
  - When prescriptions are transmitted to a pharmacy through an interoperable system, there is no question about legibility or the loss of a paper prescription.
  - Doctors can find out whether or not a patient filled or refilled a prescription.
  - There will be less opportunity for those who try to obtain multiple prescriptions from many doctors or commit other fraud.
  - Healthcare providers can rely on the same kind of safeguard as pharmacists to prevent drug interaction.

Chronic Disease and Rural Health Management

More than 125 million Americans suffer from at least one chronic medical condition.[7] Chronic conditions are a special problem for residents of rural America because of the typical distances separating patients from doctors' offices, hospitals, and emergency responders. Compared to those of patients in cities and suburbs, office visits for rural residents require more coordination, planning, and time.

Casual contact with healthcare providers is not as easy to make in rural areas as it is for patients in more-densely populated areas. This is important because seemingly minor symptoms for chronic-condition patients are often indicators of situations that need immediate attention to prevent long-term consequences. City- and suburb-dwellers can more easily contact their doctors about these "minor" symptoms and get early treatment. But the prohibitive distances and circumstances of many rural dwellers can cause them to put off seeking attention for such symptoms until the next scheduled doctor's visit. Such delays can have serious health consequences.

But a connected system would help to change that. Rural patients and their doctors would gain greater access to care because the distance from a doctor's office and the formality of a doctor's office visit would both be significantly decreased.

[7] "Thedacare, Inc. –Touchpoint Health Plan". 2005. Center for Health Transformation. August 15 2005. <http://www.healthtransformation.net/Transforming_Examples/Transforming_Examples_Resource_Center/139.cfm>

[8] Ibid.

[9] Ibid.

Administrative efficiencies

- **Many outcomes.** Connectivity leads to the creation of communication tools that were previously impossible. New ways to synthesize, share, and transmit data naturally suggest new applications to enhance administrative efficiencies.

- **Less duplication of work.** Establishing files for patients and keeping them up-to-date can require significant time and effort from both staff and patients. Time to fill out forms has to be built into appointment time, even for returning patients. A connected system of healthcare information supports individual data that can be shared by all providers. If a patient's psychiatrist orders a liver test, the general practitioner could review the results instead of ordering another test. A patient with a complete medical history on file with their doctor can make that record available to a new doctor for consultation or when the patient moves to a new town.

" ... Draw from your errors the very lessons which may enable you to avoid their repetition."

Sir William Osler, Canadian Physician (1849 – 1919)

Financial Pressures

The financial pressures on physicians are severe. Reimbursements are more tightly controlled, the rate of inflation in the medical field is higher than the overall rate of inflation, and insurance costs are soaring.

In 1999, total physicians' administrative work and costs equaled $72.6 billion, $261 per capita or 26.9 percent of physicians' gross income.[10]

The *New England Journal of Medicine* reports that 31 cents of every healthcare dollar goes toward administrative costs and other expenses.[11] These expenses are from a variety of sources, but interoperability can contribute to reducing them.

Up to $500 billion is spent on unneeded or duplicative care, which is nearly one-third of annual U.S. healthcare spending.[12]

Byproducts of Interoperability

1. Advancement of telemedicine
2. Computerized physician order entry
3. Disease registries
4. Electronic health records
5. E-prescribing
6. Monitoring of chronic diseases
7. Personal health records
8. Secure e-mail messaging

[10] S. Woolhandler, T. Campbell, and D. U. Himmelstein. "Costs of Health Care Administration in the United States and Canada." *New England Journal of Medicine* 349 (2003): 768–75.

[11] Ibid.

[12] Statement of Mike Leavitt, Secretary of the Department of Health and Human Services, before the Committee on the Budget, United States Senate, July 20, 2005.

Making IT Work for Everyone

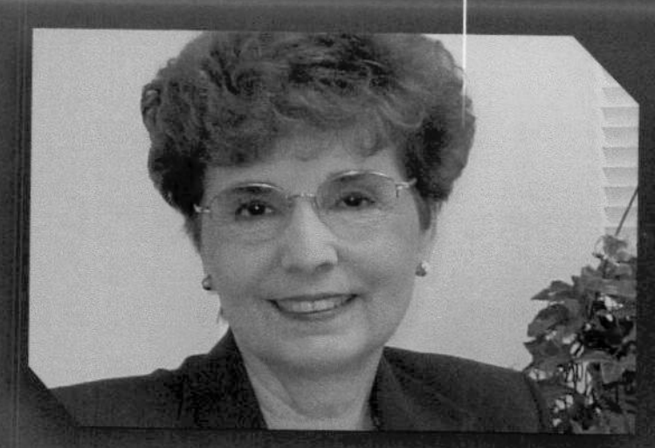

» PROFILE:

Arlowen Raygor

RNBC, MN, BCNA
VIRGINIA

~ Information Systems Director at a Non-Profit Hospital Highlights Smaller Facilities' Needs

"Gathering all essential data about a patient's situation is critical in decision-making."

– Arlowen Raygor
RNBC, MN, BCNA

Arlowen Jordan Raygor has a daunting task ahead of her. As Director of Clinical Information Systems at a not-for-profit community hospital, she is responsible for updating their current information system to an interactive, interconnected, efficient, and accessible system of patient medical records.

"We want to be able to automate more documentation and we want more integration. Currently we do not have computerized physician order entry (CPOE), but we want to implement that in the future. We also want evidence-based practice modules for physicians, nurses, and other care providers. We need vendors who are willing to work with us to create electronic health records that are available to the patient anywhere they happen to be. Currently none of the systems are truly interoperable, but that's the direction we need to go. Patients should have one seamless record."

"Gathering all essential data about a patient's situation is critical to decision-making. In our hospital, like most hospitals throughout the country, patient data resides on multiple systems. We need to have all that data integrated in such a manner that care decisions can be made safely. We also need more tools within these systems that use data to guide practice. Currently there is a lot of attention on evidence-based practice modules for physicians, but nurses and other clinicians need these tools also. Given the nursing shortage we are experiencing, most hospitals have nurses with various levels of experience. Embedded practice guidelines based on research and data specific to an individual patient will help us make better decisions about the care of our patients. This integration needs to extend outside the walls of the hospital. Many of our physicians express frustration in having some of the patient data on the electronic health record in their office and some of it on the hospital system. Interoperability is definitely needed."

"One of the biggest roadblocks to purchasing and implementing systems that meet all these needs is financial. As a single community hospital, we face numerous challenges and must make wise decisions on how we spend our money. Picking the right vendors to provide the solution that is right for us and at a price we can afford is critical. These systems cost millions. While we appreciate that there will be substantial savings for Medicare, it is the hospital that pays for the system. Part of our decision process must include not only the quality improvements but also our return on investment in terms of operational costs and efficiency gains."

Did You Know?

- A standardized, encoded, electronic healthcare information exchange would save the U.S. healthcare system $395 billion over a 10-year implementation period ... [and] save $87 billion each year thereafter.

Source: Middleton, Blackford, MD, MPH, MSc, FHIMSS, The Value of Healthcare Information Exchange and Interoperability. February 2004 Presentation: HIMSS Annual Conference & Exhibition.

Lack of Access to Health Information Kills

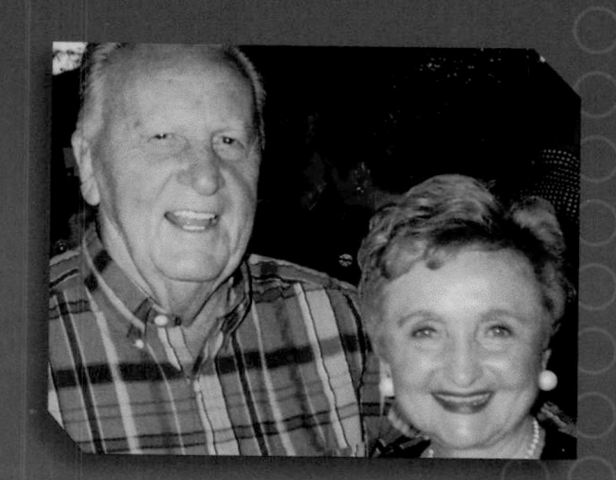

» PROFILE:

Dave and Jeanne Canfield

SOUTH CAROLINA

~ Active Elderly Couple Managing Multiple Health Conditions

"We got in the car and my husband looked at me and said, 'I could have been dead.'"

– Jeanne Canfield

Eighty-four-year-old Dave Canfield is on dialysis and has two knee replacements, two stents, and a pacemaker that his life depends on. Dave's wife, Jeanne Canfield, is thorough and proactive when it comes to his medical care. She carries a briefcase detailing all procedures and medications that apply to Dave's health to each and every medical appointment. But, unfortunately Dave is a patient who has witnessed multiple medical oversights due to a lack of electronic health information.

In April 2005, Dave had a magnetic resonance image (MRI) appointment at a local hospital. Dave and Jeanne filled out the two pieces of paper that they were handed and marked "yes" notifying the physicians of his knee replacements, stents, and pacemaker. The completed questionnaire failed to catch the attention of the hospital staff. The Canfields were escorted to a private waiting area where Jeanne vocally mentioned Dave's stent and pacemaker information to the staff members. It was at that moment that Dave and Jeanne were informed that an MRI would cause his pacemaker to stop completely, killing Dave. Had Dave's nephrologist, who manages up to 250 patients, had access to Dave's medical records from all of his specialists, this potentially fatal mistake could have been avoided.

Sadly, in May 2005, Dave experienced a similar situation regarding preparation for an operation. Jeanne was unable to read the handwriting of Dave's doctor instructing him to stop taking Plavic, a prescribed blood thinner. Plavic is dangerous to take if you are going into an operation. Dave was still taking Plavic up until the day of his operation due to Jeanne's inability to read the doctor's handwriting. The hospital staff caught this oversight and postponed the operation until Dave stopped taking the medication.

These two examples of potentially serious medical oversights could have been prevented with the use of interoperable electronic medical information. Jeanne does her best to follow Dave's care and inform medical professionals about his existing conditions and medications. However, it is not always possible for her to be in the right place at the right time, especially lacking the necessary professional medical knowledge.

FACT

~ Inadequate availability of patient information, such as the results of laboratory tests, was directly associated with 18 percent of adverse drug events.

Source: Connecting for Health ... A Public Private Collaborative. "Facts and Stats." Connecting Healthcare in the Information Age, 2003.

Connecting the Data

"We spend a lot of money and we waste a lot of time, just because we don't have access to medical information from another place."

Jorge Rangel-Meneses, M.D.

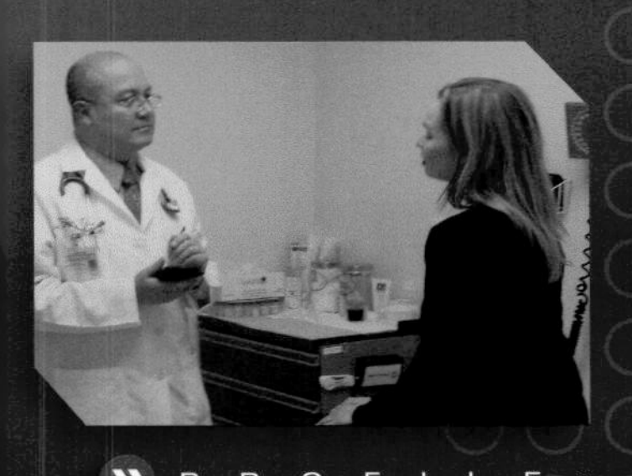

PROFILE:

Jorge Rangel-Meneses, M.D.
FLORIDA

~ Discovering the Benefits of E-Prescribing

For Dr. Jorge Rangel-Meneses, being able to connect the dots of his patients' medical information has been the missing link between providing care with limited knowledge, and providing the best possible care—with the most accurate information—for every one of his patients through the use of information technology.

Using tools and technology that already exist for doctors, Dr. Rangel is saving a significant amount of money for the community health center where he practices. He is also able to save his patients time and frustration every time they come to see him ... and help them stay healthier longer.

After only a few years of using the electronic prescribing (e-prescribing) system, he can't imagine going back to pen and paper that most doctors still cling to. He sees about 9,000 patients every year, and before he was able to use the system, he had to rely on his patients' memory to know what medications they were taking. He also had to rely on his own memory to decide if a new drug he might prescribe would interact with one that his patient was already taking. And if a patient was trying to "doctor shop" to get a drug he or she had already been prescribed by another doctor, Dr. Rangel would have no way to know. Needless to say, the pen-and-paper system was far from foolproof.

Now Dr. Rangel is empowered with the information he needs to treat his patients and improve their overall quality of life. "The system allows me to get a list of all my patients and a list of all the medications that my patients are on. It allows me to write or renew prescriptions electronically and send them directly to the patient's pharmacy of choice. And it allows me also to check for interactions and duplications. It allows me to see what other physicians have prescribed my patients. It is definitely much better than the written paper communication form."

Dr. Rangel's office is in the process of connecting the drug information they have to a new system of complete electronic health records, but for now, e-prescribing has transformed the way he practices medicine. Rather than being isolated from data and limited to a scribbled note in a paper record or his own memory, he is now able to be proactive—rather than reactive—when prescribing treatment. The e-prescribing system even lets him see immediately if a drug he has prescribed is not covered by his patient's insurance, and saves the phone tag that would normally ensue with the pharmacy.

Continued

"I can communicate clearly with the pharmacist. The pharmacist doesn't have to call me back because he or she doesn't understand what I wrote. That saves time. There is also the ability to check for interactions as I write the prescription. When I write a prescription, the system will tell me that I'm duplicating, or that there is a possible interaction with other medications that the patient is on."

"It's a big difference when one writes a prescription by hand. One has to have all the information and be cautious about what one is writing, where the system does that automatically and checks on a much bigger database than is usually available only by memory from the physician."

Dr. Rangel also has a large population of HIV-positive patients. They have been able to benefit from e-prescribing and electronically connected information more than a lot of his patients. But the doctor wishes he could do even more. He looks forward to the day when he will have their complete medical records at his fingertips whenever he needs them. "Sometimes their care can be very complicated. They can see multiple physicians for a variety of problems. They can have neurological problems, and ophthalmologic problems, and gastrointestinal problems, and dermatologic problems, and oncological problems, so they see a variety of specialists. If we all had just one record, it would be great, because we could communicate much more easily. Unfortunately, we don't get reports from every physician that sees our patient."

Looking toward the future, Dr. Rangel sees the definite need for a new way of doing business for doctors. "I can't understand how physicians can be so far behind in the use of information technology. If we don't use electronic records, if we keep using the manual records, we are basically using the same technology and communications that we've been using since the 18th century. I think that it is very, very important that we can intercommunicate. I think it's critical. Right now, we unnecessarily duplicate a lot of testing. We spend a lot of money and we waste a lot of time, just because we don't have access to medical information from another place."

Dr. Rangel also has a word of wisdom for doctors who are hesitant to start using such a system. "The system is not perfect, and I think part of the resistance of some physicians to use this system is because we expect perfection from the system. Of course it isn't perfect, and there is a learning curve, and it takes time to enter patients, and physicians are—in general—very conservative: we don't want to change our ways. But I think that as we get used to electronic systems, and we learn about how this saves some time and makes our practice safer for patients, we have to move in this direction. I don't think we have a choice. I think that there is evidence that the electronic records are going to be cheaper if you consider the direct and indirect costs."

Did You Know?

~ The Institute of Medicine states that 7,000 people die every year due to medication errors.

Source: To Err Is Human: Building a Safer Health System, Institute of Medicine, 200

- **Improved workflow and streamlined processes.** Electronic systems save time and money in standard business activities such as payroll, human resources tracking, attendance, billing, transcription, accounting, and inventory. When applied to healthcare, those benefits will expand to include:

    - Reduction of the number of documents lost in transmission, especially via fax or postal mail;
    - Reduction in spending on printing, transcription, faxing, mailing, scanning, duplicate data entry, and shredding;
    - Elimination of the problem of illegible handwriting and signatures;
    - Greater ease of sharing information with other providers;
    - Reuse of information instead of reentering; and
    - Flexible and instant reporting and tracking capabilities.

- **Easier accommodation to changes in paperwork requirements.** An electronic and interoperable system accommodates changes in regulatory filing requirements with fewer changes to procedure—the system can incorporate new filing requirements. For instance, data may be requested automatically or mined from existing information. It is even possible that a vendor could make changes needed in the office or hospital software without any administrative effort on the part of the staff in the hospital or physician's office.

- **More competitive practice benefits.** "The reality of today's healthcare environment is that providers are competing for every patient, every employee, and every dollar."[16] Healthcare providers can increase their ability to compete not only by offering benefits directly to patients, but by

Savings of Money and Time: Real-world Examples

CareGroup, a six-hospital integrated delivery system, has saved more than $1 million annually from implementing a Web-based electronic medical record retrieval system that improves workflow processes. The group anticipates a 33 percent annual increase in revenues from higher customer retention and attraction rates.[13] CareGroup has seen cost and process time reductions in a range of hospital operations: clinicians need less time to find and retrieve records, the admittance process is quicker, and the average overall stay is shorter.[14]

Savings of Money and Time: Real-world Examples

In Massachusetts, a paper-based insurance claim takes, on average, 100 days to process. New England Health EDI Network, connecting a large group of payers and providers in the region, projects that electronic data interchange could shorten this process to three to five days.[15]

[13] InterSystems Corporation. "CareGroup Healthcare System Expects System Projects Multi-million Dollar ROI from CareWeb Application Built on Caché e-DBMS Technology." Press release, April 10, 2000.

[14] Ibid.

[15] Hearing before the Subcommittee on Oversight and Investigations of the House Veterans' Affairs Committee. 108th Congress, Second Session. March 17, 2004, 108-32. "Hearing VI on the Department of Veterans' Affairs Information Technology Programs." Written testimony of John D Halamka, MD, MS, 59–68.

[16] Daniel Fell. "Seven Steps: Using Marketing in Healthcare Technology Planning." *HealthLeaders News*. May 23, 2005.

enhancing elements of the practice that will become apparent to patients over time. The return on investment in interoperable systems may appear not only as an increase in the number of patients, but also as better retention of doctors and other employees.[17]

Patient communication

- **Better interaction with patients.** Electronic networks make it easier for doctors to review patient information, find patterns in patient history, provide patients with relevant information, monitor adherence to treatment, consider patient questions and concerns in advance of visits, and prepare more thoroughly for a patient visit. This results in a savings of time and trouble for the provider and the patient, as well as a more focused and need-oriented experience for the patient.

- **Better doctor-patient relationships.** Electronic networks that operate over the Internet facilitate the frequent and relatively simple exchange of information without the need for expensive and time-consuming office visits or even phone calls. When doctors have electronic networks, they can closely monitor patient progress and more often form practical, effective partnerships with patients. Additionally, the ability of doctors to direct patients to reliable health information across such networks would provide patients with the opportunity to review important and detailed information about their condition and use that information to better care for themselves. The result can be a more engaged patient, working with a healthcare provider toward better health outcomes such as better care for chronic conditions, better initial diagnosis and treatment, and interaction focused on specific problems and solutions toward better health maintenance.

- **More time for contact with patients.** In offices and hospitals where electronic systems are in place, doctors appear to have more time for patients and spend less time performing administrative duties and waiting for information. According to a physician interviewed by Commission staff, patient e-mails have relieved his practice of numerous phone call obligations. The doctor describes the telephone as the "most expensive piece of equipment in the office."

"The two words "information" and "communication" are often used interchangeably, but they signify quite different things. Information is giving out; communication is getting through."

Sydney J. Harris,
American Journalist (1917 – 1986)

A Lack of Information

"The proportion of physicians saying they do not have enough time to spend with patients rose nearly 24 percent between 1997 and 2001."[18]

[17] Ibid.
[18] Sally Trude. *So Much to Do, So Little Time: Physician Capacity Constraints, 1997-2001*. Center for Studying Health System Change, 2003.

By using e-mail, he can answer the five to 18 messages he receives each day in about 10 minutes. Naturally, he recommends an office visit for patients whose complaint needs more attention; otherwise, an e-mail answer saves the patient the trouble of coming in.[19] Doctors, and especially patients, believe that medical errors are prevented when physicians have more time to spend with patients.[20] This suggests that doctors who effectively use information technologies in their practices will have more time to spend with patients, both in the clinical setting and through nontraditional means of communications such as e-mail. This allows doctors to direct patients to reliable health information on the Internet so patients can take time to review important and detailed information at their leisure.

Public health and security

- **Improved public health.** Right now, there is no automated tracking in the United States for patterns and locations of patient diagnoses and treatment. If this information were available, it could support medical research and medical practice. Such data are even more important for activities such as biosurveillance, quick response to outbreaks of disease or to chemical or biological attacks, and improved monitoring of adverse drug effects.[21] An electronic health information exchange would provide more thorough monitoring of adverse drug effects, and citizens could be automatically notified if their medication was no longer safe to take.

- **Tracking research and disease incidence.** Without a connected system of healthcare information, there is no way to accurately track trends of disease and injury. Tracking how a disease spreads helps health officials understand the size of the threat. By looking at how quickly diseases spread through a particular area, officials can accurately determine the number of vaccinations needed to control the disease throughout the Nation. With interoperable tools at their fingertips, public health agencies can more efficiently and effectively control and contain the spread of diseases.

> “The health of the people is really the foundation upon which all their happiness and all their powers as a state depend.”
>
> **Benjamin Disraeli, Former Prime Minister of England**

On-line Tools and Chronic Disease Management

One study noted, on-line chronic disease management tools have been shown to significantly improve patient compliance with medication regimens, from compliance rates of 34 percent to 63 percent without the tool, compared with 93 percent to 95 percent with the tool.[22]

Savings of Money and Time: Real-world Examples

With the implementation of an interoperable electronic record system in his Cummings, Georgia, clinics, Dr. James Morrow calculates a savings of $33.15 per patient visit. This savings had been invested in widening the facilities' services and medical capabilities. The result of the savings, the system, and the investment: the clinics' patients do not need to come into the office as frequently and can now find all of their care—and all of their records—in one place. In addition, patients avoid unnecessary lost days of work and improve their interaction with their doctors, thus improving their healthcare.[23]

[19] Commission on Systemic Interoperability staff interview with James Morrow, MD, February 2005.
[20] Robert J. Blendon. “Views of Practicing Physicians and the Public on Medical Errors.” *New England Journal of Medicine* 347, no. 24 (2002): 1933–40.
[21] T. Brewer and G. Colditz. “Postmarketing Surveillance and Adverse Drug Reactions: Current Perspectives and Future Needs.” *Journal of the American Medical Association* 281, no. 9 (1999): 824–29.
[21] Connecting for Health Collaborative. *Financial, Legal and Organizational Approaches to Achieving Electronic Connectivity in Healthcare.* Markle Foundation, 2004.
[23] Commission on Systemic Interoperability staff interview with James Morrow, MD, February 2005.

- **Better tools for first responders.** A connected system would also support individual responders. Emergency workers would be able to get the most up-to-date information on vaccines and treatment for biological threats. They could more efficiently coordinate with hospitals and clinics, and all healthcare providers could more easily find up-to-the-minute information to provide care and to help contain a health crisis or epidemic.

Adoption and Implementation

"Knowing is not enough; we must apply. Willing is not enough; we must do."

**Johann Wolfgang von Goethe,
German Poet, Dramatist, Novelist, and Scientist (1749 – 1832)**

Overcoming cultural barriers by phasing in the system slowly

The key to successful adoption of an interoperable system is to gradually phase in functionality. The first features should be nondisruptive and prove to be time- or cost-saving—they should enable information access without requiring redesign of work procedures and data entry. For example, access to a browsable chart—transcribed reports, lab data, scanned paper—is a fundamental yet nondisruptive change that could be the main feature of the first implementation. The next step might be to add simple intrateam messaging, then e-prescribing, then structured notes and orders.

In this way, users gain time and cost savings in the first steps, then give back some of the time in exchange for quality improvement in the latter steps. For instance, cost savings may come through improved reimbursement, either as a result of coding, participation in pay-for-performance programs, or through improved productivity.

The Four Levels of Interoperability[24]	
Level 1: **Nothing**	Traditional data-sharing: Information is either physically mailed or communicated over the phone.
Level 2: **Basic**	Very simple use of technology such as scanning paper documents and e-mailing or faxing them. No ability to update or amend electronic documents.
Level 3: **Interpreter**	Information is structured, but data standards do not exist. As a result, computer programs (often called "middleware") are used to interpret and translate data for processing.
Level 4: **Superior**	All data are standardized and coded. All systems can send and receive information using a uniform format and vocabulary.

[24] E. Pan, D. Johnston, and J. Walker. *The Value of Healthcare Information Exchange and Interoperability.* Center for Information Technology Leadership, 2004.

Making healthcare providers a part of the effort

Healthcare providers must realize that adopting interoperable electronic healthcare information is in their best interest in terms of time and professional convenience.

In particular, the rollout of the system should engage doctors, nurses, and other healthcare providers in the identification of electronic healthcare implementation priorities that will allow better use of their time while directly caring for patients.

Those in charge of implementing a system must remember that doctors currently are using procedures that work for them. Those procedures may not be particularly efficient procedures, but they get the job done; and for most managers, a proven system that is not quite perfect is worth much more than the promise of a more efficient system—especially when that system demands an intense conversion effort.

Adoption Statistics

Reported rates of adoption vary widely, and not necessarily because the rates are actually different. At this early stage of interoperability, language and definitions are not universal, so the terms in survey questions mean different things to different respondents: one clinic's "complete implementation" is another clinic's "first step."

- Only about 10 to 30 percent[25] of the more than 871,000 practicing physicians[26] in the United States use a "fully automated" system of electronic medical records.
- In the 2003 National Hospital Ambulatory Care Survey, 22 percent of physician offices, 30 percent of outpatient departments, and 40 percent of emergency rooms had adopted electronic medical records.[27]
- In the 2002 HIMSS/AstraZeneca Clinician Wireless Survey, 72 percent of respondents had no electronic medical records deployed in their facilities, eight percent of respondents had some deployment, and 21 percent had complete deployment in all departments.[28]
- In the 2003 Commonwealth Fund National Survey of Physicians and Quality of Care, 35 percent of physician offices with 10 to 49 physicians, and 57 percent of offices with 50 physicians or more had adopted electronic medical records.[29]
- In 2002, 13 percent of hospitals and 14 to 28 percent of physician's practices had electronic health records.[30]

Although statistics are not consistently reliable for the reasons mentioned above, the trends noted by the Commission indicate that adoption and implementation exist in early stages.

[25] *Advanced Studies in Medicine* 4, no. 8 (2004): 439.
[26] American Medical Association. *Physician Characteristics and Distribution in the U.S., 2005 Edition* and prior editions. <http://www.ama-assn.org/ama/pub/category/12912.html>
[27] C. Burt and E. Hing. *Use of Computerized Clinical Support Systems in Medical Settings: United States, 2001–03.* Division of Health Care Statistics of the National Center for Health Statistics, 2005.
[28] *2002 HIMSS/AstraZeneca Clinician Survey.* Healthcare Information and Management Systems Society, AstraZeneca, 2002. <http://www.himss.org/content/files/surveyresults/Final%20Final%20Report.pdf >
[29] *The Commonwealth Fund 2003 National Survey of Physicians and Quality of Care.* Harris Interactive, 2003. <http://www.cmwf.org/surveys/surveys_show.htm?doc_id=278869>
[30] *2002 HIMSS/AstraZeneca Clinician Survey.* Healthcare Information and Management Systems Society, AstraZeneca, 2002. <http://www.himss.org/content/files/surveyresults/Final%20Final%20Report.pdf >

Doctors and their staffs deserve to have their concerns addressed with clear and simply stated information about benefits, potential delays, and realistic timetables. The more quantitative data available to make the case—in terms of saved money and especially increased time made available to care for patients—the more likely providers will support the switchover to an interoperable electronic healthcare system.

Financial barriers

Even for early adopters, the shift to a connected system will be an evolutionary process that will require updates, replacements, and changes in software, hardware, and procedures as standards and practices are refined. This alone is a discouraging truth, and it is compounded by the fact that healthcare providers face competing capital demands and have relatively limited resources. Financial incentives should be considered in various forms.

"By creating national interoperability standards, we will give healthcare providers the confidence that an investment in health IT is an investment in the future."

Senator Hillary Rodham Clinton

Good news: much of the technology already exists

The necessary technology already exists and in some places is already in use. *The Washington Post* described the daily use of a system in a recent story:

> At 9 a.m., Dr. Julio Panza begins his rounds at [a] coronary care unit.... Residents and fellows review the status of the 14 patients in the unit. Panza takes notes and records his diagnoses and orders with a pen, as doctors have for centuries.
>
> Discussion turns to one particularly vexing case, a patient admitted the previous afternoon with chest pains. Panza turns to a computer screen and calls up the patient's lab results, which have been transmitted by lab machines. Another click and he can see what medicines have been dispensed from the unit's automated medicine cabinet. Yet another click and the group watches a video of what happened the day before as doctors threaded a thin wire through the patient's arteries and installed three tiny stents to keep the passageways open. Panza clicks again to find details of previous hospital visits and learns that the patient was a heavy smoker and a diabetic.

What the folks at the [facility] have discovered is that most of the makings of an electronic medical record are already available in digital form at most hospitals. By investing a relatively small amount of time and money, they've collected it all in one database and designed an easy-to-use interface that allows nurses, doctors, medical researchers, and finance staff to organize it in almost any way they want.[31]

Conversion

The transition from a paper-based system to an electronic interoperable system will require changes in the way physicians and their staffs work. Procedures that are now carried out on paper will have to be translated and modified to fit the electronic system—although the expectation is that these new procedures will be faster and simpler. Conversion will therefore require physician and employee training. It will also require the establishment and adoption of standard terminology—that is, a common language for the description and exchange of data.

While efficiency will drastically improve simply by automating much of what is painstakingly done by hand now, the full benefits of interoperability will not be realized if workflow patterns do not change with the introduction of technology.

Certification

Healthcare accounts for nearly 16 percent of the U.S. economy,[32] and as the industry embraces information technology, more and more vendors will compete to sell their products to doctors, hospitals, and clinics.

Given the complexity of the systems and the myriad choices that will be available, few if any people will be equipped to both practice medicine and study these systems well enough to make a completely informed decision best suited to their circumstances.

Implementing Interoperability Must Be Made as Simple as Possible

The new procedures and systems that make interoperability possible must be straightforward in their adoption, transparent in their influence and benefit, and in line with the priorities of the business of being a healthcare provider. The new procedures and systems should also require as little adjustment in practice as possible. The concerns of healthcare providers should be respected as they are given the opportunity to adopt more efficient and resource-saving systems into their daily practice.

American Health Information Community

On June 6, 2005, Department of Health and Human Services Secretary Mike Leavitt announced the creation of the American Health Information Community (AHIC) that will serve as a standards and policy advisory board for the healthcare industry. It will focus on accelerating the work necessary to reach widespread implementation of health data standards.[33]

[31] Steven Pearlstein. "Innovation Comes From Within." *The Washington Post*, March 4, 2005.
[32] Statement of Mike Leavitt, Secretary of Department of Health and Human Services, before the Committee on the Budget, United States Senate, July 20, 2005.
[33] Office of the National Coordinator for Health Information Technology, Department of Health and Human Services. "American Health Information Community (the Community)." August 2005. <http://www.os.dhhs.gov/healthit/ahic.html >

If price difference is not a significant factor, purchasers will most often select those products that have the imprimatur, or certification, of a trusted entity. Product certification would allow doctors to purchase information technology systems knowing that they meet minimum standards of functionality and interoperability.

Certification will increase purchasers' confidence, encourage adoption, and ensure interoperability of systems with each other, as well as facilitate compliance with laws and regulations governing the exchange of healthcare information—much in the same way consumers feel more comfortable buying a car that got a favorable rating in *Consumer Reports*.

Certification should be based on universally recognized standards.

Standards: definition and parameters

Standards are agreed-upon specifications that allow independently manufactured products, whether physical or digital, to work together, or in other words, to be interoperable. Adherence to standards is the reason that any automobile gas tank can be filled at any gas pump, that any web browser can locate any public web page, and that an e-mail sent from an IBM-compatible PC can be read by people using Apple computers and vice-versa.

Unfortunately the standards that support universal web browsing and e-mail exchange are important, but not close to sufficient for interoperable healthcare. True connectivity for healthcare requires standardization of the format and content of a wide range of health data elements so they can be understandable to computer programs as well as people.

Systems must be able to read and write standard messages to request health data, such as lab test results or complete medical records, and to return data when legitimately requested by patients and authorized healthcare providers. Many key data elements in these messages, including a patient's current problems, medications, allergies, and lab tests, must contain standard vocabulary if the full benefits of interoperability are to be realized.

Over the past five years, considerable progress has been made in selecting the base set of messaging and vocabulary standards needed for efficient exchange of healthcare information. For example, some specific kinds of healthcare data, such as lab tests results and radiology images, are routinely exchanged in standard electronic messages, but most do not yet use standardized terminology within them. Work has begun to ensure that the standard healthcare terminologies are properly aligned with the message standards and with standard code sets used in billing and statistical reporting. Vendors are beginning to incorporate standard vocabularies into new versions of their health information technology products.

Despite these significant accomplishments, the standards selected have not yet been refined to work together efficiently to create a single coordinated, comprehensive, non-overlapping set. Lacking this single set, system developers have been unable to build the standards-compliant systems that can support all the functions required by the people who will use them. The standards retain gaps that must be filled and some duplication that needs to be eliminated.

The selected standards will need to be tested in a wide range of healthcare settings in order to identify what changes must be made to ensure that these standards are helping patients and clinicians collaborate more efficiently, rather than slowing them down. One way to minimize the potential negative effects of the implementation of standards for doctors, nurses, and other health professionals is to standardize key healthcare data, such as medical devices, drug labels, and test kits at the point of manufacture.

Healthcare Data Elements

What data elements need to be standardized? Another way to ask this question is, 'What kinds of information do healthcare providers and payers need to know and computer systems need to interpret?' These items will range from basic identifying information to specific information about a patient's condition and history. Some examples will include:

1. Name, birth date, and gender of patient;
2. Family contacts;
3. Presented conditions and dates;
4. Records of allergies and reactions to medications;
5. Physicians seen; and
6. Lab test orders and results.

Why we need standards right now

Until a practical and comprehensive set of standards is in place, the United States will never be able to trade the current patchwork of electronic health records and other systems for a system of interoperable healthcare. The lack of easily implemented, usable standards is the primary barrier to creating this system, but fortunately, this is a barrier that can be overcome with focused attention and action. Recent Federal actions to provide leadership for standards completion and implementation and to support robust regional testing of health information exchange will be critical in achieving workable standards.

Standard Product Identifiers and Vocabulary. The standards and vendor products that enable the U.S. system of interoperable healthcare information must support these functions:

- Physician access to patient information, including past diagnoses and treatment, lab results, prescriptions, MRI results, and x-rays;
- Access among providers in multiple care settings;
- Systems that allow doctors to order medications and tests for patients in the hospital;
- Computerized decision-support systems, including best practices;
- Tracking for compliance to support study and revision of best-practice definitions;
- Secure electronic communication among providers and patients;
- Automated administration processes, such as scheduling;
- Automated filing of insurance claims;
- Patient access to health records, disease management tools, and health information resources; and
- Data storage and reporting for patient safety and public-health monitoring efforts.

Infrastructure Issue: Broadband Internet Access

Interoperability will require nationwide broadband connectivity—high-speed access to the Internet-among healthcare providers. This is because access to data for more than a trivial number of patients will call for significant bandwidth—the ability to accommodate many requests for large data files. Dial-up connections will be too slow to meet provider needs. (Patients, however, may be able to rely on dial-up, since they may only rarely need the bandwidth-driven ability to view detailed images and streaming audio or video.)

The level of broadband adoption has surged in the last few years. A study by the Department of Commerce shows that the number of Americans with high-speed Internet connections doubled from 2001 to 2003. Another study by the Pew Project shows a 60 percent increase between March 2003 and March 2004.[34] However, many rural areas have no broadband access and it will be an essential ingredient in fostering the development of health information technology in already underserved areas.

President Bush set a goal for universal affordable access to broadband technology by 2007. He said, "My Administration has long recognized the economic vitality that can result from broadband deployment and is working to create an environment to foster broadband deployment. All Americans should have affordable access to broadband technology by the year 2007."[35]

Federal, State, and private programs to promote the expansion of broadband may resolve this problem well before a connected healthcare system is fully deployed.

Federal preemption

Today, States can—and do—create laws that differ substantially from each other on privacy, security, and the handling of personal information.[36] In this environment, it is not possible to create a single set of procedures and systems that satisfies the regulations and statutes of all States.

This means that two physicians authorized by a patient to share information may not be able to legally do so simply because they are located in different States. Therefore, Federal jurisdiction should be superior to State jurisdiction in matters of medical privacy related to healthcare interoperability.

Legacy systems

"Legacy" systems (usually electronic medical record systems with limited interoperability capabilities) are those systems implemented prior to the introduction of common national standards. These are the healthcare systems in use today.

[34] John Horrigan. "Pew Internet Project Data Memo." Pew Internet & American Life Project. April 2004.
[35] White House. "Broadband Rights-of-Way Memorandum." Memo to the heads of executive departments and agencies, April 26, 2004.
[36] Stephen A. Stuart. *HIPAA/State Law Preemption Fact Sheet.* State of California Office of HIPAA Implementation, January 9, 2003.

Their data storage, input, and even inventory of data items are unique and often proprietary. Legacy systems present a problem because each one is built for the needs of a particular task or even a particular facility, instead of for industry-wide flexibility. Moreover, many of these systems are designed to prevent interoperability with other vendors' applications to protect market share and to encourage purchases by hospital or clinic chains.

Legacy systems will be a part of the overall connected healthcare network, either temporarily or permanently. In either case, these legacy systems will require "middleware"—software and sometimes hardware—that translates the input and output of a system so it can interact with other connected healthcare systems.

Because legacy systems are critical to the business side of medicine, they cannot be shut down while new interoperable systems are being implemented. If a legacy system is being replaced instead of adapted, it must run simultaneously with the new system for a time to ensure constant, reliable access.

Other challenges of implementation

- **Planning for the unexpected.** The transition to a connected healthcare system may not be easy, but the problems on the way to conversion will be more readily accepted by providers if they understand, from the beginning, that unexpected problems will occur, and if they understand, at least in general terms, what types of problems may arise.

- **The timeline for adoption.** Providers are more likely to embrace an interoperable system if they know how long it will take to get the system up and running. No one wants a promise of an early delivery if that promise is not likely to be kept. It is especially important to build in extra time to solve unexpected problems.

- **Education strategy.** Healthcare providers will need to be taught how to use the connected system and why its use is important. If healthcare providers simply believe the system is a new way to fill out forms, they are less likely to acquire the technical skills and knowledge needed to make full use of the new system. When healthcare providers understand the potential for making their job easier, they are far more likely to apply serious effort toward using the tools of the new interoperable system.

"If there is no struggle, there is no progress."

Frederick Douglass, American Abolitionist and Author (1818 – 1895)

"If we're not connecting, we're not getting the data on the labs, on the vital signs, or the medications that they're taking. The more information you have at your fingertips, the better."

– Robert Lamberts, M.D.

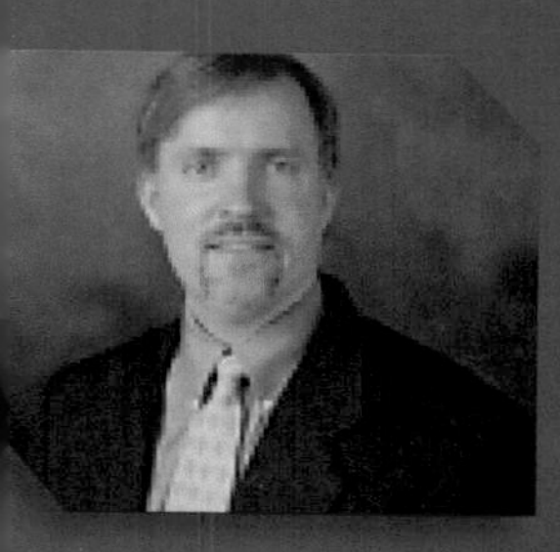

» PROFILE:

Robert Lamberts
M.D.
GEORGIA

~ Less Time Searching for Patient Information and More Time for Quality at the Point-of-Care

More Time for Quality Patient Care

Dr. Lamberts was first introduced to "computerized" medicine when he completed his residency in an Indiana hospital. They used computers to look up test results, x-rays, and patient records. After finishing his residency, he settled in Georgia to start his practice. He was shocked when he realized how behind the times they were. "I got kind of spoiled there, then I came here to Georgia to practice medicine and realized that I had gone back to the dark ages, and quickly decided I wanted to get on to electronic medical records."

The switch was not easy, but it was definitely worth it. Now, Dr. Lamberts' office is able to provide the best possible care to all his patients. "The computer doesn't cut down on the time you're talking to your patient. The computer does allow you to spend less time doing all of that other stuff. If I can have information at my fingertips, I can spend much more time caring for my patients, because I don't spend as much time looking for information."

The biggest reward for Dr. Lamberts is being able to see his patients becoming healthier. He can look at his system and find numbers for his patients with high cholesterol, diabetes, heart disease ... and see them improving. His new, larger office is now totally paperless, containing more space for patient care areas instead of paper medical records. He is also able to better monitor his patients who are on various medications. "When Vioxx® got recalled, we had a letter in the mail that same day to our patients. They were so impressed, and said 'How do you get all that to us? My other doctor never sent me anything.' I said of course they don't, they have no idea you're on Vioxx. We did because we keep track of that."

Worth the Cost

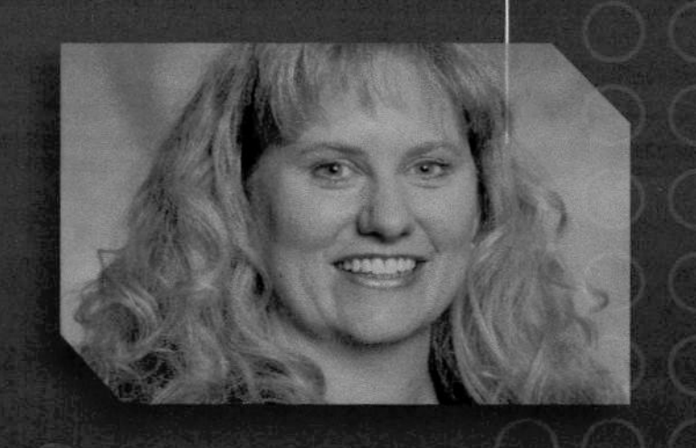

Tamara Lewis, M.D.

UTAH

~ A Medical Director in Utah Knows the Costs and Benefits of Interoperability

Dr. Tamara Lewis has a unique vantage point on what it takes to develop interoperable systems of health information. Dr. Lewis has helped to "mesh" the Utah Statewide Immunization Information System (USIIS) with her health system's electronic medical records (EMR) system. USIIS/WebKids is used by 50 pediatricians and 80 family practitioners in their health system, which covers all of Utah and parts of southern Idaho. The system allows doctors to see exactly what immunizations each child has received and "forecast" which immunizations they still need and when. The State Department of Health gathers the information from clinics and hospitals all over the State, and stores it in a secure database that doctors can access.

Being in the trenches throughout this complicated process has given Dr. Lewis a unique perspective on the many obstacles and considerations that are involved. The first major factor she cites is money. She says that money has to be available, not just to initially implement the systems, but to keep the systems up-to-date with the most recent health information and medical terminology. "It has to be constantly flexible, constantly rebuilding, and constantly changing according to new medical information."

"I think we need to have certain national standards so that systems will in the future be able to talk to each other. That's core and critical."

– Tamara Lewis, M.D.

Another major barrier to the wide use of health information technology by doctors is that government bureaucracies tend to work much slower than private sector doctors and hospital systems. The result is that when a new vaccine comes out, the computer systems have to be updated and ready to handle the new vaccine. There are layers of bureaucracy that have to "approve" the update, and the process is painfully slow. New vaccines may be ready and on the market, but doctors can't use them because they can't document them in the system.

Despite the many barriers, Dr. Lewis sees many more benefits—for patients, doctors, and even the government and the Nation's health as a whole. With Utah's system of tracking immunizations, they may someday have the capability to see, for example, how many people in the state need a smallpox vaccine in the case of a bioterrorism attack. The system has the potential to save the lives of countless men, women, and children, not only in Utah, but all across America.

Finding the Perfect Balance

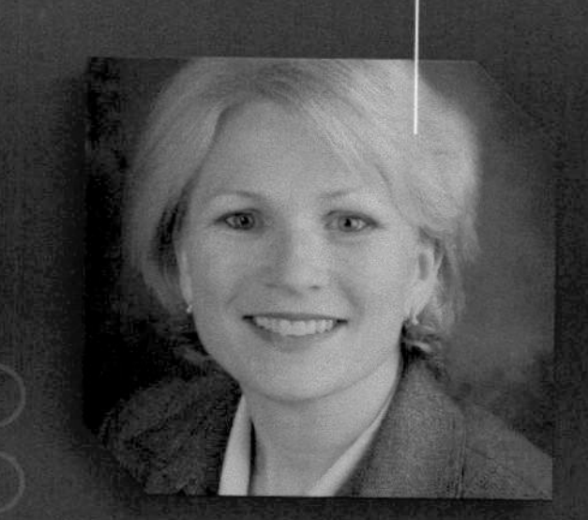

» PROFILE:

Alice Loveys, M.D.
NEW YORK

~ A Pediatrician and Working Mother Says EMRs Help Her Provide Better Care

"My motivations for doing this were not financial; it was definitely more a balance of personal and professional life, still giving good quality care and an enjoyable atmosphere."

– Alice Loveys, M.D.

Dr. Alice Loveys is a woman who values people. She values her family, her friends, and her patients. So when she saw the potential of computerized medical records, she decided to "take the plunge" and invested in an electronic medical record (EMR) system. At first, Dr. Loveys didn't know if she would be able to afford it, but she found a good basic system she could afford and has been able to make it work for her patients and her lifestyle.

While it may not be perfect, the difference the system has made in the quality of care she can provide to her patients has been amazing. She says her nurses have seen one of the greatest differences. Now, they are thrilled that they are able to spend more time doing what they love—nursing—rather than calculating growth charts or writing down medical histories.

"I think the beauty of an electronic medical record in a group practice is your partner can view the patient care record you've started. That benefit is a no-brainer. But with a paper chart, I couldn't read half my partner's handwriting and sometimes I couldn't even read my own writing. You sleep easier at night knowing that you're going to have adequate documentation."

They can also do digital imaging in the office. One time, a patient came to see Dr. Loveys' partner, and her partner took a picture of the rash. The next day Dr. Loveys was covering for her, and the little boy came in with a rash that was even worse than the day before. "I was able to look up what it looked like the day before and looked at it that day, and I could not have done that with a handwritten note. If I had to rely on a handwritten note, I know I would have made the wrong diagnosis."

"I think doctors should not be about inputting all the data, but reviewing the data that's available. And I think technology allows you to do that. Technology assembles the data. You review it, and then you make decisions based on it." The system has truly made a difference in the way she practices medicine.

A Hefty Price Tag

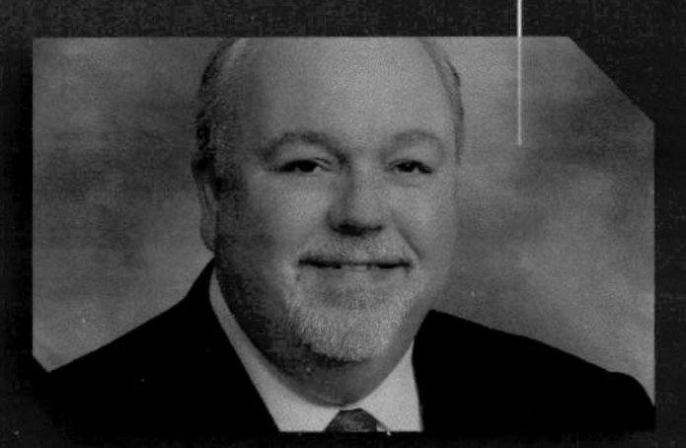

PROFILE:

Joseph Flood, M.D.
OHIO

~ An Ohio Rheumatologist Longs for an EMR System, But Like Many Solo Practices Can't Afford the Cost

Like most doctors in America, Dr. Joseph Flood is in his own practice. He is a specialist who has patients referred to him from other doctors, and as a result, has a huge amount of paperwork flowing through his office all the time: letters to doctors, patient records sent from other offices, and so on. Also, like most other doctors, Dr. Flood continues to struggle with the skyrocketing costs of healthcare and the rising costs of keeping his office up and running every day.

Dr. Flood is well aware of the enormous benefits of using an interoperable system of electronic medical records, but he has discovered that the cost of installing such a system is difficult to afford. "The situation for a solo practitioner has been increasingly difficult. We see decreases in reimbursement and increases in expenses. My malpractice insurance has gone up substantially over the last year. The cost of getting all the supplies I need for my practice has gone up considerably. The cost of health insurance in my office has gone up. Everything seems to have gone up except for my salary. When I look at the potential costs to switch over to such a system, it's something that I just would not be able to do, even if the cost were spread out over several years."

Things like subsidies, loans, or reimbursement changes that would help pay for the kind of quality healthcare an interoperable system would ensure are all things Dr. Flood thinks are good ideas. "We've heard about pay-for-performance, but we haven't seen what that really means for a practicing physician at this point in time. I do efficient care of patients with high quality. And to the extent that I might be rewarded for that, I would be happy to see that. If the use of an electronic health record is part of that measurement, then I would certainly hope that those people who are measuring me would make the reward for using that at least neutral in terms of cost."

"I think that almost every physician I know would be happy to have easily accessible data available to them, and all of us would like to see a patient who was on vacation or visiting another town have access to their medical records, so that people don't reinvent the wheel for them or put them through potentially hazardous testing that's already been done or wait while diagnostic testing is repeated."

– Joseph Flood, M.D.

Improved Care Justifies Costs

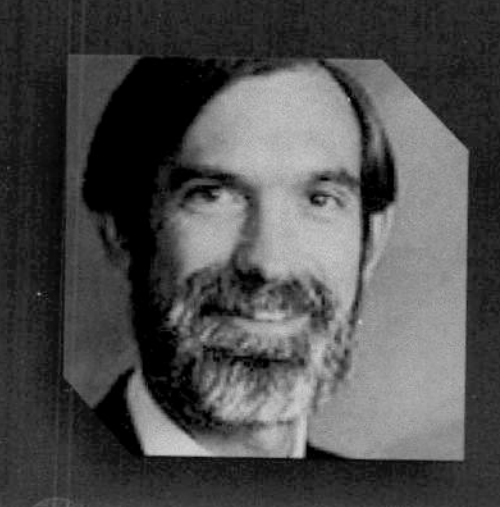

» PROFILE:

Robert Fried, M.D.

NORTH CAROLINA

~ Family Physician Focuses on Improved Quality of Care Through Use of Electronic Information

"We need a system that works for us and the workflow in our organization and gives us communication so our hospitalists and the people in our walk-in clinic, which is an urgent care after-hours, have access to the

With 9,000 patient charts and 60 patient visits per day, family physician Dr. Robert Fried is excited and mindful of the positive impact that electronic information exchange could have on his practice. Because of the need to have patient charts on hand, link with the affiliated hospital, and connect data such as x-rays, surgical reports, and lab tests, Dr. Fried is actively investigating what an electronic medical record (EMR) system will mean for his practice.

When it comes to adopting an EMR system, Dr. Fried is not concerned financially. He says, "Every year we're spending more on transcription than the system is going to cost, and we already have a couple pay-for-performance contracts. So, one of our criteria when we're looking at systems is that they can give us quality indicator reports, so we can have our own data to go by, instead of just going by the insurance company's data."

Physicians often have to monitor multiple health conditions and know necessary medications and their side effects. Doctors like Dr. Fried, must be familiar with up to 60 patients' medical histories daily. Dr. Fried explained that complicated multiple conditions and treatments can be a difficult balance. Even a small oversight can have a major impact on an individual's health.

Because of the tremendous amount of information that is needed for accurate medical care, repeated medical tests are common. They are a necessity that can become expensive for patients and would be unnecessary for doctors if access to prior results were available. Dr. Fried states, "I do labs not knowing what they [the patients] have done, and some of them are repeated. It's hard to eliminate that waste."

With the help of an electronic system that allows doctors to communicate, some medical oversights can easily be avoided. Dr. Fried says, "I'm really looking forward to having a system that helps remind me of all the things I should be doing when I've got somebody with, you know, three and four problems going on at the same time, because it's hard to juggle it all in your head."

FACT

~ In an article published in the July/August, 2004, *Annals of Family Medicine*, medical errors were studied as a chain of events rather than isolated incidents. Two-thirds of all errors in treatment and diagnosis were found to begin with errors in communication. These included missed communication between physicians, misinformation in medical records, mishandling of patient requests and messages, inaccessible records, mislabeled specimens, misfiled or missing charts, and inadequate reminder systems.

Source: Wooley, Mary. Research for Health: The Power of Advocacy. January 14, 2005. Research!America. PowerPoint. August 2005. www.nlm.nih.gov/csi/research_america_011405.pdf

Interoperability costs and benefits

Spending on interoperability is an investment, not just an expense, because it produces a return in the form of saved time, reduced paperwork, increased quality of care, reduced need for treatment, and saved lives.

Since there is no complete implementation of a connected health information system yet, the exact financial savings are only speculation. However, the extent of these returns will depend on how thoroughly the interoperable system is integrated into the facility or practice and the extent to which patients participate.

Ultimately, interoperability will enhance the "culture of care." It changes the structure of an organization by redirecting resources, step by step, toward more patient-centered services. Tasks that once required a doctor or nurse to take time away from direct caregiving become automated at best and less time-consuming at least.

Pay-for-Performance

Pay-for-performance is an initiative to promote quality care. This initiative realigns provider payment incentives to follow care guidelines based on scientific evidence about what actually helps to prevent or treat disease. Pay-for-performance is directly tied to the development of a national health information exchange because tools such as electronic prescribing and electronic information exchange help improve patient care and reduce medical errors.

Confidentiality

"We need a better way to share information. We need a better system so that physicians have at their fingertips all the information they need to do their job—including patient history, the latest research, drug interactions, and everything else they need.... Information, in the hands of the right people, at the right time, drives quality and value. We need to empower patients and healthcare providers to make the right choices. And to do that, healthcare decision-makers—providers, payers, and patients—need to have access to the right information, where and when it is needed, securely and privately."

Senator Hillary Rodham Clinton

Patient consent

Before the interoperable system goes on-line, the rules on consent must be clear. Privacy and security policies should be considered as a part of design, not as an afterthought, and should be based on current law.[37] Legislation and regulation should be regularly considered to reevaluate emerging technologies and capabilities. Policies must be widely agreed to by patients and practitioners alike on the terms and conditions for access to and dissemination of patient data.

The structure and rules of health information networks must support the exercise of patient rights under Federal privacy regulations. Although State privacy rules vary, Federal jurisdiction should be superior to State jurisdiction in matters of medical privacy related to connectivity. Health activities that are not directly covered by the Health Insurance Portability and Accountability Act (HIPAA) need to be associated with this or other privacy rules, by either regulation or statute.

[37] Some laws, such as the Health Information Portability and Accountability Act of 1996 (HIPAA) (Public Law 104-191), may need revision in light of the benefits and concerns that arise under an electronic and interoperable system.

According to HIPAA rules at the time of this writing, a patient's consent is not required:

- When emergency care is needed;
- When a provider is required by law to administer treatment;
- When substantial communication barriers exist and, in a professional's judgment, the circumstances infer the individual's consent;
- For a provider with an indirect treatment relationship to provide services (e.g., laboratories);
- For a health plan to use the information for treatment, payment, or healthcare operations; and
- For a clearinghouse to use the information for treatment, payment, or healthcare operations.

Security authorization devices

Systems of passwords and biometric devices such as fingerprint readers and voice-scanning systems should be used to help ensure data and networks are secure. These security devices and procedures will vary from application to application. For instance, it should be physically easy (but not easier in terms of data protection) to enter authorization on devices to be used primarily in emergency applications. An emergency medical technician working an accident on the side of the road should be able to log in without using a large keyboard or numerous keystrokes. A retinal or fingerprint scan would save time and, therefore, speed treatment.

Punishment for violations

The Federal government has passed laws to punish individuals guilty of identity theft.[38] Electronic information breaches of any kind should be punished at least as severely as similar offenses such as fraud, theft, and forgery. Laws should be

[38] United States. Cong. Senate. *The Identity Theft and Assumption Deterrence Act.* Public Law 105-318.

enacted with stiff criminal sanctions against individuals who purposefully access protected data without authorization. There should also be clear and comprehensive safeguards to protect anyone whose personal data was improperly accessed or released.

Patient Authentication

Creating a unique number would be the most direct way to establish a patient's identity and this approach is used throughout Europe. However, no approach to personal authentication in computer systems is free of financial costs, management issues, and privacy concerns. A direct approach would involve an administrative infrastructure that may be unacceptable to some at this time for a variety of reasons, including privacy concerns.

This approach could be modified to allow individuals to opt out of the uniform patient identifier. This compromise would let the nation provide a system benefiting individuals who recognize that their need for connected health information exceeds their privacy concerns, while not penalizing those who find privacy more valuable. However, such a compromise would sharply reduce the administrative savings because the system would have to accommodate both sets of individuals. It would also present new liability challenges, specifically involving the potential liability of providers who lacked information in the treatment of a consumer whose information was not available.

An alternative to creating unique personal identification for everyone is to define a national standard set of authenticating information required to receive healthcare. This set of data could be captured when an individual first enters the healthcare system. Such information could include a set of data such as date of birth, school, employment, and insurance policy number.

Individual Access

Medical records should be like money in a bank account: the money belongs to you, while the task of accounting belongs to the bank. By further allowing patients to add comments to specific areas within the record, they can take a proactive role in maintaining their health record while the information remains clear to the healthcare provider.

In healthcare, changes most often enter the practice of medicine in the form of new drugs and procedures for a single illness or disease. But interoperability or connectivity—the notion of a national or even global electronic health information system—is a change that will affect the overall practice of medicine. Its legion of benefits—better-educated patients, complete physician access to medical histories, and easier consultations, just to name a few—enhance patient care and provider support in all healthcare circumstances. This is a rare thing.

As the Internet affected all facets of daily life, connectivity will enhance all facets of healthcare. At last, healthcare providers will gain tools to support healthy lifestyles of patients. The information gap for providers seeing new patients will be closed. And the costly and time-consuming paperwork that burdens everyone in this field will be significantly diminished—a light at the end of the tunnel that few doctors ever imagined they would see.

Existing Efforts: Connecting the Country

Many efforts are underway to connect the country's healthcare delivery systems electronically. These efforts are important steps to a better equipped, more reliable, and more efficient healthcare system that will save lives and money.

The focus of these efforts is on making critical connections between patients and doctors, doctors and doctors, doctors and pharmacies, healthcare providers and payors, and healthcare providers and the government. These efforts to improve communication and increase safety in the healthcare system are parts of a step-by-step process involving legislation, government programs and departments, and public and private projects.

Following is a summary of existing efforts included in this section:

- **Existing Federal Legislation**
  Many members of the 109th Congress have introduced legislation that impacts electronic information exchange and healthcare. The legislation section includes a list of proposed bills organized by subject matter: electronic healthcare information exchange, prescription electronic reporting, emergency communications for first responders, and homeland security and emergency response.

- **Government Programs and Departments**
  The US government is the largest single purchaser and provider of healthcare in the country and is a leader in health IT initiatives. In 2003 government funding was nearly 46% of all the dollars spent on healthcare in the United States.[1] These organizations are leaders in implementing tools that will enable information exchange, and their efforts are described in this section.

- **Public and Private Projects**
  The section on public and private projects provides a national overview of public and private efforts taking place around the country to connect health information.

[1] "Effects of Health Care Spending in the U.S. Economy." Ed. Health and Human Services, 2005.

This is not an exhaustive list, as work is ongoing to advance healthcare delivery systems. Each description lists a point of contact as well as Web resources where more detailed information may be found. The information provided comes directly from the organizations listed and has not been independently verified by the Commission.

Existing Federal Legislation: Summary of Bills from the 109th Congress that Apply to Healthcare Interoperability

Electronic Healthcare Information Exchange:

1. **Bill Number: S.544**
   Patient Safety and Quality Improvement Act of 2005
   Introduced by: Senator James M. Jeffords (VT)

The Patient Safety and Quality Improvement Act of 2005 promotes the interoperability of healthcare information technology systems not later than 36 months after the date of enactment of this bill; the Secretary shall develop or adopt voluntary standards and provide for the ongoing review and periodic updating of the standards developed. The Secretary shall provide for the dissemination of the standards developed and updated under this section. It amends the Public Health Service Act to designate patient safety data as privileged and confidential. It permits certain disclosures of patient safety data by a provider or patient safety organization (PSO), including (1) voluntary disclosures of non-identifiable data; (2) disclosures of data containing evidence of a wanton and criminal act to directly harm the patient; (3) disclosures necessary to carry out PSO or research activities; and (4) voluntary disclosures for public health surveillance.

The Patient Safety and Quality Improvement Act of 2005 prohibits an accrediting body from (1) taking any accrediting action against a provider based on the provider's good faith participation in collecting, developing, reporting, or maintaining patient safety data; or (2) requiring a provider to reveal its communications with any PSO. It prevents a provider from taking an adverse employment action against an individual based upon the good faith reporting of information.

This bill also requires the Secretary to (1) maintain a patient safety network of databases that has the capacity to accept, aggregate, and analyze non-identifiable patient safety data voluntarily reported and that provides an interactive resource for providers and PSOs; (2) develop or adopt voluntary national standards to promote the electronic exchange of healthcare information; and (3) contract with a research organization to study the impact of medical technologies and therapies on healthcare.

2. Bill Number: S.1223
Information Technology for Health Care Quality Act
Introduced by: Senator Christopher J. Dodd (CT)

The Information Technology for Health Care Quality Act established the Office of the National Coordinator for Health IT (ONCHIT) within the Office of the President to direct all health IT activities within the Federal government and facilitate interaction between the Federal government and the private sector. It establishes specific duties and responsibilities for ONCHIT.

This bill shall provide for the adoption by the Federal government of national data and communication health IT standards. Standards adopted shall be voluntary for the private sector and shall be adopted at the conclusion of a collaborative process that includes consultation between the Federal government and private sector/IT stakeholders. To the extent practical, the Secretary shall pilot test health IT standards developed under this Act. The Secretary may license standards or use of other means to facilitate dissemination and implementation one year after adoption of standards.

The Information Technology for Health Care Quality Act shall guarantee loans to independent consortiums—community stakeholders—to implement LHII, facilitate the development of interoperability, or to facilitate the purchase and adoption of health IT. Special consideration will be given to specified entities.

It states that within six months of enactment, ONCHIT shall make recommendations on changes to Federal reimbursement and payment structures that would encourage the adoption of health IT. This bill also states that Health Insurance Portability and Accountability Act of 1996 (HIPAA) privacy, confidentiality, and security regulations shall apply to the implementation of programs and activities under this Act.

It states that a collaboration of DHHS, DoD, and VA—in consultation with Quality Interagency Coordination Taskforce—IoM, JCAHO, NCVHS, AHQA,

NQF, MedPAC, and others shall develop uniform healthcare quality measures for each of the 20 priority areas identified by IoM within 18 months of enactment. Each federally supported health delivery program may conduct pilot tests of quality measures and establish ongoing reporting and evaluations of quality measures.

3. Bill Number: S.1227
Health Information Technology Act of 2005
Introduced by: Senator Debbie Stabenow (MI)

The Health Information Technology Act of 2005 states that within two years of enactment, the Secretary shall provide for the development and adoption of national data and communication health IT standards. No later than Jan. 1, 2008, the Secretary shall implement procedures to enable DHHS to accept the optional submission of data derived from reporting requirements established after enactment using standards adopted under this section. Not later than Jan. 1, 2010, the Secretary shall implement procedures to enable DHHS to accept the optional submission of data derived from all healthcare reporting requirements using standards adopted.

This bill states that the Secretary shall develop a grant program to offset costs incurred related to clinical healthcare informatics systems and services from Jan. 1, 2005, through Sept. 29, 2010, and it states that priority in awarding grants will be given to specified entities. At least 20% of funds must be given to entities in shortage areas or rural areas. This bill states that the Secretary shall establish a methodology for making adjustments in Medicare payments to providers and suppliers who use health IT and technology services that the Secretary determines improve the quality and accuracy of clinical decision-making, compliance, healthcare delivery, and efficiency—such as EMRs, e-prescribing, clinical decision support tools, and CPOE.

The Health Information Technology Act of 2005 states that the Secretary shall conduct studies and demonstration projects to evaluate the use of clinical healthcare informatics systems and services to measure and report on quality data and demonstrate impact on improving patient care, reducing costs, and increasing efficiencies.

4. Bill Number: S.1418
The Wired for Healthcare Quality Act
Introduced by: Senator Michael B. Enzi (WY)

The Wired for Healthcare Quality Act establishes the Office of National Health Information Technology to ensure that patient health information is secure and to improve overall healthcare. It states that the DHHS Secretary shall establish a public-private cooperative American Health Information Collaborative, and asks the Secretary to advise achievable actions for the collaborative, such as recommending standards. One year after enactment, and annually, the Secretary is to recommend national policies for adoption and the collaborative shall review adoption efforts as consistent with HIPAA regulations. This bill states that standards adoption in private entities should be voluntary, but private entities with contracts with the Federal government must comply with the standards. The Secretary must then submit an annual report to the Senate Finance Committee and the HELP Committee and the House of Representatives Committee on Energy and Commerce and Committee on Ways and Means.

The Wired for Healthcare Quality Act states that the Secretary shall develop criteria for implementation and certification of a health information exchange. The Secretary may award competitive grants to eligible entities to facilitate the purchase and enhance utilization of health information technology systems, but the entities must match the grant $1 for each $3. Preference can be awarded to entities in rural, frontier, and other underserved areas. Competitive grants may also be awarded to States for development of State loan programs for health IT adoption, which must be matched by non-Federal contributions $1 for each $1. Competitive grants may also be awarded to eligible entities to implement a regional or local health information exchange or to carry out demonstration projects to develop academic curricula for clinical education of health professionals. These grants may not be used for the purchase of hardware, software, or services.

It states that the Secretary shall contract a private entity to conduct a study that examines the variation between State laws regarding licensure, registration, and certification of medical professionals and how these laws impact electronic health information exchange. This bill states that relevant Secretaries and government agencies shall develop or adopt a quality measurement system for patient care. The Wired for Healthcare Quality Act states that the Secretary shall provide an analysis of quality measures collected and the dissemination of recommendations and best practices derived from such analysis. S.1418 states that the Public Health Service Act shall be amended by added language for a Center for Best Practices.

5. Bill Number: H.R.747
National Health Information Incentive Act of 2005
Introduced by: Representative Charles A. Gonzalez (TX-20)

The National Health Information Incentive Act of 2005 states that the Secretary shall develop or adopt standards for transactions and data elements for transactions that lead to the creation of NHII. The Secretary will act through ONCHIT and CSI and recommendations from NCVHS. The Secretary shall adopt trial standards two years (or subsequent date) after enactment. Entities that voluntarily use electronic health record (EHR) systems shall comply with standards adopted or modified within 24 months of adoption or modification, and the standards shall supersede any State law or regulations relating to electronic transmission of patient history, eligibility benefit, or other information.

National Health Information Incentive Act of 2005 provides for optional financial incentives to small healthcare providers and entities to implement a national health information infrastructure. It states that the Secretary shall include additional Medicare incentives to small healthcare providers to move toward NHII by acquiring EHR systems. Types of reimbursement include add-on payments for evaluation and management services; care management fees; payments for structured e-mail consults; and other methods deemed appropriate by the Secretary. This bill amends the Internal Revenue Code to provide for a refundable credit for a portion of the expenses of or for establishing a healthcare IT system.

6. Bill Number: H.R.2234
21st Century Health Information Act of 2005
Introduced by: Representative Tim Murphy (PA-18)

The 21st Century Health Information Act of 2005 authorizes the DHHS Secretary to make grants to regional health information organizations (RHIOs) to develop and implement regional health information technology plans. This bill requires the Director of AHRQ to establish and maintain a national technical assistance center to provide assistance to physicians to facilitate adoption of health information technologies and participation in such regional plans. It requires the Secretary to establish a program of accrediting health information networks.

This bill requires the Comptroller General to report to Congress on the progress of RHIOs in realizing the purposes of this Act. The 21st Century Health Information Act of 2005 prohibits Federal funds available under this Act from being used for the purchase of a health information technology product unless such product has been certified as incorporating interoperability data standards and compliance criteria.

It allows the Secretary to make loans to any accredited RHIOs to finance investments in network infrastructure and technology acquisition, training, and workflow engineering for physicians. The 21st Century Health Information Act of 2005 amends the Social Security Act to exclude the provision of equipment or services for the development of such a regional plan from illegal remuneration provisions and limitations on physician compensation arrangements. It requires the Secretary to (1) establish a methodology for making adjustments in Medicare payments to providers participating in an accredited network; and (2) make matching Medicaid payments to States for the development and implementation of a regional plan under certain circumstances. This bill states that no Federal funds may be made for the purposes of this Act for the purchase of health IT unless the product is certified by the CCHIT and must be approved by ANSI or the Secretary if the CCHIT is not approved by ANSI or the Secretary, the Secretary shall adopt interoperability standards and compliance criteria or designate a private entity to do so.

7. **Bill Number: H.R.3010**
Department of Labor, Health and Human Services, and Education, and Related Agencies Appropriations Act, 2006
Sponsor: Representative Ralph Regula (OH-16)

The Department of Labor, Health and Human Services, and Education, and Related Agencies Appropriations Act, 2006, makes appropriations for FY 2006 to the Department of Health and Human Services (DHHS) for the Office of the National Coordinator for Health Information Technology; and the public health and social services emergency fund, for activities related to countering potential biological, disease, and chemical threats to civilian populations, and to developing and implementing rapidly expandable influenza vaccine production technologies and purchasing influenza vaccine as necessary.

It authorizes, for expenses necessary for the Office of the National Coordinator for Health Information Technology, including grants, contracts, and cooperative agreements for the development and advancement of an interoperable national health IT infrastructure, $58,100,000 (reduced by $12,000,000): provided, that in addition to amounts provided herein, $16,900,000 (increased by $12,000,000) shall be available from amounts under section 241 of the Public Health Service Act to carry out health IT network development.

8. Bill Number: Yet to be Introduced
Sponsor: Representative Nancy Johnson (CT-5)

This bill states that the National Coordinator for Health Information Technology at the Department of Health and Human Services (DHHS) shall serve as the coordinator of Federal government activities relating to health information technology. It states that the National Coordinator shall harmonize standards, provide for certification and inspection of health IT products, provide for the evaluation of variations in business policies and Federal and State laws that affect confidentiality, and provide for the development of prototypes for a national health information network.

This bill states that the Secretary shall conduct a study to determine the impact of safe harbor laws, and shall submit a report to Congress recommending changes in the safe harbors.

This bill states that the Secretary shall conduct a study of State laws and regulations relating to the security and confidentiality of health information and submit a report to Congress. This bill also includes language for Federal preemption of State laws for confidentiality and security of health information.

This bill includes language for the Secretary to issue notice for rulemaking for the adoption of updated ICD codes for HIPAA standards and Medicare. The Secretary must also provide Congress with a report on the work conducted by the American Health Information Community.

Prescription Electronic Reporting:

1. **Bill Number: S.16 Affordable Health Care Act**
   Introduced by: Senator Edward M. Kennedy (MA)

The Affordable Health Care Act allows the DHHS Secretary to require the sponsor of an approved drug to conduct one or more studies that confirm or refute a credible hypothesis of a significant safety issue. It amends the Public Health Service Act to establish the Office of Health Information Technology to improve the quality and efficiency of healthcare delivery through the use of health information technology.

The Affordable Health Care Act requires that the DHHS Secretary, the DoD Secretary, and the VA Secretary establish uniform healthcare quality measures and public reporting requirements across all federally supported health delivery programs.

2. **Bill Number: S.518**
   National All Schedules Prescription Electronic Reporting Act of 2005
   Introduced by: Senator Jeff Sessions (AL)

The National All Schedules Prescription Electronic Reporting Act of 2005 amends the Public Health Service Act to require the DHHS Secretary to award grants for terms of 18 months to each approved State to establish or improve a State controlled-substance monitoring program. It requires the Secretary to develop minimum standards for States to ensure the security of information collected and to recommend penalties for the provision or use of information in violation of applicable laws or regulations.

This bill requires each approved State to (1) require dispensers to report to the State within one week of each dispensing of a controlled substance to an ultimate user; and (2) establish and maintain an electronic searchable database containing the information reported. It allows a State to provide information from the database in response to certain requests by practitioners; law enforcement, narcotics control, licensure, disciplinary, or program authorities; the controlled substance monitoring program of another State; and agents of DHHS, State Medicaid programs, State health departments, or DEA.

It requires the Secretary to (1) specify a uniform electronic format for the reporting, sharing, and provision of information under this Act; and (2) study and report to Congress on such programs, including on interoperability between programs, the feasibility of a real-time electronic controlled substance monitoring program, privacy protections, and technological alternatives to centralized data storage.

3. **Bill Number: H.R.1132 National All Schedules Prescription Electronic Reporting Act of 2005**
   Introduced by: Representative Ed Whitfield (KY-1)

The National All Schedules Prescription Electronic Reporting Act of 2005 amends the Public Health Service Act to require the DHHS Secretary to award one-year grants to each approved State to establish or improve a State controlled-substance monitoring program. It requires the Secretary to develop minimum standards for States to ensure security of information collected and to recommend penalties for the provision or use of information in violation of applicable laws or regulations.

It requires each approved State to (1) require dispensers to report to the State within one week of each dispensing of a controlled substance to an ultimate user or research subject; and (2) establish and maintain an electronic searchable database containing the information reported. It allows a State to provide information from the database in response to certain requests by practitioners; law enforcement, narcotics control, licensure, disciplinary, or program authorities; the controlled-substance monitoring program of another State; and agents of DHHS, State Medicaid programs, State health departments, or DEA.

This bill requires the Secretary to (1) specify a uniform electronic format for the reporting, sharing, and provision of information under this Act; (2) give preference to approved States in awarding any grants related to drug abuse; and (3) study and report to Congress on such programs, including on interoperability between programs, the feasibility of a real-time electronic controlled substance monitoring program, privacy protections, and technological alternatives to centralized data storage.

Emergency Communications for First Responders:

1. **Bill Number: S.1274**
   Improve Interoperable Communications for First Responders Act of 2005
   Introduced by: Senator Joseph I. Lieberman (CT)

Improve Interoperable Communications for First Responders Act of 2005 establishes an Office for Interoperability and Compatibility (OIC), headed by a Director, within the Directorate of Science and Technology of DHS. S.1274 requires the OIC Director to (1) assist the Secretary in developing and implementing the program to enhance public safety interoperable communications at all levels of government; (2) carry out DHS responsibilities and authorities relating to the SAFECOM Program; and (3) conduct extensive, nationwide outreach and foster the development of interoperable communications systems by State, local, and tribal governments and public safety agencies, and by regional consortia thereof.

It requires the Secretary to (1) establish a comprehensive research and development program to promote communications interoperability among first responders; and (2) make grants to States and eligible regions for initiatives necessary to achieve short-term or long-term solutions to Statewide, regional, national, and, where appropriate, international interoperability.

2. **Bill Number: H.R.1251**
   The Connecting the Operations of National Networks of Emergency Communications Technologies for First Responders Act of 2005
   Introduced by: Representative Nita M. Lowey (NY-18)

The Connecting the Operations of National Networks of Emergency Communications Technologies for First Responders Act of 2005 requires the DHS Secretary, in cooperation with State and local governments, Federal agencies, public safety agencies, and the private sector, to develop a national strategy to achieve communications interoperability and to report to Congress annually on progress toward achieving such interoperability.

3. **Bill Number: H.R.1544**
   Faster and Smarter Funding for First Responders Act of 2005
   Sponsor: Representative Christopher Cox (CA-48)

The Faster and Smarter Funding for First Responders Act of 2005 amends the Homeland Security Act of 2002 to set forth provisions governing DHS grant funding for first responders pursuant to the State Homeland Security Grant Program, the Urban Area Security Initiative, and the Law Enforcement Terrorism Prevention Program. It directs the Secretary of Homeland Security to require any State applying for a covered grant to submit a three-year State homeland security plan, to be developed in consultation with local governments and first responders.

This bill directs the Secretary, in consultation with specified officials and standards organizations, to promulgate national voluntary consensus standards for grant-funded first responder equipment and training. It requires the coordination of such activities that relate to health professionals with the DHHS Secretary, and also requires the Comptroller General to report to Congress on the overall inventory and status of first responder training programs of DHS and other Federal agencies and the extent to which such programs are coordinated.

Homeland Security and Emergency Response:

1. **Bill Number: S.21**
   Homeland Security Grant Enhancement Act of 2005
   Introduced by: Senator Susan M. Collins (ME)

The Homeland Security Grant Enhancement Act of 2005 requires the Director of the Office for Domestic Preparedness to allow any State to request approval to reallocate funds received under the State Homeland Security Grant Program under specified Federal laws among the categories of equipment, training, exercises, and planning.

This bill creates the position of Executive Director to head the DHS's Office for State and Local Government Coordination and Preparedness (OSLGCP) and give it additional responsibility for managing the Homeland Security Information Clearinghouse. The Clearinghouse will provide States, local governments, and emergency response providers with information regarding (1) homeland security grants; (2) technical assistance; (3) best practices; and (4) the use of Federal funds.

It directs the DHS Secretary to support the development of, promulgate, and update as necessary national voluntary consensus standards for the performance, use, and validation of first responder equipment for purposes of assessing equipment-related grant applications.

The Homeland Security Grant Enhancement Act of 2005 establishes in DHS an International Border Community Interoperable Communication Demonstration Project to (1) address the interoperable communication needs of police officers, firefighters, emergency medical technicians, the National Guard, and other emergency response providers; (2) foster interoperable communications among domestic government agencies and their counterparts in Canada or Mexico; (3) foster standardization of interoperable communications equipment; (4) ensure that emergency response providers can communicate with one another and the public at disaster sites or in the event of a terrorist attack or other catastrophic event; and (5) provide training and equipment to enable emergency response providers to deal with environmentally varied threats and contingencies.

2. Bill Number: S.1013
Homeland Security FORWARD Funding Act of 2005
Introduced by: Senator Dianne Feinstein (CA)

The Homeland Security FORWARD Funding Act of 2005 requires the DHS Secretary to establish clearly-defined essential capabilities for State and local government preparedness for terrorism (sets forth factors to address in establishing such capabilities and lists critical infrastructure sectors and types of threats to specifically consider).

It directs the DHS Secretary to promulgate national voluntary consensus standards for grant-funded first responder equipment and training, and it expresses the sense of Congress regarding interoperable communications and Citizen Corps councils, and requires the Secretary to (1) ensure coordination of Federal efforts to prevent, prepare for, and respond to acts of terrorism and other major disasters and emergencies among DHS divisions; and (2) study the feasibility of implementing a nationwide emergency telephonic alert notification system.

3. **Bill Number: H.R.796**
   Domestic Preparedness Act of 2005
   Introduced by: Representative Carolyn McCarthy (NY-4)

The Domestic Preparedness Act of 2005 authorizes the Secretary of Homeland Security to make grants to address homeland security preparedness shortcomings of units of municipal and county government. It specifies that each grant shall be made for one of the following categories: (1) equipment and training, or (2) improving interoperability among members of a consortium of municipal and county governments. It states that the Secretary may not make a grant under this Act unless the applicant conducts an assessment of the applicant's risk and vulnerability to possible acts of terrorism, including conventional biological, nuclear, and chemical attacks.

The Domestic Preparedness Act of 2005 provides that grant amounts may be distributed to fire departments, police departments, emergency services, and public health agencies of the grantee.

4. **Bill Number: H.R.1323**
   The Public Safety Interoperability Implementation Act
   Introduced by: Representative Bart Stupak (MI-1)

The Public Safety Interoperability Implementation Act amends the National Telecommunications and Information Administration Organization Act to establish in the Treasury the Public Safety Communications Trust Fund. It requires the Administrator to make grants to implement interoperability and modernization for the communication needs for public safety, fire, emergency, law enforcement, and crisis management by State and local government agencies and instrumentalities and nonprofit organizations.

Government Programs and Departments:

American Health Information Community (AHIC)

On June 6, 2005, the Department of Health and Human Services (DHHS) Secretary Mike Leavitt announced the formation of a national collaboration, the American Health Information Community (AHIC), which will advance health IT efforts across the public and private sectors to respond to the President's call for a majority of Americans to have electronic health records within 10 years. AHIC will help the nationwide transition to electronic health records—including common standards and interoperability—to proceed in a smooth, market-led way. AHIC, which will be formed under the auspices of the Federal Advisory Committee Act, will provide input and recommendations to DHHS on how to make health records digital and interoperable, and it will ensure that the privacy and security of those records are protected.

AHIC will be initially chartered for two years, with the potential to extend its charter. Secretary Leavitt intends for AHIC to be succeeded within five years by a private sector health information community initiative that, among other things, would set additional standards, certify new health information technology, and provide long-term governance for healthcare transformation.

For more information, please contact:

The Office of the National Coordinator for Healthcare IT
ONC c/o U.S. Dept of Health and Human Services
200 Independence Avenue, S.W.
Washington, DC 20201
Phone: 866-505-3500
E-mail: onchit.request@hhs.gov
Web site: http://www.hhs.gov/healthit/

Agency for Healthcare Research and Quality (AHRQ)

Originally created in 1989 as a Public Health Service agency in the Department of Health and Human Services (DHHS), the Agency for Healthcare Research and Quality (AHRQ) was reauthorized in 1999. AHRQ's mission is to support research designed to improve the quality, safety, efficiency, and effectiveness of healthcare in America. It sponsors and conducts research and programs that provide evidence-based information on healthcare outcomes: quality as well as cost, use, and access.

AHRQ's health IT initiative in fiscal year 2005 includes $139 million in multiyear funding for more than 100 projects and contracts across the country via its Transforming Healthcare Quality Through Information Technology (THQIT) grants and State and Regional Demonstration (SRD) contracts portfolio, which impact 40 million Americans. These initiatives are exploring and testing a wide range of health IT applications with the potential to transform everyday clinical practice and help build the 21st century health IT infrastructure. AHRQ's health IT initiative encompasses three types of grants that:

- Support planning for health IT projects;
- Support implementation of health IT projects; and
- Demonstrate the value of health IT applications.

The goals of these projects are as follows:

- Using IT to improve patient safety and reduce medical errors;
- Identifying barriers and solutions to IT implementation;
- Increasing satisfaction among patients and providers through health IT;
- Making the business case for health IT by determining both the costs and the benefits; and
- Streamlining work for clinicians and enhancing efficiency.

AHRQ also maintains the National Resource Center for HIT. The Center provides technical assistance, expert advice, and best practices to a variety of organizations and entities utilizing or contemplating the utilization of health IT. Currently, AHRQ is concentrating on the support of AHRQ and Health Resources and Services Administration (HRSA) HIT grantees and contractors. However, the Center has recently begun to provide support to local, State, and regional entities developing health information exchanges/networks. To date, they supported efforts in Florida, Montana, Wyoming, and New York. The center was established through a five-year, $18.5 million contract and is a central component of AHRQ's commitment to provide assistance, project and technical insight, and the dissemination of best practices.

For more information, please contact:

Dr. Scott Young, Director for Health IT
540 Gaither Road
Rockville, MD 20850
Phone: 301-427-1500
E-mail: syoung@ahrq.gov
Web site: http://www.ahrq.gov/

Centers for Medicare and Medicaid Services (CMS)

The Centers for Medicare & Medicaid Services (CMS), an agency of the U.S. Department of Health and Human Services (DHHS), administers the Medicare program for U.S. citizens age 65 and older, the disabled, and people with end stage renal disease (ESRD), and works in partnership with the States to administer Medicaid, the State Children's Health Insurance Program (SCHIP), and health insurance portability standards. CMS also works on administrative simplification standards from the Health Insurance Portability and Accountability Act of 1996 (HIPAA) quality standards in healthcare facilities through its survey and certification activity, and clinical laboratory quality standards. Currently, about 83 million beneficiaries, or more than one in four Americans, receive healthcare coverage through Medicare, Medicaid, and SCHIP. In fiscal year 2005, CMS will spend about $519 billion.

CMS is currently supporting several initiatives to support the effective use of HIT to improve the quality and efficiency of healthcare. Through Quality Improvement Organizations, CMS offers assistance to physicians' offices in adopting and using information technology in the Doctor's Office Quality Information Technology Project (DOQ-IT). This project provides primary care physicians with information on more than 60 private electronic health record systems (EHRs) and tools to select and implement the best EHR for their practice. As a part of this effort, CMS is working with VHA to reconfigure VistA, the VHA's Electronic Healthcare Record (EHR) technology, which is a low-cost alternative for certain small physician offices or safety net providers. In another effort to accelerate the adoption of HIT, CMS is developing the Care Management Performance Demonstration program, a pay-for-performance demonstration program in which physicians will be reimbursed, in part, based on their use of HIT to improve quality of care.

CMS is also accelerating the adoption of e-prescribing by requiring sponsors of the new outpatient drug benefit to comply with standards to enable e-prescribing.

To empower Medicare beneficiaries with information about their own care, CMS has initiated the Medicare Beneficiary Portal demonstration project. This project is being implemented nationally on a rolling basis throughout 2005 and will allow beneficiaries direct Web access to their Medicare claims information, including claims type, dates of service, and procedures in a way that will protect their privacy and the security of their information.

Finally, CMS has provided funding for some State activity related to the use of information technology. New York State is planning to use approximately $200 million in savings from a Section 1115 Medicaid Waiver to promote the adoption of e-prescribing, EHRs, and regional health information programs.

For more information, please contact:

Ms. Kelly Cronin, Senior Advisor to the Administrator
Centers for Medicare and Medicaid Services
7500 Security Boulevard
Baltimore, MD 21244-1850
Phone: 202-260-6726
E-mail: kelly.cronin@cms.hhs.gov
Web site: http://www.cms.hhs.gov

The Cancer Biomedical Informatics Grid™ (caBIG™)

Aiming to speed the delivery of innovative approaches for the prevention and treatment of cancer, the cancer Biomedical Informatics Grid™ (caBIG™) was launched in February 2004 with an initial budget of $20 million from the National Cancer Institute (NCI). Currently in the second year of a three-year pilot project, caBIG™ operates with 50 NCI-designated cancer centers as well as with other organizations. caBIG™ enables clinical researchers to exchange a wide range of data, including lab tests, tissue samples, and research information using a semantically interoperable infrastructure.

caBIG™ is developing open and shared biomedical informatics tools, standards, infrastructure, and data, focusing on the following:

- Clinical trial management systems;
- Integrative cancer research;
- Tissue banks and pathology tools;
- Architecture; and
- Vocabularies and common data elements.

caBIG™ is expanding participation of both NCI- and non-NCI-designated cancer centers in the interoperable system, with the ultimate goal of supporting patient-centric molecular medicine. Discussions are also taking place regarding potential partnerships between caBIG™ and other NIH components, Federal agencies, and international initiatives.

For more information, please contact:

Dr. Kenneth Buetow, Director, NCI Center for Bioinformatics
6116 Executive Blvd., Suite 403
Rockville, MD 20852
Phone: 301-435-1520
E-mail: buetowK@mail.nih.gov
Web site: https://cabig.nci.nih.gov/

Department of Defense (DoD)

The Department of Defense (DoD) has been working on electronically coordinating healthcare information among the United States Army, Navy, and Air Force since the approval to deploy the Composite Health Care System worldwide in 1993. Since these initial efforts toward an interoperable health system in the military, DoD has invested more than $2 billion dollars toward health IT adoption. DoD's efforts toward healthcare interoperability span a wide range of methods throughout the echelons of medical care, ranging from treatment on the battlefield to the rehabilitation facilities in the various branch hospitals.

Today, DoD is investing in initiatives such as the Composite Health Care System II (CHCS II), the Pharmacy Data Transaction Service (PDTS,) telehealth, and other efforts to facilitate communication in the Military Health Services. These initiatives are often part of larger interoperable efforts such as the Executive Information/Decision Support, which provides real-time, accurate decision information that supports the Defense's TRICARE program; the Theater Medical Information Program (TMIP), which provides interoperable health information to the services during combat or contingency operations across all echelons of care; and the Clinical Information Technology Program Office (CITPO), which manages clinical information technology support for the Military Health Services.

Along with these initiatives to connect the three service branches within DoD, DoD is collaborating with VA to coordinate connected health information in the future.

For more information, please contact:

Ms. Marianne Coates, Director of Communications for OASD Health Affairs
5111 Leesburg Pike, Suite 601
Falls Church, VA 22041
Phone: 703-681-1698
E-mail: marianne.coates@ha.osd.mil
Web site: www.defenselink.mil/

HEALTHeFORCES™

Established under congressional direction in 2000 at the Walter Reed Army Medical Center (WRAMC), HEALTHeFORCES™ was created with patient involvement and communication at the heart of the delivery system. Effective communication combined with comprehensive digital records, advanced analytical tools, and Web-based access allows the medical staff to make informed decisions to reduce incidence of chronic illness, prevent clinical errors, and contain costs—all while increasing the quality of care to all patients. With the extension of this application into civilian rural underserved areas, these methods will give patients and doctors state-of-the-art information and the ability to predict and identify health threats for both the military and civilian communities.

The strength of HEALTHeFORCES™ is its modular design and universal Web-based access. HEALTHeFORCES™ uses modules such as HEALTHeSURVEYS, where patients provide valuable feedback; HEALTHeCARDS, which document clinical practice guideline data and reference Web sites for provider and/or patient education; and HEALTHeNOTES, a clinical note writer. The system has evolved from a low-cost military application into one that can be employed throughout the United States. HEALTHeFORCES™ currently operates from a $5 million annual budget, which includes an active programming effort with an eight-week release schedule.

HEALTHeSTATES™, a civilianized technology transfer of the HEALTHeFORCES™ application, focuses on rural, medically underserved areas. It launched its first program in West Virginia in 2004. The program permits real-time collection of patient health status information and allows the provider to assess identified issues immediately and to document the encounter thoroughly and appropriately.

The United States Air Force is prepared to offer HEALTHeSTATE™ as open-source software to public and private institutions through a Cooperative Research and Development Agreement (CRADA). This public/private partnership will collaborate on intellectual property, labor, licensing, patents, data sharing, and distribution to limit the risks of adoption that private sector partners face.

HEALTHeFORCES™ was the first and only civilian or military organization to receive six Disease Specific Care Certifications from the Joint Commission on Accreditation of Healthcare Organizations (JCAHO) and has been nationally recognized with the following awards:

- Disease Management Association of America's "Best Disease Management Program in the Military";
- Grace Hopper "Gracie" Technology Leadership Award for "Leadership in the Innovative Application of Information Technology Contributing to the Advancement of Scientific Knowledge and Applications";
- Emerging Technology and Healthcare Innovations Congress' "Best In Show" and Most Innovative Technology in the Hospital Community" TETHIE Awards;
- American Council for Technology (ACT)'s "Innovative Approach to Service to the Citizen" Award.

For more information, please contact:

Colonel Peter Demitry, Assistant Surgeon General, Modernization Directorate, AF/SGR
5201 Leesburg Pike, Suite 1401
Falls Church, VA 22041
Phone: 703-681-7055
E-mail: peter.demitry@pentagon.af.mil or Jill.Phillips@pentagon.af.mil
Web site: www.healtheforces.org

Indian Health Services (IHS)

The Indian Health Services (IHS) is an agency within DHHS that operates a comprehensive health service delivery system for approximately 1.8 million of the nation's estimated 3.3 million American Indians and Alaska Natives living mainly on reservations and in rural communities. IHS's annual budget for its many initiatives is $3.5 billion.

IHS has an extensive history of using IT to improve patient care and data reporting, including the following:

- Resource and Patient Management System (RPMS)—designed as a suite of more than 60 software applications, RPMS is an easy and integrated way to manage resource and patient information effectively.

- Clinical Reporting System (CRS)—a population-based software application that facilitates reporting on more than 40 clinical quality measures. CRS produces local reports that are then exported to the regional and national levels to evaluate quality of care.

- Indian Health Performance Evaluation System (IHPES, formerly ORYX)—to receive private certification for quality patient care, IHS implemented this tool to help track statistical outcome indicators of care.

- National Patient Information Reporting System (NPIRS)—building upon RPMS data, NPIRS receives, processes, and reports all patient demographics and patient care related activity for IHS on a national basis. NPIRS allows better management of individual patients, local facilities, and regional and national programs.

Currently, IHS is upgrading its systems to a National Data Warehouse (NDW), a new, state-of-the-art, enterprisewide data warehouse environment. Once established, the NDW database will continue as the source for aggregate patient and population information that facilitates compliance with administrative, accreditation, and patient care needs.

For more information, please contact:

Dr. Theresa Cullen, Senior Medical Informatics Consultant
300 West Congress
Tucson, AZ 85701
Phone: 520-670-4803
E-mail: theresa.cullen@ihs.gov
Web site: http://www.ihs.gov

Health Resources and Services Administration (HRSA)

HRSA's mission is to provide the national leadership, program resources, and services needed to improve access to culturally competent, quality healthcare. In fiscal year 2005, HRSA's budget totaled $7.4 billion to support access to primary and other health services to uninsured, underinsured, and special needs populations.

HRSA's health information technology initiatives encompass a variety of programs aimed at improving the quality and safety of health services delivered by safety net providers in rural areas, medically underserved communities, and to special populations such as those with HIV/AIDS.

- Community Health Centers—Over the past 10 years, HRSA has invested nearly $95 million in 50 networks of health centers that provide health information technology services to 410 grantees around the country, including support for electronic health records. One of these networks, the Health Choice Network in Florida provides HIT services to 14 centers in Florida, six centers in New Mexico, and seven centers in Utah. These networks will be among the major mechanisms for disseminating health information technology to other centers and safety net providers around the country.

- Health Community Access Programs (HCAP)—HRSA supports HIT through HCAP, which is funded with more than $80 million a year. This program helps safety net providers in a community reorganize their delivery systems to provide better coordinated, more efficient care for uninsured residents. Using HIT to share information on uninsured patients between hospitals and local clinic services is one common strategy supported by this program.

- HIV/AIDS Program—The Special Projects of National Significance supports demonstrations that evaluate the use of health information technology on the quality of primary care for people living with HIV. Six grantees have been funded in the four-year initiative, which will continue through 2006.

- Office for the Advancement of Telehealth—This program awards 15 grants a year totaling about $4 million for rural telemedicine and telehealth network projects.

- Chronic Disease Management and Rural Health Programs—As part of its efforts to improve healthcare quality, HRSA supports investments in HIT under its Health Disparities Collaboratives in health centers. Collaboratives are organized around a care model that uses disease registries and other clinical information systems that track patient care and patient self-management for patients with diabetes, cancer, and other chronic diseases. Similar investments are available for rural health programs such as critical access hospitals and rural health clinics.

For more information, please contact:

Dr. Dennis Williams, Deputy Administrator for HRSA
5600 Fishers Lane, Room 14-05
Rockville, MD 20857
Phone: 301-443-2194
E-mail: dwilliams1@hrsa.gov
Web site: www.hrsa.gov

National Committee on Vital and Health Statistics (NCVHS)

NCVHS was established by Congress to serve as an advisory body to DHHS on health data, health statistics, and national health information policy. Its work includes advising on the development of a National Health Information Infrastructure (NHII), the selection of health data standards and the promotion of privacy policies to ensure public trust. The NCVHS 2005 budget includes $1.3 million from DHHS, including staff costs. The overall focus of NCVHS is on identifying the information and information technologies needed to improve the health of the U.S. population.

NCVHS has delivered several reports and recommendations to the Secretary of DHHS focusing on standards identification and development, e-prescribing, and technical infrastructure.

- E-prescribing, 2004–2005—The Medicare Modernization Act directed NCVHS to identify and recommend standards for e-prescribing that could be used in implementing the new Medicare Part D benefit.

- Information for Health: A Strategy for Building the National Health Information Infrastructure, 2001—Recommended the creation of ONCHIT and proposed a vision and framework for interoperable health information technology.

- Uniform Data Standards for Patient Medical Records Information, 2000–2003—Set forth a strategy, framework, and criteria for selection of clinical data standards and recommended to DHHS specific clinical data standards that became the foundation of the Consolidated Healthcare Informatics Standards.

NCVHS continues to examine issues and make recommendations, focusing on the following:

- HIT standards and harmonization;
- Privacy and security issues and solutions;
- Developing National Health Information Networks (NHINs);
- Other HIT strategy issues such as personal health records; and
- Health and healthcare disparities.

For more information, please contact:

Marjorie S. Greenberg, Executive Secretary
National Center for Health Statistics, CDC
3311 Toledo Road, Room 2413
Hyattsville, MD 20782
Phone: 301-458-4245
E-mail: msg1@cdc.gov
Web site: www.ncvhs.hhs.gov

The Veterans Health Administration (VHA)

Since 1985, VA has been working to automate health information. In late 1996, VHA launched the Computerized Patient Record System (CPRS) to provide a single interface to allow healthcare providers to review and update a patient's medical record and use computerized order entry for a variety of services and items, including medications, special procedures, x-rays, patient care nursing orders, diets, and laboratory tests. Of the VHA's 2005 fiscal year budget, 4.86%, or approximately $78 per enrollee, is dedicated to information technology.

Today, CPRS supports one of the largest integrated health systems in the United States. CPRS serves more than five million veterans and is used in all VA Medical Centers (157 hospitals), 134 nursing homes, and 887 outpatient clinics. The Bar Code Medication Administration (BCMA) is a component of CPRS that electronically validates and documents medications for inpatients in all VA Medical Centers, handling more than 590,000 inpatient medications each day.

My HealtheVet is a Web-based personal health record that creates a new, on-line environment where veterans, family, and clinicians may come together to optimize veterans' healthcare. By the end of calendar year 2005, appointment scheduling and medication refill ordering will be added to the current functionality. The next generation, HealtheVet VistA, will move to a person-centered, fully sharable system that will improve flexibility to respond to future health needs while lowering the cost of maintenance.

HealthePeople is a collaborative strategy to increase interoperability while providing a new platform for information sharing among other healthcare providers. Since 1995, VA's budget has increased 51% while the number of patients has increased 104%. The number of employees has decreased 5%.

For more information, please contact:

Ms. Gail Graham, Director, Health Data and Informatics
Veterans Health Administration (19F2)
810 Vermont Avenue, N.W.
Washington, DC 20420
Phone: 202-273-9220
E-mail: gail.graham@va.gov
Web site: www1.va.gov/vha_oi/

Disclaimer: The contents of the digital map and HIT database are solely the responsibility of the authors and do not necessarily represent the official view of the Center for Health Information and Decision Systems or the University of Maryland. The material contained in this document is for informational purposes only. CHIDS makes no guarantees as to the accuracy and/or completeness of this information. Copyright in any third-party materials found in this document must be respected. Some webpage links are provided to other Internet sites for the convenience of users. CHIDS is not responsible for the availability or content of these external sites, nor does CHIDS endorse, warrant, or guarantee the products, services, or information described or offered at these other Internet sites.

Legend

A012	AHRQ	AHRQ HIT Projects – "Transforming Healthcare Through Information Technology"
H053	HIE	Health Information Exchanges
H024	RHIO	Health Information Exchanges which received some HRSA/OAT funding in July 2004
C5	CCIP	Center for Medicare and Medicaid (CMS) – Chronic Care Improvement Programs (CCIP)
B04	BTE	Bridges-to-Excellence - Physician Office Link, Diabetes Care Link, Cardiac Care Link
S53	DOQ	Quality Improvement Organization (QIO)/ Doctors' Office Quality IT (DOQ-IT)
P30	PHIT	Private HIT Projects and Initiatives - BCBSMA eRx in Boston, Kaiser EMR project

Note: Some projects fit multiple categories, in these instances, the item was placed in the most appropriate category. Most projects in this list have elements of Health Information Exchange.

Health IT Activity in USA as of July 2005

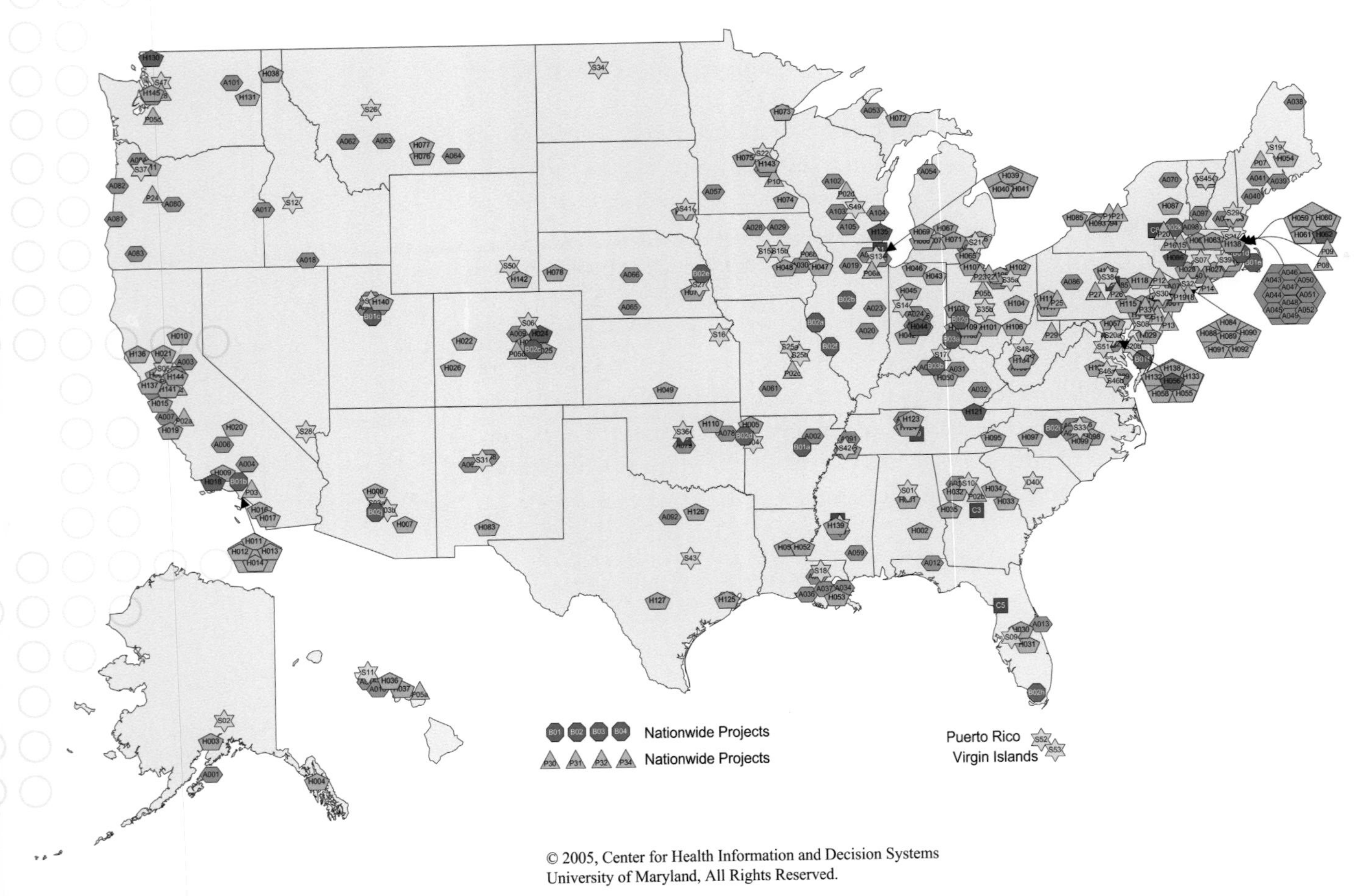

The database and digital map were compiled by the Center for Health Information and Decision Systems (CHIDS), an academia-led, health information technology research and development center located in the Robert H. Smith School of Business at the University of Maryland. The mission of CHIDS is to improve the delivery of health care by offering researched solutions in health information technology that have an impact on safety, quality, access, efficiency, and return on investment.

For more information regarding CHIDS' capabilities or to inquire about a dynamic, interactive version of the CHIDS HIT Digital Map and HIT database, please contact a CHIDS representative at 301.405.0702 or chids@rhsmith.umd.edu.

Center for Health Information and Decision Systems
Robert H. Smith School of Business
University of Maryland
College Park, MD 20742

CHIDS HIT Digital Map
Project Lead: Corey M. Angst, Associate Director, CHIDS
Other Personnel: Ken Yale, Senior Fellow, CHIDS
Ritu Agarwal, Director, CHIDS

Nation-wide	Bridges-to-Excellence (POL)	Bridges to Excellence Physician Office Link (POL) reward program - eligible physicians must demonstrate that they have implemented systematic office processes passing NCQA's office practice performance assessment program. Office practices are assessed in three critical system areas: clinical information systems, patient education and support, and care management. Enables physician office sites to qualify for bonuses based on their implementation of specific processes to reduce errors and increase quality. They can earn up to $50 per year for each patient covered by a participating employer or plan. In addition, a report card for each physician office describes its performance on the program measures and is made available to the public.	Medstat Group 1-800-224-7161 bridgestoexcellence@thomson.com	BTE_01
Nation-wide	Bridges-to-Excellence (DCL)	To obtain the rewards available through the Bridges to Excellence Diabetes Care Link (DCL) reward program, eligible physicians must demonstrate that they provide high levels of diabetes care by passing NCQA's diabetes performance assessment program. Two performance assessment options are available through NCQA: -For 1-year certification for BTE rewards-eligible physicians, physicians submit data on HbA1c, blood pressure, and lipid testing for diabetes patients. -For 3-year recognition from NCQA's Diabetes Physician Recognition Program (DPRP), physicians submit data on the same three outcome measures as needed for 1-year certification, as well as data on eye, foot, and nephropathy exams for their diabetes patients.	NCQA 2000 L Street, NW, Suite 500 Washington, DC 20036 202-955-3500, Customersupport@ncqa.org	BTE_03
Nation-wide	Bridges-to-Excellence (CCL)	To obtain the rewards available through the Bridges to Excellence Cardiac Care Link (CCL) reward program, eligible physicians must demonstrate that they provide high levels of cardiac care by passing NCQA's cardiac performance assessment program. Physicians must submit data on blood pressure, lipid and cholesterol testing, aspirin/antithrombotic use, and smoking cessation status for their cardiac patients.	NCQA 2000 L Street, NW, Suite 500 Washington, DC 20036 www.ncqa.org/hsrp, 888-275-7585	BTE_04

Nation-wide	Medem (free Personal Health Record) and Allscripts Healthcare Solutions	Medem, a for-profit company affiliated with the American Medical Association, announced it would offer patients free, personal health records. The new service, called iHealthRecord, allows patients to enter information about the medications they take, their allergies, emergency contact information and other data and share that information with physicians or other authorized users. About 100,000 physicians pay $25 a month to subscribe to Medem's other online patient communications services. Medem has partnered with EMR vendor Allscripts Healthcare Solutions its records to exchange data with the iHealthRecord.	Ed Fotsch, M.D., CEO MEDEM 649 Mission Street, 2nd Floor San Francisco, CA 94105 info@medem.com 415-644-3800	PHIT_30
Nation-wide	Kaiser Permanente and Epic Systems	A three-year research project that measures the effects of using an electronic medical record across 110 physician teams at Kaiser Permanente could have wide-ranging implications for physician practices across the country. Entitled "The Impact of Health Information Technology on Clinical Care," the project will measure the effects of staggered installation of technology developed by Epic Systems that includes an electronic medical record, provider order entry and clinical decision support. The nearly $1.5 million research initiative is designed to test the assumption that healthcare information technology can improve the quality of care and patient safety while at the same time reducing the number of visits to the doctor's office. A grant from the Agency for Healthcare Research and Quality will pay for the study.	John Hsu, Principal Investigator Kaiser Foundation Research Oakland, CA	PHIT_31
Nation-wide	Trigon, Blue Cross Blue Shield of Illinois, Blue Cross Blue Shield of Michigan, and Independence Blue Cross (PA)	Trigon, an Anthem affiliate health plan, operates a program similar to Empire's in that the health plan rewards hospitals for adopting Leapfrog standards for safe practices. Rewards are tied to patient safety improvements in the individual hospitals. Blue Cross Blue Shield of Illinois, Blue Cross Blue Shield of Michigan, and Independence Blue Cross (PA) are examples of other health plans using Leapfrog standards to encourage patient safety improvements.	Anthem Blue Cross and Blue Shield 2 Gannett Drive South Portland, ME 04106	PHIT_32
Nation-wide	MedicAlert Foundation and CapMed eHealthKey PHR Initiative	The MedicAlert® E-HealthKEY is USB-based tool that launches critical health information when plugged into a computer. It also allows people to their complete personal health record at all times.	Ramesh Srinivasan, VP Marketing MedicAlert Foundation 209-669-2407 or Wendy Angst CapMed, wangst@capmed.com 267-757-3315	PHIT_34
Region	Bridges-to-Excellence (General)	The four coalitions launching BTE-related projects are located in Illinois (two in Illinois), Colorado and Arkansas. The coalitions, through a licensing arrangement with BTE, have begun talking with employers and estimate launching customized programs in their respective markets later this year. Business coalitions are well suited to coordinating such incentive programs - by coordinating activities among employers, they can pool resources and streamline related operations, thus making the efforts more attractive to employers and physicians. All four coalitions are members of the National Business Coalition on Health (NBCH), a 70-coalition member strong organization that strongly supports pay-for-performance.	Francois de Brantes Bridges to Excellence 1-800-224-7161 bridgestoexcellence@thomson.com	BTE_02
Various	Healthcare Collaborative Network (HCN)	The goals of the Healthcare Collaborative Network (HCN) are as follows • Demonstrate both the feasibility and the value of a standards-based, interconnected, electronic model of data interchange to a wide variety of stakeholders; • Demonstrate how electronic communications using common standards can help patients receive necessary and timely medical treatment and guard against medical errors, incorrect prescriptions and adverse drug.	Bruno Nardone, CHE, Managing Consultant, Healthcare Strategy and Change Practice, IBM Business Consulting Services, Waltham, MA	HIE_138
AK	Qualis Health	Practices that participate in DOQ-IT will receive free assistance to select, implement, and optimize IT systems such as EHRs, e-prescribing, and registries. CMS has contracted with Qualis Health to provide DOQ-IT services to participating physicians in Washington, Idaho, and Alaska.	Terry Keith, BS, RHIA / Clinical Consultant 907-562-2133 800-878-7170 tkeith@qualishealth.org	DOQ_02
AK	Multi Facility Integration (MFI)	This HIE was started in 1974 under the auspices of the Indian Health Services (IHS), with data stored on microfiche. Since the mid 80s data has been stored on an IHS system called the "Resource and Patient Management System" (RPMS).	Richard Hall 4141 Ambassador Dr. Anchorage, AK 99508 907-729-2622 rhall@anthc.org	HIE_003

AK	Alaska Health Passport	This HIE was set up as a medication management program to assist avoid adverse drug interactions and allergic reactions. The program is a partnership between the Alaska State Hospital Association and the Alaska State Nursing Home Association. The program uses "smart cards" carried by patients that records medication information and basic insurance coverage info. The system is also described as a way to accurately identify individual patients.	Heidi Gosho 426 Main St. Juneau, Alaska 99801 907-586-1790 hgosho@ashnha.com	HIE_004
AK	Central Kenai Peninsula Health Collaborative Technology	Assesses current technology resources and plans implementation of area-wide electronic communications and connectivity to electronic health records and a patient-support Web-based data system.	Edward Burke, Central Peninsula General Hospital, Inc., Soldotna, AK	AHRQ_001
AL	Alabama Quality Assurance Foundation	(No specific DOQ-IT information)	205-970-1600 800-760-4550	DOQ_01
AL	Dynamic Online Event Reporting System (DOERS PRO)	DOERS is an adverse event reporting system that identifies "medication error and near miss" and reports it. The system is touted to be a medication error reporting, medication management, and medication safety education tool. The system is used by members of this HIE to assist with risk management.	Barbara Traylor 2800 University Drive, Ste. 304 Birmingham, AL 35233 250-939-7443 BTraylor@stv.org	HIE_001
AL	Montgomery Area Information Network	The Montgomery Area Community Wellness Coalition was started in 2002, and advertises itself as an HIE. Their "Shared Patient Information Network" is intended to assist with health quality, efficiency, and effectiveness improvements. In 2003 they started a database to assist with the health needs of the homeless, called "Homeless Management Information System". Currently the two initiatives are called the Montgomery Area Information Network, providing a health and social services data repository for users.	Carroll S. Nason, Dr PA 3090 Mobile Highway Montgomery, AL 36108 334-293-6504 cnason@adph.state.al.us	HIE_002
AR	Bridges-to-Excellence (POL)	CMS is looking towards the BTE Physician Office Link program as a possible element in its forthcoming Medicare Care Management Performance Demonstration project, an initiative which will promote the adoption and use of health information technology to improve the efficiency and quality of patient care for chronically ill Medicare patients. Doctors who meet or exceed performance standards established by CMS in clinical delivery systems and patient outcomes will receive performance payments for managing the care of eligible Medicare beneficiaries.	Medstat Group 1-800-224-7161 bridgestoexcellence@thomson.com	BTE_01a
AR	Bridges-to-Excellence (General) - Employers' Health Coalition	The four coalitions launching BTE-related projects are located in Illinois (two in Illinois), Colorado and Arkansas. The coalitions, through a licensing arrangement with BTE, have begun talking with employers and estimate launching customized programs in their respective markets later this year. Business coalitions are well suited to coordinating such incentive programs - by coordinating activities among employers, they can pool resources and streamline related operations, thus making the efforts more attractive to employers and physicians. All four coalitions are members of the National Business Coalition on Health (NBCH), a 70-coalition member strong organization that strongly supports pay-for-performance.	Susan Dorsey, Director NBCH 1015 18th Street N.W., Suite 730 Washington, DC 20036 Sdorsey@nbch.org 202-775-9300	BTE_02d
AR	Arkansas Foundation for Medical Care	Vision: Quicker access. Fewer errors. Improved efficiency. Electronic health records could transform your practice. But success takes time, planning and strategy. AFMC can help. As part of our commitment to improving health care in Arkansas, AFMC is taking part in a special study to help primary care offices understand and use this rapidly growing technology. We can help you analyze available options.	Nancy Archer, 501-375-5700, ext. 661 Hotline: 877-375-5700 narcher@arqio.sdps.org physicianoffice@afmc.org	DOQ_04
AR	Washington Regional HealthMedx Health Information Exchange	The Washington Regional Health Information Exchange (called HealthMedx) is designed as a patient registry with a variety of information, including medical records scanned into the system. The HIE is looking for grant funding to expand. Washington Regional Medical Center created the Arkansas Institute for Research and Education Education in August 2002.	Becky Magee 1125 N. College Ave. Fayetteville, AR 72701 bmagee@wregional.com	HIE_005

AR	Arkansas Delta Inpatient/ Outpatient Quality Improvement	Implements a computer decision-support system in a 23-county service area in both inpatient and outpatient settings, including several rural clinics; includes a training component for physicians and other health care providers as well as a hospital pharmacy component for adverse drug event management and prevention strategies.	Cinda Bates St. Bernards Medical Center Jonesboro, AR	AHRQ_002
AZ	Bridges-to-Excellence (General)	CIGNA HealthCare is licensing the Bridges to Excellence program and is working with employers to pursue a pay-for-performance effort.	Susan Dorsey, Director NBCH 1015 18th Street N.W., Suite 730 Washington, DC 20036 Sdorsey@nbch.org 202-775-9300	BTE_02j
AZ	Health Services Advisory Group	HSAG can provide the following free consulting services to a practice considering or in the process of implementing an EHR system: Assessment of your practice IT needs, practice workflows and efficiencies, staff IT competency levels, Assistance in planning and preparing your practice for an IT implementation, An evidence-based approach to helping you select the right IT solution, Help in using your IT system for better care management and improvement of your care delivery processes	Sharon Miller/Director, Health Information Technologies 602-745-6200 smiller@azqio.sdps.org	DOQ_03a
AZ	Health Care Excel	Through this initiative, Health Care Excel (HCE), the Medicare Quality Improvement Organization for Indiana, will assist primary care physicians in adopting Electronic Health Record (EHR) systems with the ultimate goal of improving office efficiency and patient outcomes. This initiative is sponsored by the Centers for Medicare & Medicaid Services (CMS).	Darlene Skelton 812-234-1499 602-441-3068	DOQ_03b
AZ	AHCCCS Health Information Exchange	This is a proposed HIE that would function as a data repository/warehouse which aggregates data from multiple sources, including but not limited to AHCCCS, Health Plans, RBHAs and PBMs. Data may include provider and member demographics, Health Plan PCP and RBHA behavioral health physician assignments by member and pharmacy data by member.	Bonnie Marsh 701 E. Jefferson Phoenix, AZ 85034 602-417-4510 BJMarsh@ahcccs.state.az.us	HIE_006
AZ	Tele-health Arizona Community Health Centers	This project is to install connectivity of tele-health videoconferencing so as to increase collaboration on DM programs among clinical staff. The project will integrate the qualified community health centers into a network to work together clinically, in management, and in educational and quality control.	NA	HIE_007
CA	Bridges-to-Excellence (POL)	CMS is also looking towards the BTE Physician Office Link program as a possible element in its forthcoming Medicare Care Management Performance Demonstration project, an initiative which will promote the adoption and use of health information technology to improve the efficiency and quality of patient care for chronically ill Medicare patients. Doctors who meet or exceed performance standards established by CMS in clinical delivery systems and patient outcomes will receive performance payments for managing the care of eligible Medicare beneficiaries.	Medstat Group 1-800-224-7161 bridgestoexcellence@thomson.com	BTE_01b
CA	Lumetra	Lumetra, assisted by key partners, is providing support to small- to medium-sized practices in implementing EHRs free of charge. Lumetra is helping physician practices: Assess practice readiness, Define EHR goals, Select an EHR vendor*, Prepare staff and office for EHRs, Conduct post implementation evaluations, Review EHR implementation and impact analysis	John Weir 415-677-2083 General: 415-677-2000 doqit-ca@caqio.sdps.org	DOQ_05
CA	Virtual Clinical Network Expansion	The Virtual Clinical Network is designed to help track uninsured, Medicaid (MediCal), and county medical services beneficiaries. The system allows identification of patients when they present to an emergency room or other facility that does not have their medical records, and reports on their medical conditions and medications. It assists with proper treatment and to ensure persons are over medicating on controlled substances or are not in compliance with their medication regimen.	Patrick Hughes 360 Campus Lane, #100 Fairfield, CA 94534 707-863-4440 PHughes@partnershiphp.org	HIE_008

CA	Healthy Fontana Online	Healthy Fontana Online is on online HIE community for residents of the city of Fontana, CA.	Mark Mayuga 8353 Sierra Avenue Fontana, CA 92335 909-350-7620 mmayuga@fontana.org	HIE_009
CA	Sierra Nevada Health Care Data Exchange	This HIE is designed to be a medical and financial record accessible by physicians. A centralized database repository may be accessed and modified by physicians over the Internet. It is not clear whether this HIE is actually operational, or just in the design stage.	Stuart Fleming MD 640 East Main Street, Suite 2 Grass Valley, CA 95945 530-271-3201 sfleming@gv.net	HIE_010
CA	Virtual Information Highway (VIH) model	This is a collaboration of stakeholders interested in developing a "federated" model of interconnected organizations that can exchange information with each other when an individual presents for treatment without their medical information. They also wish to use the system as a way to track, analyze, and study community health and disease prevalence. They will use a "VIH" model.	Frederick W. James, MD Department of Pediatrics Charles R. Drew University Los Angeles, CA 310-668-4641 frjames@cdrewu.edu	HIE_011
CA	Health-e-LA	Health-e-LA™ is going to develop the infrastructure to allow exchange of clinical information to participants in Los Angeles city and surrounding areas.	Mark S. Windisch, Esq. L.A. Care Health Plan 555 West Fifth Street, 29th floor Los Angeles, CA 90013 213-694-1250, ext. 4144 mwindisch@lacare.org	HIE_012
CA	Long Beach Networking for Health & Surveillance	This is described as a collaborative that intends to build the infrastructure to allow interconnectivity of health stakeholder databases (e.g. hospitals, physicians, laboratories, pharmacies, etc.) to exchange data to help improve healthcare of the local population.	Laura Landry 2525 Grand Avenue Long Beach, CA 90815 562-570-4148 laura_landry@longbeach.gov	HIE_013
CA	Provider-Payor Network clinical data exchange	Working on the infrastructure to allow exchange of clinical information between 20 medical groups, 20 hospitals, and a "health plan reference library" to assist with treatment of patients with diabetes, asthma, and cardiovascular diseases.	Donald Crane, President 515 S. Figueroa Street Suite 1300 Los Angeles, CA 90071 213-538-0772 DCRANE@CAPG.ORG	HIE_014
CA	HealthConnect	This project is designed to create the infrastructure to exchange clinical and administrative data over the Internet among stakeholders, including providers, payors, pharmacies, laboratories, government agencies, and patients. The platform is called "HealthConnect" and is designed to provide a common platform, reduce the cost of IT adoption, and allow for secure information exchange.	DeLeys Brandman, MD 510 Logue Ave Mountain View, CA 94043 650-962-2680 dbrandman@commerce.net	HIE_015
CA	Circle of Care	LMFC has created a coalition of technology companies, providers, a payer, and a medical information content provider to develop the Circle of Care project. The project is designed to build the infrastructure for electronic data interchange to exchange health information.	Zara Marselian, CEO 4185 Fairmount Avenue San Diego, CA 92105 619-584-1612 zaramarselian@lamaestra.org	HIE_016
CA	Clinical Information Exchange Improvement Through Direct Patient Data Entry	This is an initiative by two medical groups (with 320+ physicians) partnering to develop the infrastructure to allow information exchange between physicians and patients over the Internet. They hope to expand to 2,500 physicians.	Joseph Traube, MD 4275 Campus Point Court-CP220 San Diego, CA 92121 858-678-6087 traube.joseph@scrippshealth.org	HIE_017

CA	Santa Barbara County Care Data Exchange (CDE)	This is considered a "public utility" model for clinical information exchange, with a "federated," or peer-to-peer exchange of information between participant organizations, providers, and patients.	Philip Greene 110 Castillian Way Santa Barbara, CA 93117 805-685-9525 phil@sbrha.org	HIE_018* RHIO_018
CA	Santa Cruz County Health Information Exchange	This is designed to build the infrastructure to allow exchange of a broad range of clinical information for stakeholders within the county.	Rama Khalsa 1080 Emeline Ave. Santa Cruz, CA 95010 831-454-4474 rama.khalsa@health.co.santa-cruz.ca.us	HIE_019
CA	Tulare District Hospital Patient Care Collaborative	This HIE initiative is designed to create the infrastructure to allow sharing of clinical information between the sole, rural hospital in this community, the community clinic, and physicians.	John Clark 869 Cherry Street Tulare, CA 93274 559-685-3409 jclark@tdhs.org	HIE_020
CA	Collaborative Health Information Project (CHIP)	This project is designed to develop the infrastructure to allow secure information exchange between the health department and health organizations. They are first developing an electronic health record standard for the county. The project includes adoption of a document management system, central information repository, role-based access control (or similar protocol), and uploading of information to the central database.	David B. Nelson 10 Cottonwood Woodland, CA 95695 530-666-8958 David.Nelson@Yolocounty.org	HIE_021
CA	Redwood Mednet	Redwood MedNet seeks to Enhance the quality of health care for all residents of Mendocino and Lake Counties; Facilitate the individual and collective practice of medicine; Encourage adoption of Electronic Health Records; Interconnect all participants in the local health care community; and Collaborate with regional, State and Federal health information technology initiatives. Redwood MedNet's initial focus is interoperable health records at solo and small practices. Later plans call for community wide participation with a special focus on population level Public Health monitoring and on HIE services for the five hospital emergency rooms in our region.	Will Ross 707-272-7255 wross@openhre.org	HIE_136
CA	CalRHIO	CalRHIO's goals are to: Encourage business, healthcare, and policy leaders to create private and public policy agendas - and to make funding commitments - in support of rapid development and implementation of health information data exchange technology in CA, facilitate creation of common governance, process, technology, and other elements needed to run one or more RHIOs under the auspices of a non-profit statewide umbrella organization, initiate sponsorship of projects that demonstrate the feasibility, utility, quality and financial benefits of health information data sharing, help organizers of existing data exchange efforts in California work toward common goals and to share information, materials, technology and learnings, support safety net provider and underserved population participation in governance, financing, and data exchange development priorities and support legislation, if required, for successful implementation of an integrated statewide health data exchange network.	Ann Donovan, Project Director 415-537-6938 adonovan@healthtech.org	HIE_137
CA	Smart Health	Smart Valley is using Health Alliant to analyze the healthcare system in Silicon Valley and build a financial model.	Seth Fearey, 408-938-1511 s_fearey@jointventure.org	HIE_141
CA	California Information Exchange-Linking Partners for Quality Healthcare (CALINX)	CALINX convened work groups to establish detailed data standards and rules for data exchange in certain clinical and administrative areas. CALINX data standards were based on ANSI and other well-established national standards. CALINX also managed pilot efforts to demonstrate the cost-effectiveness of exchanging data using those standards in a secure, private way.	David Hopkins, Pacific Business Group on Health, (415) 615-6322 dhopkins@pbgh.org	HIE_144

CA	Sutter Health and Epic Systems	Sutter Health has made a commitment to deploy an electronic health record (EHR) inpatient-outpatient system network-wide over the next few years. This newest commitment expands on $154 million investment in EHR technology (EPIC). Sutter's online system will electronically connect more than 5,000 physicians, 27 hospitals and millions of patients across its not-for-profit Northern California network. Also has a patient safety initiative over the next 10 years, including bar-coding technology for safe bedside administration of medications, digital imaging and computerized physician order entry.	John Hummel, Sutter Health Sr VP, CIO or Karen Garner Communications Manager 916-286-8297 garnerk@sutterhealth.org	PHIT_01
CA	Wellpoint eRx or Paper Reduction	WellPoint is spearheading an electronic initiative at a cost of $40 million that will reach 19,000 physicians. In California, Georgia, Missouri, and Wisconsin, physicians will be given the opportunity to choose from either of two electronic packages: a Prescription Improvement Package or a Paperwork Reduction Package.	Ron J. Ponder, PhD, EVP Information Services, WellPoint or Nadia Leather – CGEY nadia.leather@capgemini.com 212-314-8233	PHIT_02a
CA	Cedars-Sinai Medical Center	Cedars-Sinai Medical Center in Los Angeles, tried to move to an electronic medical record system, with disastrous results. The hospital's computerized physician order entry (CPOE) system was suspended when physicians complained that the new system slowed down the process of filling and checking the accuracy of prescription orders and even lost some orders in the system. Cedars-Sinai plans to eventually reinstall the CPOE system when problems are resolved.	Cedars-Sinai Medical Center 8700 Beverly Blvd. Los Angeles, CA 90048 Main Switchboard 310-423-3277	PHIT_03
CA	Integrated Healthcare Association, RWJF grant, and the California Healthcare Foundation	Integrated Healthcare Association (IHA), supported through funds from its members, a Robert Wood Johnson Foundation grant (for evaluation), and the California Healthcare Foundation (for implementation), convened California's six leading health plans (Aetna, Blue Cross of California, Blue Shield of California, CIGNA HealthCare of California, Health Net, and PacifiCare with a seventh – Western Advantage - to join in 2004) to launch a program that 'pays for performance'. The IT portion of the bonus is based on the groups' ability to match multiple clinical data sets at the patient level and to deliver electronic data at the point of care (e.g., electronic lab results in the physician office, registries, EHRs).	Sheera Rosenfeld, The Health Strategies Consultancy LLC, 1350 Conn. Ave, N.W., Suite 900 Washington, DC 20036 202-207-1308 SRosenfeld@healthstrategies.net	PHIT_04
CA	El Dorado County Safety Net Technology Project	Develops a comprehensive plan for health IT implementation and integration by assessing specific clinical and organizational needs, feasibility of health IT implementation, defining project parameters, developing the implementation plan, and specifying procedures for ongoing evaluation and feedback.	Neda West, Marshall Medical Placerville, CA	AHRQ_003
CA	Crossing the Quality Chasm in Eastern Rural County	Develops a regional collaborative and business plan for implementing health IT in a rural region; also conducts a telemedicine demonstration project to assess the barriers and issues of broad health IT intervention including telemedicine/teleradiology, scan/store medical record, chronic disease registry and personal health record, and linking the region's partners.	Kiki Nocella, Tehachapi Hospital Tehachapi, CA	AHRQ_004
CA	IT Systems for Rural Indian Clinic Health Care	Integrates health services research, clinic redesign, and electronic practice management through the implementation of electronic health records and clinical decision support systems (CDSSs) by partnering with three rural Tribal Health Programs to implement electronic health records with clinical decision support systems.	Susan Dahl, California Rural Indian Health Board, Sacramento, CA	AHRQ_005
CA	Tulare District Hospital Rural Health EMR Consortium	Builds on an existing infrastructure to construct a fully integrated EMR to give clinicians real-time access to patient data through pharmacy management, laboratory management, patient scheduling, barcoding, clinical physician order entry, electronic signature, insurance eligibility, and Pyxis medication-dispensing units at nursing stations.	Paul Galloway, Healthcare Management Systems, Tulare, CA	AHRQ_006
CA	Santa Cruz County, CA Diabetes Mellitus Registry	Expands an established Web-based, interactive Diabetes Mellitus Registry that provides patient histories and needed tests at the point of care among public, private, and not-for-profit health care providers; also tracks the diabetes population to identify trends in key indicators of care.	F. Wells Shoemaker, Pajaro Valley Community Health, Watsonville, CA	AHRQ_007

CA	Impact of Health Information Technology on Clinical Care	Evaluates the effects of staggered installation of an Epic health IT system that includes an electronic medical record (EMR) with provider order entry and clinical decision support in primary care settings on quality, safety, and resource use within a large integrated delivery system on cohort of 780,000 members with chronic illnesses.	John Hsu, Kaiser Foundation Research Oakland, CA	AHRQ_008
CO	Bridges-to-Excellence (General) - Colorado Business Group on Health	The four coalitions launching BTE-related projects are located in Illinois (two in Illinois), Colorado and Arkansas. The coalitions, through a licensing arrangement with BTE, have begun talking with employers and estimate launching customized programs in their respective markets later this year. Business coalitions are well suited to coordinating such incentive programs - by coordinating activities among employers, they can pool resources and streamline related operations, thus making the efforts more attractive to employers and physicians. All four coalitions are members of the National Business Coalition on Health (NBCH), a 70-coalition member strong organization that strongly supports pay-for-performance.	Susan Dorsey, Director NBCH 1015 18th Street N.W., Suite 730 Washington, DC 20036 Sdorsey@nbch.org 202-775-9300	BTE_02c
CO	Colorado Foundation for Medical Care	CFMC conducts DOQ-IT activities in Colorado under the direction of CMS.	Cynthia King, RN, BSN, MSCIT informatics quality improvement advisor; 303-306-4483 or 1-800-950-8250 x3156 cking@coqio.sdps.org	DOQ_06
CO	Roaring Fork Valley Community Health Plan	This health plan intends to develop the infrastructure to exchange information with providers, employers, and beneficiaries.	William Hanisch 315 Oak Run Road Carbondale, CO 81623 970-963-8044 wdhresource@earthlink.net	HIE_022
CO	Colorado Access Project to Enhance Proider-Member-Plan Communications	This HIE is designed to exchange administrative information (eligibility, authorization, referral, claims, etc) with providers over the Internet. Other functions include secure email between providers, pharmacy data, educational material, health plan information, and other information useful to providers. This group is considering the inclusion of electronic medical record information from providers.	Marshall Thomas, MD 10065 E Harvard Ave. Suite 600 Denver, CO 80231 720-744-5404 marshall.thomas@coaccess.com	HIE_023
CO	Colorado Health Information Exchange (COHIE)	This is a collaborative of stakeholders with a governing body to oversee membership, security, access, maintenance, and other matters. It is designing the infrastructure for secure transmission of information based on standards being developed nationally (e.g., through the ONCHIT Standards Harmonization initiative and the NHIN program). The intention is to allow interconnectivity between various systems (not develop a central information repository) that will allow information exchange accessed by providers to facilitate point-of-care services to patients.	Matt Madison 303-724-0334 matthew.madison@UCHSC.edu	HIE_024* RHIO_024
CO	Connecting Colorado	This HIE is designed to develop the infrastructure for a "clearinghouse" function, or "federated" system that allows authenticated users to query various databases located at participating organizations. One component of the data exchange is the Continuity of Care Record (CCR) and development of a template for patients having no electronic health information.	Robert Dellavalle 4200 E. Ninth Ave., B-153 Denver, CO 80262 303-315-2957 robert.dellavalle@uchsc.edu	HIE_025
CO	Mesa County Health Information Network	This HIE will develop a clinical information record for Mesa County residents that can be shared with providers involved with their care.	Curt Hatch 2764 Compass Drive, Suite 107 Grand Junction, CO 81506 970-248-8031 CURTHATCH@aol.com	HIE_026
CO	Kaiser Permanente and Epic Systems	The Colorado region plans to go live with the new records system this fall.	Louise Liang, MD, SVP for Quality and Clinical Systems Support Kaiser Foundation Health Plan One Kaiser Plaza, Oakland, CA 94612 510 271-6317	PHIT_05c

CO	Colorado Connecting Communities—Health Information Collaborative (C3-HIC)	Contract that implements Statewide information and communications technologies to enable clinicians to access patient information from other clinical data repositories at the point of care.	Project Director: Arthur J. Davidson University of Colorado Health Sc Ctr Aurora, CO Arthur.Davidson@UCHSC.edu	AHRQ_009
CT	Qualidigm	(No specific DOQ-IT information) Qualidigm is Connecticut's Quality Improvement Organization (QIO). Under contract with the Centers for Medicare & Medicaid Services (CMS), Qualidigm works with health care providers, such as home health agencies, nursing homes, hospitals and physicians to improve the quality of care they provide. Qualidigm also focuses on educating Medicare beneficiaries about the type of care they deserve and how to stay healthy.	http://www.qualidigm.org/ who_contact.asp 860-632-2008 info@qualidigm.org	DOQ_07
CT	C-VAMS	This is a data repository at the Griffin Hospital intended to collect health record information from participating providers. The data repository also has administrative, clinical, and financial applications used by the hospital. Remote access will be provided for authorized users to help network providers in the community and facilitate health care delivery, referrals, enrollment, etc.	Susan Rosen 67 Maple Avenue Derby, CT 6418 203-732-1330 srosen@vwhcc.org	HIE_027
CT	Wellness Information Network	The WIN program was created for uninsured persons. It has an electronic medical record available through the Internet linking emergency rooms in local health facilities (Fair Haven Clinic, Hill Health Center, Yale-New Haven Hospital, Hospital of St. Raphael). It was designed to allow exchnage of clinical information for persons seeking primary care through emergency departments.	James Rawlings, Executive Director Community Health 20 York Street New Haven, CT 06504 203-688-5645 jim.rawlings@ynhh.org	HIE_028
CT	Electronic Records to Improve Care for Children	Implements and evaluates a community-wide EHR for health care providers in pediatric primary care, school health, specialty care, and emergency medicine who provide care for inner city children with asthma.	Richard Shiffman, Yale University, New Haven, CT, 203-737-5213 richard.shiffman@yale.edu	AHRQ_010
CT	Web-based Renal Transplant Patient Medication System	Develops and evaluates Web-enabled education tools in hospitals and homes for renal transplant patients to reduce medication errors and improve safety and compliance using wireless portable computers.	Amy Freidman, Yale University New Haven, CT 203-785-2565 amy.friedman@yale.edu	AHRQ_011
DC	American Healthways	American Healthways will provide services directly to beneficiaries in Maryland and the District of Columbia and in collaboration with CIGNA HealthCare in Georgia.	American Healthways, Inc. 3841 Green Hills Village Drive Nashville, TN 37215 800-327-3822	CCIP_2
DC	Connecting Visiting Nurses, Patients and Physicians	This Telehealth project extends the reach and scope of MedStar's visiting nurses and facilitates timely and secure communications among nurses, physicians and patients.	Allison Stover 100 Irving Street, NW, Suite EB-6106 Washington, DC 20010 703-780-4942 allison.stover@medstar.net	HIE_132
DC	Evidence-Based Medicine (EBM) Online	This HIE proposes to offer three online EBM workshops that will be interactive and learner-centered. These workshops will focus on helping practicing clinicians become more efficient knowledge managers.	Karen Lencoski 2501 M Street NW, Suite 575 Washington, DC 20037 202-887-5150 lencoskik@sgim.org	HIE_133
DC	CareFirst BlueCross BlueShield's Bridges To Excellence (BTE) program	A continuing effort to enhance quality care for its policyholders led CareFirst BlueCross BlueShield (CareFirst) to expand its partnership with Bridges To Excellence (BTE), which provides recognition and financial rewards to physicians who implement specific steps to deliver safe, high quality care. CareFirst expanded the innovative pay-for-performance pilot program to include 94 physicians in 29 practices that serve nearly 60,000 CareFirst members. CareFirst estimates that nearly $1.3 million in rewards will be paid out in 2005.	William L. Jews, CareFirst 10455 and 10453 Mill Run Circle Owings Mills, MD 21117 410-581-3000	BTE_01f

DC	Delmarva Foundation for Medical Care	Delmarva Foundation, the Quality Improvement Organization (QIO) for Maryland and the District of Columbia will provide technical assistance and support free of charge to adult primary care physician practices	Carmen Tyler Winston Director, DOQ-IT Program 202-496-6559 Corporate HQ: 410-822-0697 doqitdelmarva@dfmc.org	DOQ_51
DE	Quality Insights of Delaware	Quality Insights of Delaware is an affiliate of the West Virginia Medical Institute (WVMI), a nonprofit physician sponsored organization dedicated to improving the health of the people we serve. As part of the project, Quality Insights will help participants to assess their information technology readiness and to select an Electronic Health Record (EHR) vendor. We will help physicians implement the new technology and offer strategies to optimize office efficiency.	Beth Schindele DOQ-IT Project Manager 302-478-3600 ext.114 1-866-475-9669 ext.114 bschindele@wvmi.org	DOQ_08
DE	Delaware Health Information Network	The DHIN is a participant in the Patient Safety Institute HIE project designed to provide governance with consumer input, and the infrastructure to allow data transmission with patient consent to authenticated providers. The DHIN intends to make clinical information available to providers at the point-of-care.	A. Herbert Nehrling Delaware Health Information Network 540 S. DuPont Highway, Suite 8 Dover, DE 19901 302-744-1220 Robin.Lawrence@state.de.us	HIE_029
FL	Bridges-to-Excellence (General)	In July 2004, United Healthcare became the first health care company to license the BTE model, working with employers in Omaha, St Louis, Dayton and South Florida to offer network doctors certain incentives for earning NCQA recognition.	Susan Dorsey, Director NBCH 1015 18th Street N.W., Suite 730 Washington, DC 20036 Sdorsey@nbch.org 202-775-9300	BTE_02h
FL	Humana /Pfizer	Pfizer Health Solutions partners with Humana and healthcare and community organizations to implement patient-centered programs that focus on prevention, disease management and care coordination.	Tom Noland Humana Corporate Comm. 502-580-3674 tnoland@humana.com	CCIP_5
FL	Florida Medical Quality Assurance	(No specific DOQ-IT information) Florida Medical Quality Assurance, Inc. (FMQAI), a subsidiary of Health Services Holdings (HSH), is Florida's Medicare Quality Improvement Organization (QIO) and the End Stage Renal Disease (ESRD) Network of Florida. FMQAI is federally funded and under contract with the Centers for Medicare & Medicaid Services (CMS) at the U.S. Department of Health and Human Services (HHS).	John Kupkovits /Health Information Technology Consultant 813-354-9111 ext. 3542 hit-fl@flqio.sdps.org	DOQ_09
FL	Improving Health and Communication with the Patient Centric Record	This organization states they have an electronic data repository that allows secure access to medical information. To be fully operational, they indicate a need to create "additional system modules" and educate the health industry and the public about health information exchange.	John Principato 460 Timber Ridge Drive Longwood, FL 32779 407-389-4442 jprincipato@cfl.rr.com	HIE_030
FL	Healthcare Access Demonstration	This is a coalition of healthcare stakeholders in Orange County who intend to host a disease management service targeted to uninsured persons with chronic illnesses. The members of the organization intend to develop a technology infrastructure for secure communication, and hope to realize savings in the cost of care by reducing hospital stays and emergency room use.	James Kragh / Mark Brewer 1411 Edgewater Dr. Orlando, FL 32804 407-629-0304 jkragh@amnetwork.com	HIE_031
FL	HIT for Medication Safety in Critical Access Hospitals	Develops an implementation plan for pharmacy health information systems in critical access hospitals to include an onsite survey of health IT, flowcharting the medication use system, and an assessment of resources.	Abraham Hartzema, Doctor's Memorial Hospital, Bonifay, FL	AHRQ_012

FL	Promoting Patient Safety with Web-based Patient Profiles	Explores the feasibility of a community-wide strategic implementation plan for Web-based standardized patient care to provide point-of-care access to patient information across acute and long-term care systems and services.	Rosemary Laird, Health First, Inc. Cocoa Beach, FL 321-868-7641	AHRQ_013
GA	Cigna HealthCare (w/ American Healthways)	By partnering with American Healthways, CIGNA can extend collaboration efforts and develop industry-leading DM capabilities.	Amy Turkington, CIGNA 1-860-226-3489	CCIP_3
GA	Georgia Medical Care Foundation	gmcf will provide the following services: Analysis of practice processes, Recommendations for improved office efficiencies, Assistance with EHR vendor selection, Development/Analysis of Request for Proposal (RFP), Assistance with EHR implementation, Post-implementation monitoring	678-527-3448 doqit@gmcf.org	DOQ_10
GA	Georgia EMR	This is a coalition of rural community health centers who intend to install electronic medical records in 13 of the member organizations. The project includes training, disease reporting, quality improvement, and standardizing data elements and clinical workflow.	Bruce M. Whyte, M.D. The Grant Building 44 Broad St, Suite 410 Atlanta, GA 30303 404-659-2861 bmwhyte@bellsouth.net	HIE_032
GA	OrderComm	This is a home-grown, order entry system using scanner technology intended to be used by the health system to transmit information from clinical areas to other areas of the health system to improve workflow and patient safety and lower administrative costs. MCG Health System believes it also meets JCAHO standards of care.	Julie Trackman 1120 15th Street Augusta, GA 30909 706-721-5585 jtrackman@mail.mcg.edu	HIE_033
GA	Tri-County Plus Rural Health Network (TCPRHN)	The Tri-County Plus Rural Health Network is implementing health information exchange to help coordinate care for a rural, underserved area of the State of Georgia. They are focusing on care management, admissions, discharge, improved patient safety, provider satisfaction, and lower costs.	Max E Stachura, MD 1120-15th Street (EA100) Augusta, Georgia 30912 706-721-6616 maxs@mcg.edu	HIE_034
GA	West Georgia Health Information Exchange	This HIE intends to tie together the three hospitals in the Tanner group and physician offices in this rural section of the States of Georgia and Alabama. This will include medical records as well as administrative information (e.g., insurance information and patient demographics) as well as lab orders and results.	Denise L. Taylor, President & CEO 303 Ambulance Drive Carrollton, GA 30117 770-836-9871 dtaylor@tanner.org	HIE_035
GA	Wellpoint eRx or Paper Reduction	WellPoint is spearheading an electronic initiative at a cost of $40 million that will reach 19,000 physicians. In California, Georgia, Missouri, and Wisconsin, physicians will be given the opportunity to choose from either of two electronic packages: a Prescription Improvement Package or a Paperwork Reduction Package.	Ron J. Ponder, PhD, EVP, Information Services, WellPoint or Nadia Leather - CGEY nadia.leather@capgemini.com 212-314-8234	PHIT_02b
GA	Comprehensive IT Solution for Quality and Patient Safety	Implements a series of new health information technologies in carefully staged processes over 2 years to include an Inpatient Pharmacy System, Electronic Medication Administration Record, Bar Coding System, and a CPOE System; evaluates the impact of these systems on safety, quality and efficiency.	Ann Beach Children's Healthcare of Atlanta, GA 404-785-7463	AHRQ_014
HI	Mountain-Pacific Quality Health Foundation	(No specific DOQ-IT information) Mountain-Pacific Quality Health Foundation is the quality improvement organization (QIO) for Montana, Wyoming, Hawaii, and the territories of Guam, the Commonwealth of the Northern Marianas and American Samoa. The Foundation operates out of offices in Helena, Montana; Cheyenne, Wyoming; and Honolulu, Hawaii. As a QIO, we receive funding from the federal government to enact programs that help ensure people with Medicare receive appropriate, high-quality care. We also hold contracts with other government agencies and private insurance companies.	808-545-2550 pacific@mpqhf.org	DOQ_11

HI	Hawaii Health Information Exchange	HHIC is a coalition of healthcare industry organizations that has worked in the past to coordinate initiatives such as HIPAA, and is now involved with development of health information exchanges. They have developed a couple of data sets for inpatient services and and emergency departments. They are looking to expand into other areas, such as assisting with the conversion from ICD-9 to ICD-10, and focusing on community health centers.	Susan Forbes, MPH, DrPH 600 Kapiolani Blvd, Suite 406 Honolulu, HI 96813 808-534-0288 sforbes@hhic.org	HIE_036
HI	Quality Healthcare Alliance Health Information Exchange	This is a broad alliance of healthcare stakeholders, including employers, bridges to excellence, and government representatives, intended to develop and HIE. They are looking to work on a patient identifier, electronic prescribing, lab results, evidence based decision support tools, patient portal, electronic health records, and education.	Mr. Gary Allen Executive Director, Hawaii Business Health Council 3814 Pukalani Place Honolulu, HI 96816 808-372-9576 garyallen@hbhc.biz	HIE_037
HI	Kaiser Permanente and Epic Systems	Three Kaiser Permanente care centers in Hawaii introduced a new outpatient electronic medical records system. The Hawaii implementations represent more than just three additional providers embracing the latest technology—they are the first step in Kaiser's $1.8 billion initiative to automate records for its 8.4 million members nationwide. The project is called HealthConnect.	Louise Liang, MD, SVP for Quality and Clinical Systems Support Kaiser Foundation Health Plan One Kaiser Plaza, Oakland, CA 94612 510-271-6317	PHIT_05a
HI	Holomua Project-Improving Patient Hand-Offs in Hawaii	Develops approaches to share data on patient clinical and diagnostic information across systems and creates an implementation plan for systems integration.	Christine M. Sakuda, Hawaii Primary Care Association, Honolulu, HI 808-536-8442, csakuda@hawaiipca.net	AHRQ_015
HI	Quality Focused Connectivity	Implements an HIE to the three rural islands of the State of Hawaii: Maui, Kauai, and the island of Hawaii that focuses on preventive health care providing an opportunity for care to be addressed in a comprehensive manner so that the responsibility of health improvement shifts from the current physician focus on illness to a patient-centered focus on wellness.	Daniel Heslinga, Quality Healthcare Alliance, Honolulu, HI	AHRQ_016
IA	Iowa Foundation for Medical Care	The Iowa Foundation for Medical Care (IFMC) is the Quality Improvement Organization (QIO) for Iowa. QIOs work with physicians and health care professionals to promote high quality medical care for Medicare consumers. IFMC is contracted by the Centers for Medicare & Medicaid Services (CMS), an agency of the U.S. Department of Health and Human Services. (No specific DOQ-IT information)	515-223-2900 1-800-383-2856	DOQ_15a
IA	Health Care Excel	Through this initiative, Health Care Excel (HCE), the Medicare Quality Improvement Organization for Indiana, will assist primary care physicians in adopting Electronic Health Record (EHR) systems with the ultimate goal of improving office efficiency and patient outcomes. This initiative is sponsored by the Centers for Medicare & Medicaid Services (CMS).	Darlene Skelton 812-234-1499 515-725-1245	DOQ_15b
IA	Telehealth	This is an HIE concept based in the local, county visiting nurses association and designed to develop home monitoring of home health patients. A variety of "telehealth" services are envisioned to monitor and report vital signs to a central repository.	Gail Coughlin 1225 E. River Drive Davenport, IA 52803 563-421-5256 coughling@genesishealth.com	HIE_047
IA	Using Physician-Patient Online Messaging to Improve Outcomes	This HIE proposes to use web-based communications between physicians and their patients to improve patient compliance. Using a series of automated messages from the physicians, the system is designed to educate patients about their condition and medications. Participants in this HIE include Columbia University, ConnectiCare (a Connecticut-based health plan) and the University of Iowa.	Michael Kienzle, MD 200 Hawkins Drive Iowa City, IA 52242 319-335-9788 michael-kienzle@uiowa.edu	HIE_048

IA	EMR Planning to Improve North Iowa Health Care	Designs a system-wide patient-centered planning process and an EHR implementation plan that will securely exchange patient information within and across diverse healthcare settings for the Hancock County Memorial Hospital and 21 affiliated physician health organization clinics.	Toni Ebeling, Hancock County Health Services, Britt, IA	AHRQ_028
IA	Rural Iowa Redesign of Care Delivery with EHR Functions	Implements a comprehensive, integrated, EHR system with CPOE and clinical decision-support tools in hospital inpatient units, ambulatory care, primary care and specialty clinics, home health, and hospice care; also evaluates medical errors and near misses, use of evidence-based practices, responsiveness to adverse drug alerts, and patient/provider satisfaction.	Donald Crandall, Mercy Medical Center—North Iowa, Mason City, IA	AHRQ_029
IA	Health Information Technology Value in Rural Hospitals	Documents the patient safety and healthcare quality challenges in critical access to rural hospitals, and assesses health IT capacity in these rural hospitals and how they would use health IT to improve safety and quality; develops a decision-making health IT toolkits for other rural hospitals.	Marcia Ward, University of Iowa Iowa City, IA 319-384-5131 marcia-m-ward@uiowa.edu	AHRQ_030
IA	Microsoft and Health Alliance Medical Plans	Health Alliance Medical Plans - Health Insurance Provider Migrates to Microsoft Integration Solution and Reduces TCO , Health Alliance Medical Plans chose to evaluate a Microsoft® solution based on Microsoft BizTalk® Server 2004 and Microsoft BizTalk Accelerator for HIPAA. Microsoft recommended that the company work with Washington Publishing Company (WPC)—a Microsoft Certified Partner and publisher of HIPAA Implementation Guides—to complete a two-week proof-of-concept (POC) study at the Microsoft Technology Center (MTC) in Chicago.	Health Alliance Medical Plans 800-851-3379 www.healthalliance.org	PHIT_06b
ID	Qualis Health	Practices that participate in DOQ-IT will receive free assistance to select, implement, and optimize IT systems such as EHRs, e-prescribing, and registries. CMS has contracted with Qualis Health to provide DOQ-IT services to participating physicians in Washington, Idaho, and Alaska.	Helen Stroebel, RN MPH 800-488-1118, ext. 5053 helens@qualishealth.org	DOQ_12
ID	North Idaho Community Connections (NICC)	This is a consortium of hospitals in northern Idaho that has already implemented a number of technologies, including interactive video, wide area network, and telemedicine related. They are working to connect with individual physicians. They are now working to develop and launch an EMR.	Sue Fox, MPH P.O. Box 1448, Sandpoint, ID 83864 208-265-3390, suefox@sandpoint.net	HIE_038
ID	Rural Connection: Strengthening Care Through Technology	Explores health IT as a method of sharing patient information and develops an electronic health record for patients who utilize rural, urban, acute, and rehabilitation facilities.	Anne Oglevie, Weiser Memorial Hospital, Weiser, ID	AHRQ_017
IL	Bridges-to-Excellence (General) - Tri-State Health Care Coalition	The four coalitions launching BTE-related projects are located in Illinois (two in Illinois), Colorado and Arkansas. The coalitions, through a licensing arrangement with BTE, have begun talking with employers and estimate launching customized programs in their respective markets later this year. Business coalitions are well suited to coordinating such incentive programs - by coordinating activities among employers, they can pool resources and streamline related operations, thus making the efforts more attractive to employers and physicians. All four coalitions are members of the National Business Coalition on Health (NBCH), a 70-coalition member strong organization that strongly supports pay-for-performance.	Susan Dorsey, Director NBCH 1015 18th Street N.W., Suite 730 Washington, DC 20036 Sdorsey@nbch.org 202-775-9300	BTE_02a
IL	Bridges-to-Excellence (General) - Heartland Healthcare Coalition	The four coalitions launching BTE-related projects are located in Illinois (two in Illinois), Colorado and Arkansas. The coalitions, through a licensing arrangement with BTE, have begun talking with employers and estimate launching customized programs in their respective markets later this year. Business coalitions are well suited to coordinating such incentive programs - by coordinating activities among employers, they can pool resources and streamline related operations, thus making the efforts more attractive to employers and physicians. All four coalitions are members of the National Business Coalition on Health (NBCH), a 70-coalition member strong organization that strongly supports pay-for-performance.	Susan Dorsey, Director NBCH 1015 18th Street N.W., Suite 730 Washington, DC 20036 Sdorsey@nbch.org 202-775-9300	BTE_02b

IL	Aetna Health Management (partnered with LifeMasters)	Aetna was awarded a CCIP for Chicago (20,000 Medicare beneficiaries to be involved). Effort to identify health risks among Medicare+Choice members and to help manage those risks through targeted case management, DM and educational programs.	Susan Millerick, 860-273-0536 Clinical/Quality Programs PR millericks@aetna.com	CCIP_1
IL	Illinois Foundation for Quality Health Care	Participating practices will receive free consultative services from the Illinois Foundation for Quality Health Care (IFQHC) throughout the process of selecting and implementing an EHR system. IFQHC provides resources with expertise on: Culture change and leadership, EHR planning and implementation. Workflow analysis and preparing practices for EHR readiness. Increased patient safety.	Grace Martos Jeanette Kebisek, 630-928-5808 630-928-5867 gmartos@ilqio.sdps.org jkebisek@ilqio.sdps.org	DOQ_13
IL	Advancing an HIE for Cardiovascular Care	This is a proposed HIE targeted to persons with cardiovascular disease, including CAD, CHF, and/or HTN. The proposal focuses on technical infrastructure and tools, performance metrics, and reports.	Karen Kmetik, PhD 515 N. State Street Chicago, IL 60610 312-464-4221 karen_kmetik@ama-assn.org	HIE_039
IL	ePrescribing HIE	This is a consortium of organizations with a concept for an HIE that allows exchange, analysis, and use of pharmaceutical information at 2 pilot facilities affiliated with the Cleveland Clinic. The consortium includes RxHub, VisionShare. The project also proposes researching the impact of electronic prescribing at Scripps Mercy Clinic and the underserved in San Diego County who use Mercy hospital.	Thomas M. Leary 230 E Ohio Street, Suite 500 Chicago, IL 60611 571-331-2486 tleary@himss.org	HIE_040
IL	Electronic Cancer Reporting	This HIE focuses on cancer diagnosis and reporting using the College of American Pathologists cancer checklist. The concept is to communicate the cancer diagnosis protocols to pathologists and facilitate electronic reporting.	Diane J. Aschman 325 Waukegan Road Northfield, Illinois 60093 847-832-7250 daschma@cap.org	HIE_041
IL	Microsoft and Health Alliance Medical Plans	Health Alliance Medical Plans - Health Insurance Provider Migrates to Microsoft Integration Solution and Reduces TCO , Health Alliance Medical Plans chose to evaluate a Microsoft® solution based on Microsoft BizTalk® Server 2004 and Microsoft BizTalk Accelerator for HIPAA. After talking with Health Alliance about its needs, Microsoft recommended that the company work with Washington Publishing Company (WPC)—a Microsoft Certified Partner and publisher of HIPAA Implementation Guides—to complete a two-week proof-of-concept (POC) study at the Microsoft Technology Center (MTC) in Chicago.	Health Alliance Medical Plans 800-851-3379 www.healthalliance.org	PHIT_06a
IL	Rural Community Partnerships—EMR Implementation Project	Implements an ambulatory EMR in multiple rural primary and specialist care provider settings and measures the impact of health information technology on clinical practice, organizational structure, and financial benefits; integrates ambulatory electronic medical record case scenarios into the curricula of the Health Science and Human Services Department to ensure that future healthcare providers have adequate training and exposure to ambulatory EMR technology.	R'Nee Mullen, Magic Valley Memorial Hospital, Twin Falls, ID	AHRQ_018
IL	Linking Rural Providers to Improve Patient Care and Health	Develops a central electronic health record system that will allow sharing of health information between a hospital, medical group, county health department, and behavioral health organization for rural economically disadvantaged, ethnic/racial minority residents, the elderly, and persons with special/complex health care needs.	Timothy Broos, Katherine Shaw Bethea Hospital, Dixon, IL 815-285-5509	AHRQ_019
IL	Sharing Patient Record Access in Rural Health Settings	Develops an implementation plan for an ambulatory EMR in a medically underserved region that will electronically connect physician offices, the regional hospital, ancillary services, and other community health services; identifies indicators to track measurable improvements in patient safety, quality of care, clinician and patient satisfaction, and operational efficiency.	Michael DeLuca, Sarah Bush Lincoln Health Center, Mattoon, IL	AHRQ_020

IL	Enhancing Quality in Patient Care (EQUIP) Project	Implements an electronic health records system in a network of community health centers and develops a data warehouse to monitor, aggregate, and provide data for quality improvement.	Alex Lippitt, Erie Family Health Center Chicago, IL	AHRQ_021
IL	Toward an Optimal Patient Safety Information System	Promotes and evaluates the interchange of patient safety information and the reporting of adverse events and close calls among public and private voluntary incident reporting systems being used at U.S. hospitals.	Andrew Chang, Joint Commission on Accreditation of Healthcare Organizations (JCAHO), Oakbrook Terrace, IL	AHRQ_022
IL	Value of Technology to Transfer Discharge Information	Assesses the value of software applications to facilitate information transfer during the high-risk transition from hospital to home at discharge and compares health information technology to usual care for benefits outcomes, adverse events, effectiveness, costs, and satisfaction among patients and physicians.	James Graumlich, Board of Trustees of the University of Illinois, Chicago, IL 309-655-2730	AHRQ_023
IN	Health Care Excel	Through this initiative, Health Care Excel (HCE), the Medicare Quality Improvement Organization for Indiana, will assist primary care physicians in adopting Electronic Health Record (EHR) systems with the ultimate goal of improving office efficiency and patient outcomes. This initiative is sponsored by the Centers for Medicare & Medicaid Services (CMS).	Darlene Skelton, 812-234-1499 1-800-300-8190 317-347-4500	DOQ_14
IN	South-Central Indiana E-prescribing Network	This is a collaboration of providers and vendors to implement an e-prescribing system. Their not-for-profit organization is called ScriptNet, which is designed to develop a central data repository, educate on data standards, provide related services, interoperate with other applications, and share costs.	Michael Sullivan, MD 501 N. Morton Street Suite 209 Bloomington, IN 47404 812-331-2208 sullivan@xylor.com	HIE_042
IN	Allen County Connections for Care Network	This consortium of federally qualified health centers, other safety net providers, hospitals and vendors proposes to develop a centralized electronic medical record (called "WebChart"), link it to an established, limited wide area network (called MED-WEB), and expand the service to safety net providers (starting with a three clinic pilot). The MED-WEB network already links hospitals and physicians in the county. Safety net clinics and local hospital emergency rooms are seeking funding so they may link into this network with the proposed electronic medical record. Curently they are operating with resources donated by the participating organizations. The goals of the group are to reduce duplication of services, improve quality and management of care, increase efficiencies and lower costs.	Mary Haupert, President P.O. Box 11949, 1717 S. Calhoun St. Fort Wayne, IN 46862 260-458-2644 mshaupert@nhci.net	HIE_043
IN	Indiana Health Information Exchange/Indianapolis Network for Patient Care (INPC)	This HIE has an existing, "population-based" electronic medical record used by providers, public health agencies, health services researchers, and other stakeholders. The EMR uses standardized data, a central data repository, and data mining capabilities.	Dr. J. Marc Overhage 1050 Wishard Blvd Indianapolis, IN 46202 317-630-8685 moverhage@regenstrief.org	HIE_044* RHIO_044
IN	Connecting Cass County for Better Health	This is a county government based coalition of government agency, provider, and academic stakeholders interested in health matters of this rural community. The coalition proposes to create the infrastructure for the electronic exchange of health information, building on the local hospital's recent acquisition of DSL technology. They are looking to put in place hardware, software, and an electronic network.	Brian T. Shockney 1101 Michigan Avenue Logansport, IN 46947 574-753-1385 bshockney@mhlogan.org	HIE_045
IN	South Bend Community HealthLinks	The South Bend Community HealthLinks HIE is a utility model data exchange using a centralized repository for clinical information. The system is designed to interface with physician practice, personal health record, and clinical decision support software. A related entity, the Michiana Health Information Network, is a collaboration of local medical specialty physician practices, formed within the South Bend Medical Foundation (SBMF) to develop the infrastructure for a data repository for clinical information exchange.	Michiana Health Info. Network 215 West Madison Street South Bend, IN 46601 574-968-1001 Robert King 531 North Lafayette Blvd. South Bend, IN 46601 574-234-4176 Bking@sbmflab.org	HIE_046

IN	An Evolving Statewide Indiana Information Infrastructure	Contract that develops and implements HIE using an established technical infrastructure and interconnects local health information infrastructures; also implements a Statewide public health surveillance network that links all hospitals to share emergency department data	Project Director: Marc Overhage Indiana University School of Medicine Indianapolis, IN 317-630-7070 joverhag@iupui.edu	AHRQ_024
IN	Improving Health Care through HIT in Morgan County, IN	Creates a secure infrastructure for communication among providers to allow electronic sharing of patient clinical info with hospitals and other physicians/ health providers in the county, region, and State; also assesses the effectiveness of the system in improving workflow, timeliness & completeness of information, patient safety, continuity of care, health outcomes.	Paul Clippinger, Morgan Hospital and Medical Center, Martinsville, IN	AHRQ_025
IN	Value of Health Information Exchange (HIE) in Ambulatory Care	Assesses the value of HIE in ambulatory care by modifying an existing economic model of HIE and tests the model in a randomized controlled trial.	Marc Overhage, Indiana University Indianapolis, IN 317-630-7070 joverhag@iupui.edu	AHRQ_026
IN	Value of New Drug Labeling Knowledge for e-Prescribing	Creates a prescribing tool with decision support (checking dosage, contraindications, and drug interactions) that can be easily integrated into a provider's practices; implements and pilot tests the tool to evaluate its benefits and costs.	Gunther Schadow, Indiana University, Indianapolis, IN 317-278-4636 gschadow@iupui.edu	AHRQ_027
KS	Kansas Foundation for Medical Care	The Kansas Foundation for Medical Care, Inc., in support of the proposed work for the CMS 8th Scope of Work contract, will be providing free assistance to Physician Offices that desire to move to an Electronic Health Record environment.	800-432-0407 785-273-2552 relations@kfmc.org	DOQ_16
KS	Jayhawk P.O.C.	This is a hospital based (Pratt Regional Medical Center) HIE tying together all of the hospital departments in a central data repository. The system is used to communicate patient information. The hospital is proposing to expand the system to allow practitioners to access patient information from anywhere in the region. Information proposed to be made available includes: medical history, lab results, diagnostic imaging, medication and immunization records, insurance information, and other personal information.	DeWayne Bryan 200 Commodore Pratt, KS 67124 620-450-1485 dbryan@prmc.org	HIE_049
KY	Bridges-to-Excellence (DCL)	Enables physicians to achieve one-year or three-year recognition for high performance in diabetes care. Qualifying physicians receive up to $80 for each diabetic patient covered by a participating employer and plan. In addition, the program offers a suite of products and tools to help diabetic patients get engaged in their care, achieve better outcomes, and identify local physicians that meet the high performance measures.	NCQA 2000 L Street, NW, Suite 500 Washington, DC 20036 202-955-3500 Customersupport@ncqa.org	BTE_03b
KY	Health Care Excel	Through this initiative, Health Care Excel (HCE), the Medicare Quality Improvement Organization for Indiana, will assist primary care physicians in adopting Electronic Health Record (EHR) systems with the ultimate goal of improving office efficiency and patient outcomes. This initiative is sponsored by the Centers for Medicare & Medicaid Services (CMS).	Darlene Skelton, 812-234-1499 502-339-7442	DOQ_17
KY	Connecting Healthcare in Central Appalachia	As an integrated, not-for-profit rural healthcare system serving Eastern Kentucky and Southern West Virginia, Appalachian Regional Healthcare, Inc. (ARH) is an integrated health collaboration consisting of hospitals, clinics, and home health agencies serving rural eastern Kentucky and southern West Virginia. They are proposing to develop a web-based, centralized patient information repository and portal for providers, and are looking to obtain hardware and staff to implement. Information proposed to be collected and stored in the repository includes encounter, demographic, and financial data.	Amanda Fryman, Appalachian Regional Healthcare, Inc. 1220 Harrodsburg Road P.O. Box 8086 Lexington, Kentucky 40533 859-226-2433 afryman@arh.org	HIE_050
KY	Meeting Information Needs of Referrals Electronically	Identifies essential technological needs for accessing and sharing data and information between patients and health care providers; develops an implementation plan to expand the transmission of referral information electronically in a closed health system to an open system.	Carol Ireson, University of Kentucky Research Foundation, Lexington, KY 859-257-5678 clireso@email.uky.edu	AHRQ_031

KY	Connecting Healthcare in Central Appalachia	Implements and trains staff on the use of an EMR system in a rural integrated health care delivery system in an integrated rural healthcare delivery system serving approximately 20 counties throughout Eastern Kentucky and Southern West Virginia.	Polly Bentley, Appalachian Regional Health, Hazard, KY	AHRQ_032
KY	ED Information Systems—Kentucky & Indiana Hospitals	Implements and trains users of a Web-based electronic record system in the emergency departments of two small community hospitals, one medium-sized community hospital, one rural hospital, and three private primary care physician practices; evaluates the reduction in medical errors, waiting time, and costs as well as patient and physician satisfaction.	David Pecoraro, Jewish Hospital Health Care, Louisville, KY	AHRQ_033
LA	Louisiana Health Care Review	Louisiana Health Care Review, Inc. (LHCR) is working with the Centers for Medicare & Medicaid Services (CMS) to help primary care physician offices adopt electronic health records (EHRs) to improve office efficiencies and quality of care. Project Objectives: Facilitate the adoption of Electronic Health Records EHRs in small to medium-sized primary care practices, Ensure that practices are using EHRs and IT to the fullest capability to improve office efficiency, Use clinical data reports for improved practice performance and patient outcomes	Chris Williams, Team Leader Jack Olden, 225-248-7078 225-926-6353 cwilliams@lhcr.org jolden@lhcr.org	DOQ_18
LA	Catahoula Consortium on Health Information Exchange	This is a collaboration between a rural hospital, university, state public health department to develop an HIE for clinical information sharing to improve care provided to uninsured persons in a rural area. The goal is to connect a majority (75%) of local providers, share information, and instigate continuous improvement by measuring outcomes and providing results to the participants for quality improvement purposes. The participants would like to replicate throughout the State the model they are building for a rural health clinic and HIE.	Holly Purvis, MHA P.O. Box 2078 Jena, Louisiana 71342 318-992-9200 hpurvis@lasallegeneralhospital.com	HIE_051
LA	Catahoula Parish Consortium	This proposed HIE is a collaboration between a rural hospital, university, and state public health department to serve Medicaid beneficiaries in a rural area, and other patients of participating providers. The project is designed to exchange clinical information, track referrals, and allow for eligibility checks and prior authorizations.	Holly Purvis, MHA P.O. Box 2780 Jena, Louisiana 71342 318-992-9200 hpurvis@lasallegeneralhospital.com	HIE_052
LA	Project Overcoming Isolation	This HIE is targeted to cystic fibrosis patients and uses a "smart card" and web-based site to access a centralized data repository with clinical and treatment information. It also is designed to provide an online support community for patients, and includes privacy controls.	Hank Fanberg 2424 Edenborn Avenue, Suite 290 Metairie, LA 70001 504-838-1550 hank.fanberg@christushealth.org	HIE_053
LA	Cardiovascular Care Disparities: Safety-Net HIT Strategy	Designs the implementation of a longitudinal cardiovascular disease information system platform to address disparities viewed as a lifelong disease process, and examines the impact of health IT on quality improvement, medical and financial effectiveness, and increased value.	Bruce Ferguson, LSU Health Sciences Center, New Orleans, LA	AHRQ_034
LA	Distance Management of High-Risk Obstetrical Patients	Develops a technology plan to improve access to maternal-fetal medicine services throughout the State and guides the implementation of telemedicine capabilities to provide real-time remote diagnostic ultrasound and consultative services to women with high-risk pregnancies.	Helene Kurtz, Woman's Hospital Baton Rouge, LA	AHRQ_035
LA	HIT Service Integration	Creates a detailed assessment of the feasibility of health IT implementation including the development of an implementation plan, specification of clinical and organizational needs, identification of goals, and identifying barriers and ways to address those barriers.	Michelle Lemming, Franklin Foundation Hospital, Franklin, LA	AHRQ_036

LA	Louisiana Rural Health Information Technology Partnership	Implements a Complete Medical Record (a computerized emergency department communication, documentation, passive tracking, and medical records system) in an emergency department and evaluates the use of this technology toward improving patient safety and quality of care.	Paul Salles, Assumption Community Hospital, Napoleonville, LA	AHRQ_037
MA	Bridges-to-Excellence (POL)	CMS is also looking towards the BTE Physician Office Link program as a possible element in its forthcoming Medicare Care Management Performance Demonstration project, an initiative which will promote the adoption and use of health information technology to improve the efficiency and quality of patient care for chronically ill Medicare patients. Doctors who meet or exceed performance standards established by CMS in clinical delivery systems and patient outcomes will receive performance payments for managing the care of eligible Medicare beneficiaries.	Medstat Group 1-800-224-7161 bridgestoexcellence@thomson.com	BTE_01d
MA	Bridges-to-Excellence (POL)	A pay-for-performance initiatives offered by the Bridges coalition in Boston and Schenectady/Albany in which 35 medical groups split $800,000 in incentives. These were rewards earned by meeting criteria established by the National Committee for Quality Assurance (NCQA) related to the adoption of technology-based care management systems.	Medstat Group 1-800-224-7161 bridgestoexcellence@thomson.com	BTE_01e
MA	MassPRO	Electronic health records could transform your practice. But success takes time, planning and strategy. MassPRO can help.MassPRO is recruiting 150 adult primary care (FP, GP, IM) practice sites. Priority will be given to those sites with 8 or fewer physicians. During this 15-month project starting in fall 2004, MassPRO will use seminars, conference calls, group e-mail, and one-on-one consultation to help practices prepare for and successfully implement EMRs. MassPRO, as part of a national pilot project, is able to offer these services at no cost.	Chuck Parker /Director Complete List: http://www.masspro.org/doqit/index htm#contacts, 781-419-2790 781-890-0011 Hotline: 800-252-5533 cparker@maqio.sdps.org	DOQ_21
MA	The Boston Community Health Information for Improvement (CHII) Project	This is an alliance of community health and academic medical centers serving poor and homeless persons. It proposes to interoperate between 11 outpatient databases to share clinical information, specifically to assist with disease management and prevention. Components in the project include: outcomes data, reporting, quality improvement, and integrating with administrative information.	Larry Culpepper, MD, MPH, Chairman Dowling 5 Boston, MA 617-414-6225 larry.culpepper@bmc.org	HIE_059
MA	Statewide EHR Adoption and Health Data Exchange in Massachusetts	This is a collaboration of physician groups, employers, and academic medical institutions that promotes use of electronic medical records in the State of Massachusetts. The group is designed to support and educate physicians, and assist with setting standards and sharing data.	David Bates, MD, MSc Brigham and Women's Hospital, 75 Francis St., Boston, MA 21115 617-732-5650 dbates@partners.org	HIE_060
MA	Connecting Consumer Communities to Healthcare Providers	This is a proposal to develop "use cases" for health information exchange and research the exchange of information between and among patients, providers, provider groups, and hospitals to foster a better understanding of information exchange, especially from the consumer perspective.	Daniel B. Hoch VBK 830 Mass General Hospital Boston, MA 21114 617-726-3311 dhoch@partners.org	HIE_061
MA	MA-SHARE MedsInfo e-Prescribing Initiative	This HIE proposes to demonstrate the value of e-prescribing, focusing on emergency department and point-of-care my measuring error reduction, workflow improvements, outcomes, and the impact on costs. This is seen as the first step towards development of a comprehensive clinical information exchange.	Elliot M. Stone, CEO 460 Totten Pond Road, Suite 385 Waltham, MA 02451 781-890-6042 EStone@mahealthdata.org	HIE_062* RHIO_062
MA	SAFE Health - Central Massachusetts	This is a collaboration of three health plans, a health system, and a vendor (Hewelitt-Packard) to develop a prototype to exchange clinical information in emergency rooms and outpatient care settings. They have developed a clinical information architecture in a "federated," or decentralized configuration allowing interoperability between different systems. The design includes a master patient index, secure information transmission, and interoperability between systems having different information technologies.	Mark Fisher, Chief Operating Officer Fallon Community Health Plan 10 Chestnut Street Worcester, MA 01608 508-368-9303 mark.fisher@fchp.org	HIE_063

MA	Medication Administration Program	This is a health system medication management platform. It is designed to track, document, manage, screen for potential drug interactions, and reduce adverse events through an information system and barcoding technology.	Sharron Finlay 11 Shattuck Street Worcester, MA 01605 508-334-1485 finlays@UMMHC.org	HIE_064
MA	Tufts Health Plan and Blue Cross Blue Shield Massachusetts (BCBSMA) and Zix Corp	Seeking to boost generic drug utilization and increase quality of service, Tufts Health Plan (Waltham, Mass.) and Blue Cross Blue Shield Massachusetts (BCBSMA, Boston) are joining in a $3 million initiative to offer physicians a comprehensive e-prescribing program. The companies will provide approximately 3,400 physicians hand-held devices equipped with Zix Corp.'s PocketScript e-prescribing software.	Robert Mandel, BCBSMA VP, Provider enrollment and services or Philip Boulter, M.D., Tufts Health Plan	PHIT_08
MA	Blue Cross Blue Shield of Massachusetts (BCBSMA)	Backed by $50 million from Blue Cross Blue Shield of Massachusetts (BCBSMA), a group of healthcare insurers, doctors, hospitals and others in the state plan early next year to wire one community with interoperable electronic medical records. The collaboration includes more than 30 organizations, including health-related state agencies and large employers that pay for health insurance. John Halamka of Healthcare System (Boston), which operates five Boston-area hospitals and is part of the cooperative, estimates a statewide e-records project could cost $1 billion, but still believes statewide adoption could happen in as few as five years. Projects are being led by the Massachusetts eHealth Collaborative, a nonprofit coalition launched last year by 34 health-care providers, health plans, and insurers in the state, which picked the three communities in March 05 from more than 35 that had applied to participate in the two- to three-year study.	John Halamka, CIO at CareGroup Healthcare System jhalamka@caregroup.harvard.edu or Carl Ascenzo, CIO of BCBSMA	PHIT_09
MA	Statewide Implementation of Electronic Health Records	Performs a rigorous evaluation of the impact of a Statewide implementation program on EHR adoption by rural and non-rural ambulatory care practices and its impact on medication errors and the quality of ambulatory care as a collaborative effort among providers, insurers, and businesses in cooperation with the State government.	David Bates, Brigham and Women's Hospital, Boston, MA 617-732-6040	AHRQ_043
MA	SAFEHealth—Secure Architecture for Exchanging Health Information	Creates a local heath information exchange infrastructure that integrates workflow and improves communication for patients, healthcare providers, payers, and public health agencies.	Lawrence Garber, Fallon Clinic, Inc. Worcester, MA	AHRQ_044
MA	EMS Based TIPI-IS Cardiac Care QI-Error Reduction System	Implements the time-insensitive predictive instruments built into the computerized electrocardiograph in emergency medical service settings and emergency departments; also evaluates its impact on reducing errors and avoidable delays in emergency care.	Harry Selker, New England Medical Center, Boston, MA 617-636-5009 HSelker@tufts-nemc.org	AHRQ_045
MA	Improving Pediatric Safety and Quality with Health Care IT	Systematically assess improvements in patient safety and experience of care associated with implementation of four decision support function embedded in an electronic health record: 1) the influence of weight based dosing on pediatric adverse drug events; 2) the influence of a test result tracking system on appropriate followup of ordered tests; 3) the influence of automated reminders on symptom monitoring and medications for children with asthma and attention deficit disorder.	Timothy Ferris, Massachusetts General Hospital, Boston, MA	AHRQ_046
MA	Improving Safety and Quality with Outpatient Order Entry	Examines the impact of integrating ambulatory CPOE with advanced CDSS on safety and quality in the ambulatory setting, its organizational efficiency, workflow, and satisfaction, and conducts a cost-benefit analysis.	Tejal Gandhi, Brigham and Women's Hospital, Boston, MA	AHRQ_047
MA	Value of Imaging-Related Information Technology	Assesses the impact of Medical Imaging Informatics on health care costs and quality and develops a business case related to the acquisition and implementation of automated radiology systems; develops a financial model to demonstrate the impact of these systems on provider systems and healthcare quality.	Scott Gazelle, Massachusetts General Hospital, Boston, MA	AHRQ_048

MA	Health Information Technology in the Nursing Home	Assesses the effects of clinical decision support systems in nursing homes on medication ordering and monitoring for residents in long term care setting; also tracks costs and assesses productivity, impact, and nursing home culture and organization.	Jerry Gurwitz, University of Massachusetts, Worcester, MA	AHRQ_049
MA	Evaluating Smart Forms and Quality Dashboards in an EHR	Assesses the value of health IT to clinicians through creation of CDSS tools integrated with clinical documentation workflow and physician performance feedback, its impact on clinical decision support and quality assessment, and its cost-effectiveness.	Blackford Middleton, Brigham and Women's Hospital, Boston, MA 617-732-6040	AHRQ_050
MA	ParentLink: Better and Safer Emergency Care for Children	Evaluates the completeness and accuracy of information on symptoms, disease conditions, medications, and allergies generated by parents using a patient-centered health technology called ParentLink compared to information documented by emergency department physicians and nurses; ParentLink's impact on patient safety and quality.	Stephen Porter, Children's Hospital Corporation, Boston, MA 617-355-2136	AHRQ_051
MA	E-Prescribing Impact on Patient Safety, Use, and Cost	Assesses the impact of a Statewide rollout of e-prescribing using PocketScript® software and its effect on safety, quality, cost, formulary compliance and outcomes.	Joel Weissman, Massachusetts General Hospital, Boston, MA	AHRQ_052
MD	Lumetra	Lumetra, assisted by key partners, is providing support to small- to medium-sized practices in implementing EHRs free of charge. Lumetra is helping physician practices: Assess practice readiness, Define EHR goals, Select an EHR vendor*, Prepare staff and office for EHRs, Conduct post implementation evaluations, Review EHR implementation and impact analysis	410-740-8756 doqit-ca@caqio.sdps.org	DOQ_20a
MD	Delmarva Foundation for Medical Care	Delmarva Foundation, the Quality Improvement Organization (QIO) for Maryland and the District of Columbia will provide technical assistance and support free of charge to adult primary care physician practices	Carmen Tyler Winston Director, DOQ-IT Program 202-496-6559 Corporate HQ: 410-822-0697 doqitdelmarva@dfmc.org	DOQ_20b
MD	Community Based Intervention System (CBIS)	Johns Hopkins Bloomberg School of Public Health and the Center for Communication Programs is working with Appalachian Regional Healthcare, Inc. to provide assistance in connecting and improving the healthcare services provided to the residents of Central Appalachia by creating elements of a Clinical Information System.	Amanda Fryman Appalachian Regional Healthcare, Inc. 1220 Harrodsburg Road, P.O. Box 8086 Lexington, KY 40533 859-226-2433 afryman@arh.org	HIE_055
MD	MD/DC Collaborative for Health Information Technology	This is an alliance of physician group practices, hospitals, health plans, and academic medical centers proposing to design and implement a regional health information organization (RHIO). It is a non-profit, incorporated entity intended to link all parts of the healthcare delivery system for health information exchange.	Victor Plavner, MD 10420 Little Patuxent Parkway Suite 400, Columbia, MD 21044 410-992-1880 vplavner@collaborativeforhit.org	HIE_056* RHIO_056
MD	Smart E-Records across Continuum of Health (SERCH)	This HIE proposes to assist with continuity of care for elderly persons by developing the infrastructure for interoperability between healthcare delivery system participants, and specifically by using a "Smart E-Records" electronic medical record.	Dr. Michael Gloth 210 Business Center Dr Reisterstown, MD 21136 410-526-1490 mgloth@victorysprings.com	HIE_057
MD	HHCC Practice Patterns and Outcomes	This HIE proposes to develop a system that will collect, store, and analyze home health care, based on the Home Health Care Classification (HHCC) System.	Ruth G. Irwin, RN MS 509 Quaint Acres Dr. Silver Spring, MD 20904 301-622-9595 ruthgirwin@aol.com	HIE_058

MD	Community HealthLink Care: Regional EMR	Develops a secure, comprehensive, virtual health record for medically underserved patients that will lead to the implementation of a health IT infrastructure necessary to support a single, shared EMR application to promote the community-wide exchange of patient information for clinical decision support, research, and disease management on behalf of low-income, uninsured people.	Thomas Lewis, Primary Care Coalition of Montgomery County Silver Spring, MD	AHRQ_042
ME	Northeast Health Care Quality Foundation	(No specific DOQ-IT information) Mission is to encourage and promote improvement in health care for the Medicare beneficiaries in our service region. We provide educational materials and tools for identified quality improvement projects, and conduct reviews to ensure quality of care for beneficiaries and protect the Medicare Trust Fund.	1-800-772-0151 603-749-1641 info@nhcqf.org	DOQ_19
ME	Regional Picture Archiving Communication System for Northern Maine	This is a proposal for a hospital-based, regional diagnostic imaging data repository based around an existing picture archiving and communications system (PACS). The current, single site system is also linked with other information systems within the hospital. The proposal is to extend the existing PACS to include all ten participating hospitals in the region through a virtual private network.	Deborah Sanford P.O. Box 404 Bangor, Maine 44020404 207-973-7058 dsanford@emh.org	HIE_054
ME	Anthem Blue Cross Blue Shield of Maine	Anthem Blue Cross Blue Shield of Maine administers a program that resembles the Bridges for Excellence model. The health plan's program uses payment differentials and rewards specific physicians for improving health outcomes by implementing technology improvements.	Anthem Blue Cross and Blue Shield 2 Gannett Drive South Portland, ME 04106	PHIT_07
ME	The Chronic Care Technology Planning Project	Plans for standard exchange of clinical information for patients with chronic disease when transitioning from acute to non-acute care settings between primary care physicians, outpatient specialists, home health providers, nursing homes, and hospitals; creates an Institute for Healthcare Improvement Breakthrough Series Learning Collaborative to build on their work implementing the Chronic Care Model by enhancing the use of IT.	John Branscombe, The Aroostook Medical Center, Presque Isle, ME	AHRQ_038
ME	Midcoast Maine Patient Safety with IT Integration	Develops new systems and a high level of integration and cooperation in four significant areas: medication management, patient discharge, high-level integration of information, and the development of a new paradigm for evaluating, selecting, and implementing new technologies.	Maureen Buckley, Northeast Health Foundation, Rockland, ME	AHRQ_039
ME	Improving Care in a Rural Region with Consolidated Imaging	Implements and evaluates the results of the Consolidated Imaging—Picture Archiving and Communication System (a shared, standards-based, interoperable health information technology) that makes radiology images available for review within minutes of when they are acquired.	Robert Coleman, Maine Medical Center, Portland, ME	AHRQ_040
ME	Improving HIT Implementation in a Rural Health System	Implements an outpatient EMR in a rural health system using distinct phases to match the expected learning curve and to reduce the potential loss of practice productivity often associated with the implementation of an EMR; also collects data about patient safety, quality, access, cost, and productivity.	Daniel Mingle, Maine General Medical Center, Augusta, ME	AHRQ_041
MI	Michigan Peer Review Organization	MPRO offers assistance at each stage of the electronic health record adoption process including assessment, planning, selection, implementation, and post implementation. MPRO can help offices maximize efficiencies while documenting quality improvement, using information technology. MPRO, Michigan's Medicare Quality Improvement Organization, is conducting a survey on the topic of health information technology (HIT). The intent of the survey is to collect information about how physicians in Michigan are using HIT in their office.	Marie Beisel, RN, MSN, CPHQ Project Director 248-465-7338 mbeisel@mpro.org	DOQ_22
MI	Inter-Plan Guideline Adherence	This is an alliance of health plans, hospitals, and employers to evaluate performance of health plans. They propose to take their evaluation tool and provide information to the provider/physician level to improve performance and adherence to treatment guidelines.	Dennis White 1709 Pontiac Trail Ann Arbor, MI 48105 734-741-0333 dcwhite@umich.edu	HIE_065

MI	Voices of Detroit Initiative	This is an alliance of local health systems and safety net providers to provide free services to uninsured persons. They are now proposing to fully automate the administrative functions needed to provide care to this population, including specialist referrals and exchanging patient medical histories. They will use a web-based platform for enrollment, disenrollment, referral, prevention, outcomes measuring, and other administrative functions. The system is also designed to identify co-morbidities early and assist with patient compliance with treatments.	Lucille Smith 4201 St. Antoine Detroit, MI 48323 313-832-4246 slucille@med.wayne.edu	HIE_066
MI	Implementing Interorganizational EMR to Improve Care for Disadvantaged Populations	The HIE is a collaboration between a local university, hospitals, and the state health department to develop a an electronic medical record tied to a network allowing secure exchange of clinical information. The university already has an HIE network in place in 32 clinics at 11 sites in Lansing Michigan using an existing electronic medical record system. They are currently networked with some local physician practices for purposes of treating Medicaid patients.	Michael H. Zaroukian, MD, PhD, FACP EMR Medical Director B-325 Clinical Center East Lansing, MI 48824 517-353-4811 michael.zaroukian@ht.msu.edu	HIE_067
MI	Use of Smart Card Technology to Promote Community-Wide Diabetic Quality Improvement	This HIE is a broad collaboration of diabetes health stakeholders proposing to implement "smart card" technology to help diabetes patients and providers. The technology is used to access medical records, treatment protocols, and evidence-based medical practices.	Kent Bottles, MD 1000 Monroe Ave NW Grand Rapids, MI 49503 616-732-6206 kent_bottles@grmerc.net	HIE_068
MI	CLEAN: Communities Leveraging e-Health for Asthma Needs	This is a broad collaboration of asthma health stakeholders using a web-based application to exchange personal health information on pediatric asthma patients. Participants are in the process of implementing information system platforms to integrate with the web-based application for diagnostic, treatment, documentation, and scheduling purposes. They are proposing to demonstrate measurable improvements in outcomes as a result of using their system.	Angela R. Tiberio, MD 100 Michigan Ave. NE - MC 843 Grand Rapids, MI 49503 616-391-9811 angela.tiberio@spectrum-health.org	HIE_069
MI	Picture Archiving and Communications Systems	The HIE is a collaboration of hospitals, radiology specialists, and physician practices to implement an diagnostic imaging data repository. There is an existing picture archiving and communication system at one of the hospitals. They propose to implement a PACS system throughout the region to allow hospitals and physicians to improve access to diagnostic imaging information and lower the cost of care.	Dean R Feldpausch 1210 W Saginaw St. Lansing, MI 48915 517-364-6445 dean.Feldpausch@sparrow.org	HIE_070
MI	The Health Care Interchange of Michigan Care Data Exchange	This HIE is an alliance of major health plans, hospitals, a vendor and a physician group in the region. They use a "federated," or "peer-to-peer" approach to exchange both clinical and administrative information. The focus of their pilot is Medicaid beneficiaries enrolled in managed care. The goal is to improve continuity of care, enhance patient compliance, and allow communication of patient information when transient Medicaid beneficiaries change providers.	Clyde Hanks, COO P.O. Box 80745 Lansing, MI 48908 517-886-8380 chanks@hcim.org	HIE_071
MI	Upper Peninsula Health Data Repository	This is a collaboration of rural health systems and hospitals that has come together to share common services over the Internet. Currently they provide services such as eligibility verification, claims processing, clinic scheduling, physician billing, and other administrative services. Other collaborative services include telemedicine and access to immunization and other state health records. They are also developing an electronic medical record to serve as an archive and repository of information.	Sally Davis 580 West College Avenue Marquette, MI 49855 906-225-3120 sdavis@mgh.org	HIE_072
MI	HIT Planning for a Critical Access Hospital Partnership	Plans, develops, and implements health IT to assist local rural communities in improving health care access, building local and regional resources to monitor the quality of healthcare, and expanding the use of health IT educational, communication, and clinical applications.	Donald Wheeler, Baraga County Memorial Hospital, L'Anse, MI	AHRQ_053
MI	Bar Coding for Patient Safety in Northern Michigan	Implements a bar-coding application to an existing integrated health IT network that alerts providers to potential drug interactions and allergic reactions, tracks "near misses," and provides a permanent record of the patient's medication history that is accessible by providers at any site.	Randi Oehlers, Munson Medical Center, Traverse City, MI 231-935-5199 oehlerr@trinity-health.org	AHRQ_054

MI	HIT Support for Safe Nursing Care	Examines the use of the HANDS software system, an health IT-supported care planning process for nursing care, and its ability to be transferable between nurses, units, and health care settings.	Gail Keenan, Regents of the University of Michigan, Ann Arbor, MI 734-763-3705 gkeenan@umich.edu	AHRQ_055
MN	Stratis Health	(No specific DOQ-IT information) Mission: Stratis Health is a non-profit independent quality improvement organization that collaborates with providers and consumers to improve health care., Vision: Stratis Health's vision is that of a health care system that supports an informed, activated consumer and competent, satisfied health care professionals working in settings that promote optimum care and reduce chance of error.	952.854.3306 1-877-STRATIS info@stratishealth.org	DOQ_23
MN	Patient Management System for Emergency Health Preparedness	This HIE is a collaboration of hospitals and clinics in an 18 county region of the State. They provide a number of services, including immunization registry, eligibility verification, and claims processing. They are looking to expand into automated reporting to public health agencies.	Cheryl M. Stephens 404 W. Superior St., Suite 250 Duluth, MN 55802 218-625-5515 cstephens@medinfosystems.org	HIE_073
MN	MN Collaborative Health Information Exchange System	This HIE is a collaboration between health plans, health systems, and the State health department to develop a benefit eligibility verification and claims status system.	Dave Moertel 200 1st Street SW Rochester, MN 55905 507-284-1762 moertel.david@mayo.edu	HIE_074
MN	Central Minnesota Health Information Network	This HIE proposes to install a hybrid paper medical and computer-based information system based on open system software to better coordinate clinical records and administrative functions to better analyze outcomes and resource use from clinical data.	Jeffrey L. Blair 500 Aberdeen Drive Waite Park, MN 56387 320-252-8550 cmhin@cloudnet.com	HIE_075
MN	PKI Model & MedNet (This project is potentially inactive)	MCHEC worked with HealthKey to build a PKI model in Minnesota to support healthcare data exchange. The organization also initiated MedNet, a private, non-proprietary, statewide, public-private health care telecommunications network in Minnesota, which is exchanging both administrative data and an exchange of certain kinds of public health data. They are also continuing to exchange and standardize clinical data between public health and providers. They are also looking at building the business case for clinical data exchange.	Walter G. Suarez, MD Executive Director, MHDI 651-917-6700 walter.suarez@mhdi.org	HIE_143
MN	Microsoft and University of Minnesota Physicians (UMPhysicians)	University of Minnesota Physicians (UMPhysicians) wanted to find a way of reducing the cost and complexity of paper-based medical records. Used Allscripts Healthcare Solutions to deploy a Microsoft® Windows®-based EMR solution that includes the deployment of nearly 500 wirelessly enabled Windows Mobile™-based Pocket PC devices that are used by UMP staff for dictation, reviewing patient medical records, and other daily activities.	Todd Carlon Chief Administrative Officer University of Minnesota Physicians 651-603-5320	PHIT_10
MN	A Community-Shared Clinical Abstract to Improve Care	Plans the use of IT to enhance communication at care transitions and develops an implementation plan for a community- and patient-shared EMR abstract that will be available at the point of care.	Barry Bershow, Fairview Health Services, Minneapolis, MN	AHRQ_056
MN	HIT Strategic Plan of SW Minnesota Health Providers	Develops a regional health IT strategic plan between 28 healthcare providers including a comprehensive needs assessment of all of the participating organizations, prioritization of needs, identification of health IT solutions to prioritized needs, and development of appropriate implementation plans.	Charles Ness, Granite Falls Municipal Hospital, Granite Falls, MN	AHRQ_057

MN	HIT-based Regional Medication Management Pharmacy System	Implements an interactive video-conferencing system at rural hospitals to provide continuing education for pharmacist and pharmacy technicians as well as a model for bedside verification of medication administration and medication bar coding; also evaluates structure, process, and outcomes related to improvement of patient safety and more effective patient medication management.	Mark Schmidt, Clouquet Community Memorial, Clouquet, MN	AHRQ_058
MO	Bridges-to-Excellence (General)	In July 2004, United Healthcare became the first health care company to license the BTE model, working with employers in Omaha, St Louis, Dayton and South Florida to offer network doctors certain incentives for earning NCQA recognition.	Susan Dorsey, Director NBCH 1015 18th Street N.W., Suite 730 Washington, DC 20036 Sdorsey@nbch.org 202-775-9300	BTE_02f
MO	Primaris	Primaris offers primary care physicians free consultation on how to select and implement the correct EHR for their office. All we ask in return is your commitment within the next 12 to 18 months. If you are already utilizing an EHR, we will show you how to achieve full benefit from the system. This includes quality improvement and pay for performance functions.	Sandra Pogones 800-735-6776 ext. 1158 Mobile: 573-230-9801 spogones@moqio.sdps.org	DOQ_25a
MO	Health Care Excel	Through this initiative, Health Care Excel (HCE), the Medicare Quality Improvement Organization for Indiana, will assist primary care physicians in adopting Electronic Health Record (EHR) systems with the ultimate goal of improving office efficiency and patient outcomes. This initiative is sponsored by the Centers for Medicare & Medicaid Services (CMS).	Darlene Skelton, 812-234-1499 573-634-3639	DOQ_25b
MO	Wellpoint eRx or Paper Reduction	WellPoint is spearheading an electronic initiative at a cost of $40 million that will reach 19,000 physicians. In California, Georgia, Missouri, and Wisconsin, physicians will be given the opportunity to choose from either of two electronic packages: a Prescription Improvement Package or a Paperwork Reduction Package.	Ron J. Ponder, PhD, EVP, Information Services, WellPoint or Nadia Leather - CGEY nadia.leather@capgemini.com 212-314-8235	PHIT_02c
MO	Project InfoCare	Creates a community-wide EMR with integrated clinical decision support that is available across the continuum of care including a rural hospital, a home health agency, 14 physician clinics, and 5 long-term care facilities.	Peggy Esch, Citizens Memorial Hospital, Bolivar, MO	AHRQ_061
MS	McKesson Health Solutions	Chosen to provide disease management services to Mississippi Medicare fee-for-service beneficiaries with heart failure and diabetes. Partnering with Joslin Diabetes Center, Boston, MA. Approximately 20,000 beneficiaries will be eligible for the program.	Dr. Sandeep Wadhwa, VP Care Management Services, McKesson Health Solutions	CCIP_7
MS	Mississippi Information and Quality Healthcare	Information & Quality Healthcare, IQH, is the Medicare Quality Improvement Organization for Mississippi. By serving as a resource to the state's healthcare providers and to the Medicare beneficiaries, IQH seeks to fulfill its vision to be a leader in promoting a quality and cost-effective healthcare system.	601-957-1575 1-800-633-4227	DOQ_24
MS	Mississippi U Project	TheraDoc, a Salt Lake City-based vendor of clinical decision support software, is installing software at the University of Mississippi Medical Center (UMC) to collect and analyze data in real time from information systems in admissions, the emergency department, surgical units, the pharmacy, laboratory and other departments dealing with infectious diseases.	Stanley W. Chapman, M.D., Director of the Department of Infectious Diseases Department of Health, UMC	HIE_139
MS	Creating Online NICU Networks to Educate, Consult & Team	Develops, implements, and evaluates a cooperative effort using health IT to facilitate a continuum of appropriate medical and developmental care from the time infants are admitted to Neonatal Intensive Care Units through the transition process to community-based health care services for infants most at-risk for long-term neurodevelopmental problems.	Jane Siders, The University of Southern Mississippi, Hattiesburg, MS	AHRQ_059

MS	Detecting Med Errors in Rural Hospitals Using Technology	Implements and evaluates a voluntary system for reporting medical errors and adverse drug events in eight small rural hospitals; identifies barriers to technology, describes the epidemiology and root causes of the errors, formulates quality-improvement interventions, and disseminates the results.	Andrew Brown, University of Mississippi, Jackson, MS 601-984-6850 abrown@medicine.umsmed.edu	AHRQ_060
MT	Mountain-Pacific Quality Health Foundation	(No specific DOQ-IT information) Mountain-Pacific Quality Health Foundation is the quality improvement organization (QIO) for Montana, Wyoming, Hawaii, and the territories of Guam, the Commonwealth of the Northern Marianas and American Samoa. The Foundation operates out of offices in Helena, Montana; Cheyenne, Wyoming; and Honolulu, Hawaii.	406-443-4020 800-497-8232 montana@mpqhf.org	DOQ_26
MT	Using Health Information Exchange to Reduce Medication Errors in the Rural Healthcare Setting	This HIE proposes to install a medical management system in a hospital and clinic to identify medication errors. This will include the infrastructure for recording of medications, clinical decision support tools and prompts, and adverse drug interactions and reactions.	Patricia Jay Coon, MD P.O. Box 37000 Billings, MT 59107 406-238-2287 pcoon@billingsclinic.org	HIE_076
MT	Community Health Access Partnership	The Community Health Access Partnership (CHAP), an alliance of public health programs and local hospitals and clinics serving uninsured and indigents, received a grant from HRSA to implement a "community medical record" which tracks patient demographic data, sodial data, and referrals. The system does not currently track other medical information and they are looking to expand and create an electronic medical record. They plan to install an "integration engine" to identify information that can be entered into a web-based application that will track patients domicile, services, medications, and physician office visits.	Judy Stewart P.O. Box 35033 Billings, MT 59107 406-247-3290 judys@ycchd.org	HIE_077
MT	Planning the Implementation of HIT in a Rural Setting	Plans the development and implementation of a health IT infrastructure throughout three rural counties including high-speed Internet access, CPOE, CDSS, EHR, and continuity of care record templates.	William Reiter, Community Hospital of Anaconda, Inc., Anaconda, MT	AHRQ_062
MT	Decreasing ADEs in Montana Frontier Critical Access Hospitals through HIT	Assesses opportunities to decrease adverse drug events and medication errors in frontier Montana Critical Access Hospitals; identifies appropriate, cost effective health IT solutions to challenges in medication use.	Kipman Smith, Townsend Health Systems, Inc., Townsend, MT	AHRQ_063
MT	Home Heart Failure (HF) Care Comparing Patient-Driven Technology Models	Assesses the impact of health IT on clinical and financial outcomes for patients with symptomatic congestive heart failure living in a rural area, including telemonitoring of vital signs and symptoms, evaluation of Technology Supported Case Management, and Technology Support Self Management.	Lee Goldberg, St. Vincent Healthcare Foundation, Billings, MT	AHRQ_064
NC	Bridges-to-Excellence (General)	CIGNA HealthCare is licensing the Bridges to Excellence program and is working with employers to pursue a pay-for-performance effort.	Susan Dorsey, Director NBCH 1015 18th Street N.W., Suite 730 Washington, DC 20036 Sdorsey@nbch.org 202-775-9300	BTE_02i
NC	Medical Review of North Carolina	(No specific DOQ-IT information)	919-380-9860 800-682-2650	DOQ_33
NC	WNC Health Network	This HIE is a collaboration of hospitals to develop an electronic medical information system between the hospitals and their affiliated provider organizations.	Gary Bowers, JD WNC Health Network, 501 Biltmore Avenue, Asheville, NC 28801 828-257-2983 Gary.Bowers@wnchn.org	HIE_095

NC	Perinatal EMR	This HIE is at the University of North Carolina medical center. It has a standard, paper-based prenatal medical tracking record. They propose to develop and electronic version of a prenatal medical record, including software that allows patient access available over the Internet.	Dr. Raj Gopalan MD., MSIS 101 Manning Drive Chapel Hill, NC 27514 919-966-3950 rgopalan@unch.unc.edu	HIE_096
NC	Patient Safety Net for Heart Failure Disease Management	This HIE is based in a hospital and proposes to establish a disease management program for congestive heart failure patients.	Van J. Stitt, Jr., MD, PhD, VP, CMO 2525 Court Drive Gastonia, NC 28053 704-834-2768 stittv@gmh.org	HIE_097
NC	North Carolina Health Information Exchange Consortium (NCHIEC)	This HIE is a partnership between a health system, medical group practices, the State health department, and a software vendor. They have implemented a pilot project for health surveillance that has been used to exchange clinical information between hospitals in the partnership. They wish to expand the service to study the impact on patient safety and public health and to involve other hospitals and health systems.	Judy O'Neal 3000 New Bern Avenue Raleigh, NC 27610 919-350-8205 JONeal@wakemed.org	HIE_098
NC	NC Community Medication Management Project	This HIE is an alliance of hospitals, group practices, health departments, employers and other stakeholders that is implementing a web-based medication history record, e-prescribing and refill system.	Holt Anderson POB 13048, Research Triangle Park NC 27709-3048 919-558-9258 holt@nchica.org	HIE_099
NC	Automated Adverse Drug Events Detection and Intervention	Establishes an automated surveillance system for detecting, reporting, and intervening as well as measuring the incidence and nature of adverse drug events suffered by patients.	Peter Kilbridge, Duke University Durham, NC	AHRQ_074
NC	Showing Health Information Value in a Community Network	Assesses the costs and benefits of health IT in an established community-wide network of academic, private and public healthcare facilities created to share clinical information for the purpose of population-based care management of Medicaid beneficiaries.	David Lobach, Duke University Durham, NC	AHRQ_075
ND	North Dakota Health Care Review	NDHCRI is participating in Doctors' Office Quality Information Technology (DOQ-IT) with small-to-medium sized physician offices. This initiative promotes the adoption of electronic health record (EHR) systems and information technology (IT). The vision is to enhance access to patient information, decision support, and reference data, as well as improving patient-clinician communications.	1-800-472- 2902 701-852-4231 lmalchose@ndqio.sdps.org	DOQ_34
NE	Bridges-to-Excellence (General)	In July 2004, United Healthcare became the first health care company to license the BTE model, working with employers in Omaha, St Louis, Dayton and South Florida to offer network doctors certain incentives for earning NCQA recognition.	Susan Dorsey, Director NBCH 1015 18th Street N.W., Suite 730 Washington, DC 20036 Sdorsey@nbch.org 202-775-9300	BTE_02e
NE	CIMRO of Nebraska	(No specific DOQ-IT information)	1-800-458-4262 402-476-1399 webmaster@cimronebraska.org	DOQ_27
NE	Nebraska Panhandle Regional Health Record Planning	This RHIO is a collaboration between the Rural Healthcare Cooperative Network, Panhandle Partnership for Health and Human Services, Panhandle Public Health District, and the University of Nebraska Public Policy Center. It is implementing the infrastructure for an electronic health record to serve the region. The infrastructure will use existing networks that connect hospitals, clinics, providers, and other health stakeholders in a rural area.	Joan Frances, Executive Director Rural Healthcare Cooperative Network, 601 High School Street Kimball NE 69145 308-235-4211 pphhsvision@earthlink.net	HIE_078

NE	Behavioral Health MIS Integration Project	This HIE proposes acquisition of hardware and software to link information system among behavioral health providers in the county.	Wende Baker, Executive Director P.O. Box 30205 Lincoln, NE 68503 402-441-8144	HIE_079
NE	HIT Plan for Region V Behavioral Health Care Providers	Plans, develops, and implements a methodology for behavioral health care providers to standardize core shared data elements; designs an integrated management information system for the sharing of health care data and information among rural and urban health care providers; connects rural providers to urban providers; and develops messaging capabilities between primary care and behavioral health care providers.	Wende Baker, Heartland Health Alliance, Holbrook, NE	AHRQ_065
NE	Regional Health Records for Frontier Communities	Plans for the implementation of a regional health record system within established networks of rural hospitals, clinics, public health providers, behavioral health providers, and others across a 14,000 sq mile remote area.	Nancy Shank, Chadron Community Hospital, Lincoln, NE	AHRQ_066
NH	Northeast Health Care Quality Foundation	(No specific DOQ-IT information) Mission is to encourage and promote improvement in health care for the Medicare beneficiaries in our service region. We provide educational materials and tools for identified quality improvement projects, and conduct reviews to ensure quality of care for beneficiaries and protect the Medicare Trust Fund.	1-800-772-0151 603-749-1641 info@nhcqf.org	DOQ_29
NH	Furthering User-Friendly Systems for Informatics and Patient Online. (FUSION)	This HIE has an established, web-based patient portal allowing appointment scheduling requests, medication refills, emails to providers, updating patient and insurance information, and downloading forms. They are proposing to link the patient portal with existing electronic medical record systems at three separate provider locations.	Barbara Walters, DO MBA Dartmouth Hitchcock Clinic 1 Bedford Farms, Bedford, NH 03110 603-629-1101 Barbara.A.Walters@Hitchcock.org	HIE_080
NH	Electronic Communications Across Provider Settings	Integrates an office-based EMR within an acute care hospital, rural community health centers, a community mental health center, a family medicine residency, private physician practices, and a home nursing service to improve use of the EMR as a clinical tool, integrate clinical data, and increase access to the data.	Deane Morrison, Concord Hospital, Concord, NH	AHRQ_067
NJ	Peer Review Organization of NJ	PRONJ Role: • Sponsor recruitment activities for physicians interested in participating in DOQ-IT project, • Select participating physicians • Work with physician office staff to conduct an assessment of the practice to identify barriers and opportunities, and develop a business case for successful EHR implementation, • Launch continuous quality improvement (QI) activities, based on EHR capabilities and data reporting • Help identify EHR systems that meet practice needs	Carolyn Hezekiah Hoitela, MLS 732-238-5570 ext. 2012	DOQ_30
NJ	Medication Information Network Exchange, (MINE)	The HIE is set up to establish a medication management system among the participants that will reduce errors. It will also give providers access to patients' histories.	Linda Woods, CIO 727 North Beers Street Holmdel, NJ 07733 732-739-5957 linda.woods@bchs.com	HIE_081
NJ	NJ Primary Care Association EMR Project	This HIE is a collaboration of federally qualified health centers proposing to develop a state-wide medical record data repository tying together all health centers in the State.	Katherine Grant-Davis 14 Washington Road, Building Two Princeton Junction, NJ 8550 609-275-8886 njpca2@aol.com	HIE_082

NJ	Virtua Health, GE Healthcare	Virtua Health is a multi-hospital healthcare system. Hospitals will be digitally based with complete electronic medical records, computerized patient rooms featuring technologies such as beds that monitor patient vital signs and the ability to convert from a medical room to an intensive care room and back without ever having to move the patient. In 2004 Virtua partnered with General Electric to position itself at the forefront of technology and the delivery of high quality care. The comprehensive strategic alliance with GE Healthcare encompasses technology optimization, leadership development, and clinical and operational excellence.	Richard P. Miller, president and CEO of Virtua Health, 888-Virtua-3	PHIT_11
NJ	NJ Department of Banking and Insurance	The NJ Department of Banking and Insurance launched an effort Wednesday to create a statewide electronic medical records system. The system would allow physicians to share patients' medical records statewide. The Department and Healthcare Information Networks and Technologies (HINT) and Health Insurance Portability and Accountability Act (HIPAA) Task Force will spearhead the project.	Donald Bryan, Acting Commissioner NJ Dept of Banking and Insurance 20 West State St., Trenton, NJ 08625 commissioner@dobi.state.nj.us	PHIT_12
NJ	Horizon Blue Cross Blue Shield of NJ	Horizon will be rolling out a similar, albeit smaller, [electronic] initiative by the end of the year. The Horizon initiative earmarks $5 million for providers to receive a free desktop computer or PDA. The Horizon effort will also have multipayer abilities, so that other health plans' formularies, and patient eligibility data are available to the provider for review.	Jay Patel, Horizon BCBS, Horizon Healthcare of New Jersey P.O. Box 820, Newark, NJ 07101 1-800-355-2583	PHIT_13
NM	New Mexico Medical Review Association	(No specific DOQ-IT information) under development	Marcia Tarasenko, RN, BSN, MBA/HC/ Quality Improvement Manager-DOQ-IT Project, 505-998-9735, 1-800-663-6351 mtarasenko@nmqio.sdps.org	DOQ_31
NM	eMS Health	This is a consortium of multiple sclerosis centers around the country that have established the eMS project as a telehealth program designed to better educate health professionals, patients and their caregivers by allowing remote access to information.	Peggy Swoveland, Ph.D. 1438 Fischer Road Las Cruces, NM 88007 505-541-5955 ptswo@aol.com	HIE_083
NM	Project ECHO—Extension for Community Healthcare Outcomes	Connects urban medical center disease experts with rural general practitioners and community health representatives over a telehealth network to effectively treat patients with chronic, common and complex diseases who do not have direct access to specialty healthcare providers.	Sanjeev Arora University of New Mexico, Albuquerque, NM SArora@salud.unm.edu	AHRQ_068
NM	New Mexico Health Information Collaborative	Develops a community-wide HIE collaborative in a rural area that will give patients and providers access to comprehensive clinical data on the Internet; develops disease-management prototypes on diabetes, pediatric asthma, depression, and low back pain and evaluates the development, implementation, and outcomes of the collaborative.	Martin Hickey, Lovelace Clinic Foundation, Albuquerque, NM	AHRQ_069
NV	HealthInsight	HealthInsight is a private, non-profit QIO whose mission is to be a catalyst in the transformation and improvement of the health care system. In our thirty-year history, HealthInsight staff has worked with the health care community on initiatives to improve the quality of care delivered in Nevada and Utah. The goal being to: Educate physician offices on EHR system solutions and alternatives, Provide implementation and quality improvement assistance, Assist physician offices in migrating from paper-based health records to EHR systems that suit their clinics' needs, Assist those currently using an EHR in using their system more effectively.	Sharon Donnelly (Medicare Beneficiaries) http://www.healthinsight.org/contact.html 702-385-9933 http://www.healthinsight.org/contact.html	DOQ_28
NY	Bridges-to-Excellence (General)	(POL, DCL, CCL)	Susan Dorsey, Director NBCH 1015 18th Street N.W., Suite 730 Washington, DC 20036 Sdorsey@nbch.org 202-775-9300	BTE_02k

NY	UnitedHealthcare Services	UHS was chosen to provide DM in NY area. They will identify how to most effectively and efficiently improve performance measurement, data aggregation and reporting in the ambulatory care setting.	www.unitedhealthcare.com	CCIP_8
NY	IPRO	(No specific DOQ-IT information)	Alan Silver, MD, MPH, Medical Officer Susan Hollander, Assistant Director 516-326-7767 asilver2@nyqio.sdps.org shollander@nyqio.sdps.org	DOQ_32
NY	Implementing the EMR into the Pediatric Subspecialty areas of the Ambulatory Health Network.	This HIE has an adult, outpatient electronic medical record installed using the NextGen product, which they are expanding to serve their pediatric clinics and physician practices.	Joan Evanzia MIS Dept, 1045 39th Street Brooklyn, New York 11219 718-283-1892 jevanzia@maimonidesmed.org	HIE_084
NY	Western New York Emergency Department Triage Surveillance Project (WNYEDTSP)	This HIE is a consortium of health departments, academic medical centers, and hospitals that has developed a health surveillance system for emergency departments that reports infectious disease and other illnesses useful for biodefense and other epidemiology projects. In addition to public health information, the system is designed to provide eligibility, benefits, and claims information.	David G. Ellis, MD ECMC, 462 Grider Street Buffalo, NY 14215 716-898-5347 dellis@ecmc.edu	HIE_085
NY	Taconic Health Information Network and Community (THINC)	This HIE is based in an IPA with 500 physician practices. Their existing information exchange system has been in service for three years and networks physicians with a common set of services. Their proposed expansion would increase the number of physician practices, hospitals, clinical labs, and payer and use a standard electronic health record, email messaging, e-prescribing, and other services.	A. John Blair, III, MD, CEO / THINC Project Director One Summit Court, Suite 200 Fishkill, NY 12524 845-897-6359 jblair@taconicipa.com	HIE_086* RHIO_086
NY	AMI Online Network (AMION)	The HIE is an alliance of health stakeholders serving an unserved population in a rural area. They propose an electronic information exchange to allow provider access to medical information and educational resources using teleconferencing. Future expansion is envisioned to allow patient, employer and public health agency access.	Patricia L. Hale Ph.D., M.D., F.A.C.P. P.O. Box 452 Glens Falls, NY 12801 518-743-1993 screengem9@aol.com	HIE_087
NY	Continuum Health Partners - MedMined Virtual Surveillance Project	This HIE is a consortium of hospitals and medical group practices to establish the infrastructure for clinical support, biosurveillance, quality improvement, and outcomes measurement using proprietary data mining and artificial intelligence technology.	Beth Raucher, MD 1st Ave at 16th St New York, NY 10003 212-420-2853 braucher@bethisraelny.org	HIE_088
NY	NYC Syndromic Surveillance	This HIE is a collaboration between the New York City health department, hospital association, and Quest Diagnostics that has implemented a health syndrome surveillance system. They plan to expand and enhance the system to include standardized architecture and emergency departments.	Farzad Mostashari 125 Worth Street, Rm 315, CN-6 New York, NY 10013 212-788-5384 fmostash@health.nyc.gov	HIE_089
NY	Anti-Coagulation Lab results through Open standards Technology (ACLOT)	This HIE is a collaboration among health systems and academic medical centers to demonstrate a model for sharing clinical information with patients and practitioners. They are using a "federated," or peer-to-peer model of system interconnectivity and data sharing.	David Liss, Vice President, Govt. Relations & Strategic Initiatives 161 Fort Washington Avenue New York, NY 10032 212-305-1190, david.liss@nyp.org	HIE_090

NY	Advancing Therapeutics in Parkinson's (APT)	This HIE is a Parkinson's-specific disease community to increase participation and retention in clinical trials. They are also proposing to develop a disease management program for their target population, including distance learning and a central repository to acquire and distribute content.	Lucy Sargent 710 West 168th Street New York, NY 10032 800-457-6676 lsargent@pdf.org	HIE_091
NY	Community Health Center HIE Consortium	This HIE is a consortium of health systems and safety net providers focusing on development of an EMR serve community health centers in New York and New Mexico. They envision an EMR that would allow use by all parties involved in care of health center patients, and decision support tools to educate on medical errors and best practices. They also will create a disease management program for diabetes, asthma, and hypertension.	Feygele Jacobs 555 West 57th Street NY, NY 10019 212-939-9192 fjacobs@rchn.org	HIE_092
NY	Rochester HealthNet	This HIE is a collaboration between medical group practices, payers, and health systems to develop a patient registry for population tracking and quality improvement using evidence-based decision support tools for small and large medical practices, and educational materials for patients.	Albert Charbonneau 1150 University Avenue Rochester, NY 14607 585-442-0030 ac@rhealth.org	HIE_093
NY	Health-e-Access	This HIE is a collaboration between pediatric medical practices, health plans, academic medical centers, and preschool child care services to provide access to resources for disadvantaged and underserved preschool children. This will expand the existing Health-e-Access model for large child care facilities into smaller and home-based facilities. They will us a number of different methods, including mobile telehealth units.	Kenneth McConnochie, MD, MPH 601 Elmwood Avenue Pediatrics Box 777 Rochester, NY 14642 585-273-4119 Ken_McConnochie@urmc.rochester.edu	HIE_094
NY	University Physicians at Stony Brook (UPSB) and PatientKeeper ePrescription(TM) (Powered by DrFirst)	University Physicians at Stony Brook, the coordinating entity for a faculty practice of 500 physicians in Stony Brook, New York, is implementing PatientKeeper ePrescription (Powered by DrFirst) on behalf of its Practices as part of a mobile healthcare initiative to improve quality of care and patient safety. UPSB doctors are already using PatientKeeper Charge Capture to streamline the charge capture and billing processes. Electronic charge capture is a major advance over a paper system in recording the services and procedures the physicians provide to their patients.	Stephen S. Hau, PatientKeeper shau@patientkeeper.com 617-987-0304 or Ellen Dank Cohen ellen.cohen@stonybrook.edu 631-444-2055	PHIT_14
NY	Taconic Health Information Network and Community (THINC). Partners included: MedAllies, Taconic IPA, Healthvision, SureScripts, NextGen, Allscripts Healthcare Solutions, IBM	The Taconic Health Information Network and Community (THINC) is a multi-stakeholder, community-wide data exchange among community physicians, hospitals, reference laboratories, pharmacies, payers, employers, and consumers. Unique to THINC is the local, ongoing support provided by MedAllies, which provides training and support to community clinicians and their office staff to drive adoption. Project Participants: The Taconic IPA, a 2,300 independent practice association (IPA), is the lead organization of the THINC initiative. Other stakeholders include: Benedictine Hospital, Kingston Hospital, LabCorp, St. Francis Hospital, and Vassar Brothers Medical Center.	A. John Blair, III, MD 845-897-6359 jblair@taconicipa.com	PHIT_15
NY	Taconic IPA (TIPA) and MVP Health Plan	MVP Health Plan teamed with one exclusively contracted IPA, TIPA, which has strong provider group relationships and expertise in the local physician market. Taconic IPA (TIPA) operates a combined quality and HIT incentive program in which bonus payments are based on daily technology usage and patient outcomes. Physicians' bonuses are determined by their performance per member per month, and are based on 40% HIT usage and 60% quality outcomes. Shared a common desire— to change care from an organization-centric model to a community-oriented model through improvements in continuity of care and connectivity across providers. The two groups created MedAllies, a separate organization, providing general technical assistance, training, and IT and local vendor support to physician groups to move towards a highly integrated community data exchange.	Jerry Salkowe, MD Senior Medical Director for Quality Improvement jsalkowe@taconicipa.com John Blair, MD, President & CEO Taconic IPA, Inc.	PHIT_16

NY	Excellus BlueCross BlueShield health plan	Excellus health plan in New York operates a program similar to MedAllies in that it brings together a coalition including the health plan, an IPA, and an independent community group to focus on improving quality through the use of bonus payments. Under this program, the coalition pays out incentive bonuses to individual providers for their performance in meeting community-wide clinical guidelines for chronic conditions including diabetes, asthma, and coronary artery disease.	Kathleen Curtin, VP, Q & I Excellus Health Plan 205 Park Club Lane Buffalo, NY 14221 716-857-6204 Kathleen.Curtin@Excellus.com	PHIT_17
NY	Empire Blue Cross Blue Shield	Empire Blue Cross Blue Shield of New York paired with four other major, self-funded employers who purchase health care services in the NY area (IBM; Verizon Communications; PepsiCo, Inc.; and Xerox Corporation) to reward hospitals that adhere to Leapfrog standards around CPOE adoption and intensive care unit (ICU) staffing. Rather than directly fund technology investments, financial incentives are calculated based on hospital claims.	Deborah Bohren Empire BCBS, VP of Public Affairs 212-476-3552	PHIT_18
NY	New York-Presbyterian Hospital Partners With GE Medical Systems	New York-Presbyterian Hospital will implement leading edge tools for improving management, service quality and operational effectiveness. Employees will be trained in GE's quality and process improvement programs. This balanced approach is comprised of Six Sigma statistical methodologies, change-management strategies (Change Acceleration Process) and team-based problem solving techniques (Work-Out™).	Dr. Michael Berman, EVP and hospital director of NewYork-Presbyterian Hospital, 622 West 168th Street New York, NY 10032 212-305-2500	PHIT_19
NY	Capital District Physicians' Health Plan, Inc. (CDPHP) and Community Care Physicians, P.C. and Northeast Health	Data Sharing Initiative Improves the Delivery of Health Care Services. Expanding its efforts to support physicians by providing real-time patient information essential to the delivery of quality care, CDPHP has piloted data sharing initiatives with two area leading health care organizations—Community Care Physicians, P.C. and Northeast Health.	William J. Cromie, MD, MBA, President and CEO, CDPHP	PHIT_20
NY	Mayo Clinic and IBM	IBM and the Mayo Clinic embarked on a collaboration to realize a shared vision of information-based medicine. As a first step, IBM and Mayo Clinic have integrated 4.4 million patient records that were in non-integrated formats, into a unified system based on a standard technology platform that incorporates robust security and privacy features. This will allow physicians and researchers access to a comprehensive set of records that can be analyzed with the security and privacy needed to protect patient confidentiality and meet government standards.	Matthew McMahon IBM 914-766-4164 mattm@us.ibm.com	PHIT_21
NY	Planning Implementation of an EMR in a Rural Area	Researches the implementation of an EMR in the medical community and the use of electronic ordering; identifies a system that will allow for the seamless exchange of clinical information throughout the medical community.	Jay Federaman, Adirondack Medical Center, Saranac Lake, NY	AHRQ_070
NY	Creating an Evidence Base for Vision Rehabilitation	Implements the newly developed Electronic Vision Rehabilitation Record and its tools to evaluate the effectiveness of current best practices and help refine practice as the evidence indicates.	Betty Bird, Lighthouse International New York, NY BBIRD@lighthouse.org	AHRQ_071
NY	Taconic Health Information Network and Community	Adds a healthcare portal to the existing community-wide electronic data exchange which will allow for use of the current electronic messaging system along with migration to a full EMR; evaluates physician office efficiency improvement and cost reduction, payer return on investment, and safety and quality improvement.	John Blair III, Taconic IPA, Fishkill, NY jblair@taconicipa.com	AHRQ_072
NY	Valuation of Primary Care-Integrated Telehealth	Assesses the impact of a telehealth program on primary care utilization and cost for remote assessment and treatment of ill children in childcare and school sites.	Kenneth McConnochie, University of Rochester, Rochester, NY ken_mcconnochie@urmc.rochester.edu	AHRQ_073
OH	Bridges-to-Excellence (General)	In July 2004, United Healthcare became the first health care company to license the BTE model, working with employers in Omaha, St Louis, Dayton and South Florida to offer network doctors certain incentives for earning NCQA recognition.	Susan Dorsey, Director NBCH 1015 18th Street N.W., Suite 730 Washington, DC 20036 Sdorsey@nbch.org, 202-775-9300	BTE_02g

OH	Bridges-to-Excellence (DCL)	Enables physicians to achieve one-year or three-year recognition for high performance in diabetes care. Qualifying physicians receive up to $80 for each diabetic patient covered by a participating employer and plan. In addition, the program offers a suite of products and tools to help diabetic patients get engaged in their care, achieve better outcomes, and identify local physicians that meet the high performance measures.	NCQA 2000 L Street, NW, Suite 500 Washington, DC 20036 202-955-3500 Customersupport@ncqa.org	BTE_03a
OH	Ohio KePRO	n/a	216-447-9604 1-800-385-5080 droffice@ohqio.sdps.org	DOQ_35a
OH	Health Care Excel	Through this initiative, Health Care Excel (HCE), the Medicare Quality Improvement Organization for Indiana, will assist primary care physicians in adopting Electronic Health Record (EHR) systems with the ultimate goal of improving office efficiency and patient outcomes. This initiative is sponsored by the Centers for Medicare & Medicaid Services (CMS).	Darlene Skelton, 812-234-1499 614-752-9854	DOQ_35b
OH	HealthBridge	This HIE is a collaboration of health systems, payers, group practices, employers, and other stakeholders who have come together to develop an Internet portal for clinical information. Their platform includes secure connections to physician practices and hospitals, access to data at hospitals, and a clinical messaging system. They are looking to enhance their system by improving the speed of delivery of information needed for clinical decision making, aggregation of population health data, and cost reduction through use of a single infrastructure.	Robert Steffel 11300 Cornell Park Drive Suite 360 Cincinnati, OH 45242 513-469-7222 ext. 20 rsteffel@healthbridge.org Keith Hepp, VP of Business Development, 513-469-7222 x12 khepp@healthbridge.org	HIE_100
OH	Berger Health System CPOE	Pickaway County, a rural community served by a single hospital through Berger Health System's is investigating CPOE.	Andy Chileski 600 North Pickaway St. Circleville, OH 43113 740-420-8284 andy.chileski@bergerhealth.com	HIE_101
OH	Pathways to Medication Safety	The goal of this HIE initiative is improved patient safety and treatment through reduction in medication errors. This is a multi-stakeholder group consisting of two community based hospitals (RHH and Bedford), an academic medical center (UHC) based within an umbrella health care system (UHHS), and a private industry sponsor (MDG Medical). They will establish critical metrics to evaluate and implement automated medication delivery system designed for small to medium size community based hospitals.	Carol Fedor, ND, CCRC Center for Clinical Research University Hospitals of Cleveland 11100 Euclid Avenue, LKSD 1400 Cleveland, OH 44106 216-844-5524 carol.fedor@uhhs.com	HIE_102
OH	HealthLink Miami Valley	Increasing access to health and human services is the goal of this HIE. The Center for Healthy Communities (CHC) at Wright State University School of Medicine is a community academic partnership.	Katherine L. Cauley, Ph.D. 140 E. Monument Ave. Dayton, OH 45402 937-775-1114 katherine.cauley@wright.edu	HIE_103
OH	Connecting Rural North East Ohio For Better Health	Twin City Hospital will be the focal point of this HIE which seeks to distribute real-time information to the network of providers caring for a patient. Partners include the Red Cross and local Health Departments.	Marge Jentes 819 N. First St. Dennison, OH 44621 740-922-2800 mjentes@twincityhospital.org	HIE_104
OH	Women & Children Data Exchange	Women of childbearing age and their newborns are the target of this HIE in Lorain County, OH. Having an electronic chart would facilitate all pieces of relevant information being accessible at the point of care. This would dramatically enhance the effectiveness and the efficiency of health care providers. The HIE will include all patients treated by EMH ob/gyns, the ECHD, OB/GYN Clinic, EMH, pediatricians, and tertiary care providers (MetroHealth and Fairview) and Home Health.	Patricia G. Egan 630 East River Street Elyria, OH 44035 440-329-7591 PEgan@emhrhs.org	HIE_105

OH	Rural Health Exchange	This is a system expansion that adds an exchange of clinical information to include bar coding of lab specimens, laboratory results reporting, shared patient registration demographics, online ordering of lab tests and prescriptions by physicians, and electronic signature.	Walt Newlon, MHSA 1106 Colegate Drive Marietta, OH 45750 740-568-2262 wnewlon@selbygeneralhospital.com	HIE_106
OH	Coordinated Patient Record System	This is a multi-stakeholder, not-for-profit, 501(c)3 organization serving the greater Toledo, Ohio area with the focus of improving the quality of healthcare in the community. The HIE is both clinically-focused and patient-focused. Key components of the system are the consistent identification of each patient across institutional boundaries, and the automatic distribution of information between care sites according to privacy-protected routing rules.	Duane Gainsburg, MD Chairman, CHANWO 5600 Monroe Street Suite A101 Sylvania, OH 43560 419-882-8401 dgains@macconnect.com	HIE_107
OH	Laboratory Information System	This is an integrated Laboratory Information System. It can be used onsite or via the Internet for physicians to place orders and look at test results. The hospital lab will also use the system to request tests of contracted reference labs for processing and as a posting mechanism for results. Lab results from both the hospital and the contracted reference labs will be available on a single website.	Phil Frohriep 610 West Main Street, P.O. Box 600 Wilmington, OH 45177 937-283-9657 phfroehreip@cmhregional.com	HIE_108
OH	Radiology Information System	The HIE will be an integrated Radiology Information System and Picture Archiving and Communications System accessible from on-site or via Internet for physicians to view radiological images or reports.	Phil Frohriep 610 West Main Street, P.O. Box 600 Wilmington, OH 45177 937-283-9657 phfroehreip@cmhregional.com	HIE_109
OH	Kaiser Permanente and Epic Systems	Kaiser's other regions are preparing to follow Hawaii's lead on the HealthConnect implementation. Ohio, for example, is now implementing the billing and appointment scheduling applications.	Louise Liang, MD, SVP for Quality and Clinical Systems Support Kaiser Foundation Health Plan One Kaiser Plaza, Oakland, CA 94612 510-271-6317	PHIT_05b
OH	SureScripts and The Cleveland Clinic and Epic Systems	SureScripts is working with The Cleveland Clinic's physician and technology staff to connect its EpicCare EMR system with the SureScripts network, allowing the Clinic's nearly 1,000 physicians currently using EpicCare to exchange renewal requests and authorizations with pharmacists and process new prescriptions completely electronically.	Michelle Bolek, Cleveland Clinic 216-444-0333 bolekm@ccf.org	PHIT_22
OH	Cleveland Clinic and IBM	Cleveland Clinic and IBM are collaborating to provide the clinic's patients with more customized treatments by allowing doctors to electronically tap into research discoveries at the bedside. IBM and Cleveland Clinic will develop a "translational medicine platform," or infrastructure that ties together patients' electronic health-record data with the clinic's clinical, genetic, and other research data. The work between IBM and Cleveland Clinic follows a similar customized medicine collaboration revealed in Aug between IBM and Mayo.	Mike Svinte, IBM's VP of information-based medicine or Michelle Bolek Cleveland Clinic, 216-444-0333 bolekm@ccf.org	PHIT_23
OH	CCHS-East Huron Hospital CPOE Project	Creates an information management environment that integrates patient care data, standardizes practice variation and use of best practices, and supports the delivery of a seamless continuum of patient care throughout the health system through CPOE.	Greg Kall, Meridia Health System East Cleveland, OH KallG@ccf.org	AHRQ_076
OH	Trial of Decision Support to Improve Diabetes Outcomes	Evaluates the effects of a Web portal-based patient empowerment program and EMR system on quality of care, patient safety, and utilization for patients with diabetes and physicians in primary care practices.	Randall Cebul, Case Western Reserve University, 216-778-3901 rdc@case.edu	AHRQ_077
OK	LifeMasters Supported SelfCare	Deployment of project will begin in Sep 05. Will be using this call center for monitoring approx 135,000 members of Bluegrass Family Health.	Denise Apcar, LifeMasters 650-829-6217 dapcar@lifemasters.com	CCIP_6

OK	Oklahoma Foundation for Medical Quality	As part of its commitment to improving health care in our state, OFMQ is helping primary care practices understand and use health IT through the Doctor's Office Quality - Information Technology (DOQ-IT) initiative. OFMQ understands that different practices have different needs and is offering support to practices implementing clinical IT solutions or improving efficiencies of current systems through DOQ-IT.	Lisa Wynn 405-840-2891 lwynn@okqio.sdps.org	DOQ_36
OK	Saint Francis Heart Hospital HIE	The technical foundation of this HIE is the Saint Francis Heart Hospital. The cardiovascular network encompasses ambulatory clinics, outpatient diagnostic centers, tertiary care centers and independent physician practices. The network will capture historical data for cardiovascular-compromised patients, with the objective of impacting outcomes in a positive manner by eliminating paper-based problems.	Tom Cooper 6585 South Yale Ave Suite 1040 Tulsa, OK 74136 918-481-7911 tcooper@saintfrancis.com	HIE_110
OK	Health Improvement Collaboration in Cherokee County, Oklahoma	Creates a plan for developing an integrated, multifunctional, HIPAA-compliant Community Health Information Network; developing a telephonic comprehensive nurse line service and triage function; and investigating and implementing improvements for streamlining of existing appointment systems.	Mark Jones, Tahlequah City Hospital Tahlequah, OK	AHRQ_078
OK	INTEGRIS Telewoundcare Network	Demonstrates and evaluates the clinical effectiveness and cost-savings of utilizing telehealth technology to reduce the days to healing for chronic wounds by improving access to caregivers, point of care processes, and dissemination of best practice information.	Charles Bryant, INTEGRIS Health, Inc. Oklahoma City, OK	AHRQ_079
OR	Oregon Medical Professional Review Organization (OMPRO)	During the current pilot phase of the project, OMPRO is working with a small number of Oregon medical practices that are currently implementing EHR systems or preparing to select a vendor. OMPRO is assisting the practices in evaluating vendors and products and in designing improved workflows for documenting patient care. OMPRO will work with a larger number of practices when the full DOQ–IT project commences in fall 2005. The full project includes quality improvement and measurement components.	Margene Bortel /Quality Improvement Specialist 503-382-3963	DOQ_37
OR	Portland Emergency Surveillance System	The proposed HIE is a real time population-based database that includes the discharge and admission diagnosis from all major area emergency departments in Portland, Oregon. This database is designed to be queried automatically for syndromic surveillance. The data will be analyzed according to GIS data and diagnosis to detect spatial and temporal clustering of diagnoses.	Jerris Hedges, MD 3181 SW Sam Jackson Park Road Portland, OR 97201 503-494-7500 hedgesj@ohsu.edu	HIE_111
OR	Oregon Senate	A plan approved by the Senate Monday, Senate Bill 541, creates a task force to make recommendations on implementing a state electronic medical records system and address necessary patient security issues. Senate Bill 541 brings together hospitals of varying sizes, representatives of physicians' clinics and vendors that can provide electronic medical record services to establish a road map toward better information sharing.	Senator Frank Morse (R-Albany/ Corvallis, OR) or Senator Ben Westlund (R-Bend, OR)	PHIT_24
OR	Improving the Quality of Healthcare in Central Oregon	Develops an integrated health IT to improve rural access to healthcare, and identifies key issues to improve patient safety and quality of care, including analyzing the cost-benefit of technical solutions.	Diane Audiss, St. Charles Medical Center, Bend, OR daudiss@scmc.org	AHRQ_080
OR	Bay Area Community Informatics Project	Plans the implementation of an HIE using a secure fiber optic connection between community care providers to share patient demographic, medical records, laboratory results and radiographic images.	Jeffery Givens, Bay Area Hospital Coos Bay, OR	AHRQ_081
OR	Using IT to Improve Medication Safety for Rural Elders	Implements a Patient-Centered Medication Information System (PCMIS) to provide secure access to accurate, complete, and current medication information for patients, clinicians, pharmacists, and nurses, reconcile differences in medication information, and provide a platform for evidence-based decision support; assess the benefits and costs of the system.	Paul Gorman, Samaritan North Lincoln Hospital, Lincoln City, OR gormanp@ohsu.edu	AHRQ_082

OR	Medication Management: A Closed Computerized Loop	Implements health IT specifically related to medication administration and management and assesses the extent to which these technologies contribute to measurable and sustainable improvements in patient safety and quality of care.	Mark Hetz, Three Rivers Community Hospital, Grants Pass, OR 541-608-5960	AHRQ_083
OR	Improving Safety and Quality with Integrated Technology	Demonstrates the value of an integrated outpatient and inpatient health information system by assessing adherence to evidence-based treatment guidelines for women who are group B streptococcus positive including inappropriate antibiotic use and screening in the outpatient setting, and cost-benefit analysis.	Jeanne-Marie Guise, Oregon Health and Sciences University, Portland, OR 503-494-3107	AHRQ_084
PA	Health Dialog Services Corp.	Health Dialog will demonstrate its approach to chronic care management by providing care management services over the next 3 years to at least 20,000 fee-for-service Medicare beneficiaries in PA with congestive heart failure and/or complex diabetes.	George Bennett, Chairman and CEO Health Dialog, Sixty State Street, 11th Floor, Boston, MA 02109, 617-406-5200	CCIP_4
PA	Quality Insights of Pennsylvania	Quality Insights of Pennsylvania is the Medicare Quality Improvement Organization (QIO) for the Commonwealth. The Centers for Medicare & Medicaid Services (CMS) contract runs from August 1, 2002 to July 31, 2005. Quality Insights: Partnering to Achieve Health Care Excellence with Information Technology.	717-671-5425 877-346-6180 http://www.qipa.org/Feedback.asp	DOQ_38
PA	SVRHP Regional Remote Pharmacy System	This proposal is for the establishment of a fully integrated remote pharmacy system between all network members using common clinical application systems. The SVRHP is developing a regional rural integrated electronic information system to enhance and support local healthcare delivery. By establishing this system, all network members will have 24 hour, 7 day a week services of licensed pharmacist.	Susan Browning, Executive Director 1020 Thompson Street Jersey Shore, PA 17740 570-321-3000 sbrowning@shscares.org	HIE_112
PA	HIE to Prevent Blindness in four Specific Blinding Disorders	This is a remote imaging HIE in which retinal images are captured, stored and forwarded via internet to qualified specialists for analysis. Diagnosis and management information is then transmitted to the patient's managing physician.	Jay L Federman, MD 501 N. Essex Ave. Narberth, PA 19072 610-949-9789 jfederbeck@aol.com	HIE_113
PA	Mercy Circle of Care Exchange Model	This program will affiliate with churches and neighborhood organizations to do insurance outreach and referral to primary care and maintain a shared data system to profile and track uninsured individuals over time. Using a web-based information management system, "ServicePoint" by Bowman Internet Systems, LLC, they will link all of the participating Mercy Circle of Care providers via the Internet and will be operated as a web-based, on-line transactional system. The database will provide the Mercy Health Partners with the capability of capturing and sharing real-time data throughout the network to facilitate patient eligibility, patient registration, patient tracking, referrals, and care and outcomes management.	William Bithoney, MD 501 South 54th Street Philadelphia, PA 19143 215-748-9420 wbithoney@mercyhealth.org	HIE_114
PA	Service Point	ServicePoint coordinates and electronically automates client intake and screening for eligibility in the HealthRight program. ServicePoint also maintains a brief history of the client's medical conditions and medical services provided, allowing HealthRight and the participating providers to identify, monitor, and case manage appropriate patients to move towards improving their health status.	Linnette Black 801 Market St., 7th Floor, Suite 7100 Philadelphia, PA 19107 215-413-8591 lblack@hfedu.org	HIE_115
PA	The Pittsburgh Health Information Network (PHIN)	The PHIN is designed to be a central repository which will collect claims data on diabetic and depressed patients as well as lab test results on 7 datapoints related to diabetes care. This central database can then be accessed by physicians on-demand and at the point of care in order to easily track available data on treatment for these chronic diseases from a single source no matter what health insurance coverage a patient has.	Ed Harrison Centre City Tower, Suite 2150 650 Smithfield St. Pittsburgh, PA 15222 412-535-0292 x 107 eharrison@prhi.org	HIE_116

PA	Patient/Physician Information Exchange (P2P)	UPMC's proposal model is to provide tools that are integrated into the physician workflow that enable communication (physician to physician, patient to physician and physician to patient). The Patient/Physician Information Exchange is a secured interactive suite of software tools that enable a variety of communication paths with physicians and patients. It supports bi-directional communication to the patient and physician with all available modalities.	Robert J. Schwartz, MD, MPH Medical Director, UPMC HS Office of Physician Relations 200 Lothrop Street Pittsburgh, PA 15213 412-647-7346 schwartzrj@upmc.edu	HIE_117
PA	Scranton Temple HIE (STHIE)	STRP Inc.goal is to plan and implement a feasible, sustainable and effective HIE system in the community that will allow authorized providers and consumers timely and efficient access to complete patient health information.	Robert E. Wright, MD 746 Jefferson Avenue Scranton, PA 18510 570-343-2383 rwrigth@mhs-nepa.com	HIE_118
PA	IBM and the University of Pittsburgh Medical Center	IBM and the University of Pittsburgh Medical Center have announced that they will spend at least $50 million over eight years to develop computer technology for health care, the Pittsburgh Post-Gazette reports. Officials hope the computer infrastructure will serve as a model for other hospitals that want to develop electronic health records, creating commercial opportunities for IBM and UPMC.	UPMC President Jeffrey Romoff 200 Lothrop St. Pittsburgh, PA 15213-2582 800-533-8762	PHIT_25
PA	Geisinger Health System and Central Penn Health Information Collaborative	A group of 24 community hospitals from across central and eastern Pennsylvania began May 11, 2005 an initiative to create a system for sharing electronic patient records between the hospitals. Mount Nittany Medical Center, and Philipsburg and Tyrone hospitals are part of the Central Penn Health Information Collaborative. The effort being spearheaded by Geisinger includes hospitals from across the state, including Altoona, Huntingdon, Scranton, Wilkes-Barre, Montrose and Lewistown. The initiative doesn't have the heavy financial backing others nationwide have had. It does have a $200,000 federal grant and has applied for an additional $3 million in funding.	Jim Walker, CMIO Geisinger Health System jmwalker@geisinger.edu 570-271-6750	PHIT_26
PA	Highmark Blue Cross Blue Shield (PA)	Highmark Blue Cross Blue Shield (PA) also operates a similar program [to the Bridges for Excellence model] which awards tiered bonuses based on performance and IT implementation for physicians in at least the 50th percentile.	Highmark Fifth Avenue Place 120 Fifth Avenue Pittsburgh, PA 15222-3099 412-544-7000	PHIT_27
PA	CapMed PHR and NextGen Healthcare	The PHR will work in conjunction with NextGen® EMR to enable the secure communication of health information between patients and providers. The PHR allows patients to keep personal health data electronically on their personal computer and exchange data with their physicians and other care providers.	Wendy Angst, CapMed wangst@capmed.com 267-757-3315	PHIT_33
PA	Regional Approach for THQIT in Rural Settings	Conducts a formal clinical information and technical needs assessment to identify the optimal technical model for information sharing as well as actions required to overcome barriers; develops a project plan that will promote implementation of cost-effective clinical information services.	James Walker, Geisinger Clinic Danville, PA	AHRQ_085
PA	Enhancing Patient Safety through a Universal EMR System	Implements an EMR system that allows 24-hour data sharing across 7 rural health care delivery sites for clinicians to access current and complete patient information using either Personal Digital Assistants or a Web portal.	Thomas Johnson, Dubois Regional Medical Center, DuBois, PA	AHRQ_086
PR	Quality Improvement Professional Research Organization (QIPRO)	n/a	n/a	DOQ_52
RI	State and Regional Demonstrations in Health Information Technology	Contract that plans, develops, implements, and evaluates a Master Patient Index to facilitate interoperability and sharing patient data between public and private health care sectors.	Project Director: Patricia Nolan State of Rhode Island, Providence, RI	AHRQ_087

RI	Quality Partners of Rhode Island	(No specific DOQ-IT information)	Lauren Pond /Physician Office 401-528-3204 lpond@riqio.sdps.org	DOQ_39
RI	Rhode Island/HealthAlliant Project	RIQI is implementing a statewide initiative in cooperation with SureScripts, Inc., a collaborative effort of independent and chain pharmacies across the nation to implement state-wide electronic connectivity between all retail pharmacies and all prescribers in the state.	Laura Adams One Union Station Providence, RI 02903 401-274-4564 ladams@riqi.org	HIE_119
SC	Carolina Medical Review	(No specific DOQ-IT information)	803-731-8225 800-922-3089	DOQ_40
SD	South Dakota Foundation for Medical Care	(No specific DOQ-IT information)	605-336-3505 800-658-2285	DOQ_41
SD	Sioux Valley Clinical Information System	Sioux Valley Hospitals and Health System has developed a plan for implementing a Clinical Information system across its entire health system. These clinical Information systems will form an electronic medical record that will be used to share appropriate clinical information between clinicians across the health system.	Arlyn Broekhuis 1305 W. 18th Street Sioux Falls, SD 57117-5039 605-333-7329 broekhua@siouxvalley.org	HIE_120
TN	XL Health	XL Health chosen to provide disease management services in Tennessee. Responsible for recruiting and offering DM services to Medicare fee-for-service beneficiaries in Tennessee with diabetes, congestive heart failure and all related co-morbidities.	XLHealth, The Warehouse at Camden Yards 351 West Camden Street, Suite 100, Baltimore, MD 21201	CCIP_9
TN	Center for Healthcare Quality	QSource, the Medicare Quality Improvement Organization for Tennessee, is embarking on a project to provide support to small and medium primary care practices in implementing EHRs. We are not a vendor of EHR products, nor do we endorse any vendor. What we do is help you and your staff identify which of the existing systems would best meet your practice's needs, look at what needs to be put in place to successfully implement it into your office structure, and what changes need to occur in your office's workflow to ensure that the EHR functions in such a way as to be effective and not to cause unnecessary issues or duplication of work.	Jennifer McAnally /EHR Implementation Advisor 1-800-528-2655 (2635)	DOQ_42
TN	Tri-Cities TN-VA Care Data Exchange Project	Our HIE is diverse collaboration of health service institutions which seek to improve health outcomes for patients through linkage of their health information. The HIE will be a peer to peer network allowing existing EMR systems to retain and maintain data while a search interface handles security, record identification, and distribution.	Liesa Jo Jenkins P.O. Box 980 Kingsport, Tennessee 37662 423-246-2017 ljenkins@kingsporttomorrow.org	HIE_121* RHIO_121
TN	Memphis Metro Area Technology Collaborative for Health (MATCH)	MATCH is a technical infrastructure for a common enterprise-wide master patient index (eMPI), becoming the foundation for a regional health information exchange network and electronic medical record system. The system will be designed so that authorized healthcare providers at any facility will have the ability to log on, find the correct patient, and immediately access all relevant health information including transcribed reports, laboratory, radiology, etc.	Chuck Fitch, Vice President and Chief Information Officer / Co-PIs: Karen Fox and Mary McCain 66 N. Pauline Street, Suite 232 Memphis, TN 38105 901-448-6683 Chuck.Fitch@utmg.org	HIE_122
TN	Volunteer eHealth Initiative	Designed to establish regional data-sharing agreements and to implement clinical data exchange, the Volunteer eHealth Initiative will provide a framework for hospitals, physician groups, clinics, health plans and other healthcare stakeholders to work together. It focuses initially on Shelby, Fayette and Tipton counties.	Mark Frisse, MD Vanderbilt Center for Better Health 3401 West End Avenue, Suite 290 Nashville, TN 615-343-1528 Mark.Frisse@Vanderbilt.edu	HIE_123

TN	Williamson-Wired Health Exchange for Kids	This HIE program will enroll parents of underinsured kids through school and church outreach, educate them via classes, assign a caregiver for web-based coaching, link the children's health to providers in the Mercy Children's Clinic and to community based providers, and monitor improvements in health outcomes and community-based care for this population. The "wired" resource network will include schools, churches and physicians in the community, with the goal of improving access to basic primary care services and, through the use of web-based technology, to improve health status in the prevention and treatment of prevalent childhood diseases and conditions.	Paul H. Keckley, Ph.D. Executive Director MCN D3300 Nashville, TN 37232 615-343-3922 paul.keckley@vandervilt.edu	HIE_124
TN	State and Regional Demonstrations in Health Information Technology	Contract that plans, implements, and evaluates a State-based regional data sharing and interoperability service interconnecting the health care entities in three counties including needs assessment for healthcare improvement and reforming TennCare.	Project Director: Mark E. Frisse Vanderbilt University Medical Center Nashville, TN	AHRQ_088
TN	Improving the Quality and Safety of Regional Surgical Patient Care.	Through the Creation of a Multi-institutional Partnership for the Implementation and Support of Perioperative Informatics Tools, this project develops a detailed plan for the implementation and support of informatics tools in regional health centers including the creation of informatics tools to manage institutional surgical care information, creation of a multi-institutional partnership to manage both the informatics and surgical quality improvement programs, and the development of an economic model related to the business and safety benefits.	Michael Higgins, Vanderbilt University Medical Center, Nashville, TN	AHRQ_089
TN	Improving Quality Care for Children with Special Needs	Develops a database that includes diagnoses, health records, and educational information on Children with Special Health Care Needs with emphasis on children with genetic conditions and developmental disabilities; makes this information available to physicians via a secure Web-based system.	Carmen Lozzio, University of Tennessee Health Sciences Center Memphis, TN	AHRQ_090
TN	Technology Exchange for Cancer Health Network (TECH-Net)	Implements a systematic care program to improve cancer management in rural communities by building upon an innovative approach to total clinical decision support to provide access to oncology, hematology, and other specialists through a dedicated telehealth network.	Karen Fox, University of Tennessee Health Sciences Center, Memphis, TN kfox@utmem.edu	AHRQ_091
TX	Rural Hospital Collaborative for Excellence Using IT	Implements advanced information technology in rural and small community hospitals including Web-based business intelligence tools, Internet connectivity, and standardized national measures of patient safety and quality; also provides education intervention to support implementation efforts and evaluate its effects on patient safety and quality.	Patricia Dorris, Palo Pinto General Hospital, Mineral Wells, TX	AHRQ_092
TX	Measuring the Value of Remote ICU Monitoring	Examines the effect of tele-ICU monitoring on mortality, complications, length of stay, cost-effectiveness, provider attitudes, and human factors issues in ICUs and 7 community hospitals.	Eric Thomas, University of TX-Houston Eric.Thomas@uth.tmc.edu	AHRQ_093
TX	TX Medical Foundation	TX Medical Foundation, under contract with the Centers for Medicare & Medicaid Services, is providing support for a limited time to small- and medium-sized primary care practices in implementing an EHR system through an initiative called Doctor's Office Quality - Information Technology (DOQ-IT). We are not a vendor of EHR products and we do not endorse any vendor.	Tara Frease, 800-725-9216 tfrease@txqio.sdps.org bstephenson@txqio.sdps.org	DOQ_43
TX	Integrated Clinical Information System	TCH is launching a major initiative to transform multiple, disparate information systems into an integrated pediatric information management portal. TCH and its other entities and partners are committed to providing an integrated electronic medical record; point of care review and capture of vital signs, medication administration, and data from biomedical equipment; improved quality of life by utilization of telemedicine and remote capture of data from new sources; and data warehouse to support clinical research and education.	David Finn, VP Information Services 1102 Bates, Suite 650, MC 3-4221 Houston, TX 77030 832-824-2062 dsfinn@texaschildrenhospital.org	HIE_125

TX	National Data Source Connectivity	PSI is deploying a communication network based on existing technology that provides patient-centric clinical information. The network backbone is based on a community-driven, patient-centric model. To facilitate expansion of PSI nationwide, PSI will offer access to the system through publicly available, open-standard technology. PSI is platform and software independent, making access to its inexpensive and trusted network service open to all communities that join the network and agree to abide by PSI's principles. PSI has been designed to be a national, rather than regional model.	Johnny Walker, PSI CEO / Executive Director, 972-444-9800 jwalker@ptsafety.org	HIE_126
TX	UHS HIE	This is a web-based patient health indicator database. The HIE will provide for a collection and exchange of patient-monitored health indicators and a sharing of these indicators with assigned clinicians.	Tim Geryk 4502 Medical Drive San Antonio, TX 78229 210-358-1392 tim.geryk@uhs-sa.com	HIE_127
UT	Bridges-to-Excellence (POL)	CMS is also looking towards the BTE Physician Office Link program as a possible element in its forthcoming Medicare Care Management Performance Demonstration project, an initiative which will promote the adoption and use of health information technology to improve the efficiency and quality of patient care for chronically ill Medicare patients. Doctors who meet or exceed performance standards established by CMS in clinical delivery systems and patient outcomes will receive performance payments for managing the care of eligible Medicare beneficiaries. The effort, scheduled to begin later this year, will involve hundreds of doctors in medical practices in Arkansas, California, Utah and Massachusetts. In many of these States, CMS will collaborate with BTE and other private pay-for-performance initiatives.	Medstat Group 1-800-224-7161 bridgestoexcellence@thomson.com	BTE_01c
UT	HealthInsight	HealthInsight is a private, non-profit QIO whose mission is to be a catalyst in the transformation and improvement of the health care system. In our thirty-year history, HealthInsight staff has worked with the health care community on initiatives to improve the quality of care delivered in Nevada and Utah. The goal being to: Educate physician offices on EHR system solutions and alternatives, Provide implementation and quality improvement assistance, Assist physician offices in migrating from paper-based health records to EHR systems that suit their clinics' needs. Assist those currently using an EHR in using their system more effectively.	Sharon Donnelly (Medicare Beneficiaries) http://www.healthinsight.org/contact.html 801-892-6668 Hotline: 800-483-0932 801-892-0155 sdonnelly@healthinsight.org	DOQ_44
UT	Utah Health Information Network (UHIN)	The Utah Health Information Network (UHIN) is a broad-based coalition of health care insurers, providers, and other interested parties, including State government. UHIN participants have come together for the common goal of reducing health care administrative costs through data standardization of administrative health data and electronic commerce (EC). UHIN has a centralized health data transaction system and is the hub for this system.	801-466-7705 Fax: 801-466-7169 Washington Building, Suite 320, 151 East 5600 South Murray, UT 84107	HIE_140
UT	Improving Communication Between Health Care Providers Via a Statewide Infrastructure: UHIN	Contract that expands and enhances current Statewide network for the electronic exchange of patient administrative and clinical data and will support the adoption of EMRs.	Project Director: Jan Root, Utah Health Information Network Murray, UT	AHRQ_094
UT	Nursing Home IT: Optimal Medication and Care Delivery	Implements an health IT system with added best-practices decision support modules in 7 nursing homes and evaluates the impact on care processes, resident health outcomes, and staff efficiency and satisfaction.	Susan Horn, International Severity Information Systems, Inc. Salt Lake City, UT	AHRQ_095
UT	Rural Trial of Clinic Order Entry with Decision Support	Assesses the value of a computerized clinic order entry tool in rural primary care practices for appropriateness of antimicrobial therapy for acute respiratory infections, frequency of hemoglobin A1c in diabetics, incidence of outpatient adverse drug events, and influenza vaccine immunizations.	Matthew Samore, University of Utah Salt Lake City, UT	AHRQ_096

VA	Virginia Health Quality Center	Through the Doctors' Office Quality-Information Technology (DOQ-IT) project, sponsored by CMS, the VHQC is working to support the adoption and effective use of information technology by physicians' offices in Virginia, along with all Quality Improvement Organizations (QIOs) across the nation.	Project Manager: David Collins, M.H.A., CPHQ; Medical Director: Kevin Fergusson, M.D., M.S.H.A. 804-289-5320 dcollins@vaqio.sdps.org, kfergusson@vaqio.sdps.org	DOQ_46a
VA	West Virginia Medical Institute	(No specific DOQ-IT information)	804-343-9776 1-800-951-3530 http://www.wvmi.org/Feedback.asp	DOQ_46b
VA	CenVaNet	Using a common web portal that enables physicians, hospitals, commercial laboratories, payers and eventually consumers to communicate in a secure and confidential environment, CenVaNet has organized the creation of a community-wide data and information interchange to allow providers to transfer critical clinical and administrative data.	Michael Matthews, CEO 2001 West Broad St., Suite 202 Richmond, VA 23220-2022 804-359-4500 x225 mmatthews@CVHN.com	HIE_129
VA	Rural Virginia e-Health Collaborative	Examines automation of the continuity of care record for use in patient referrals, hospital admission, and hospital discharge; e-prescribing in physician practices, hospital discharge medications, and long-term care facilities with links to community pharmacies; and disease registries for managing preventive care interventions and chronic diseases.	Michael Matthews, Rappahannock General Hospital, Kilmarnock, VA	AHRQ_099
VI	Virgin Islands Medical Institute	(No specific DOQ-IT information)	340-712-2400 askvimi@viqio.sdps.org	DOQ_53
VT	Northeast Health Care Quality Foundation	(No specific DOQ-IT information) Mission is to encourage and promote improvement in health care for the Medicare beneficiaries in our service region. We provide educational materials and tools for identified quality improvement projects, and conduct reviews to ensure quality of care for beneficiaries and protect the Medicare Trust Fund.	1-800-772-0151 603-749-1641 info@nhcqf.org	DOQ_45
VT	Community Electronic Health Record	Goal is to create a patient record integrated with CVH's EMR and to make it available immediately to all providers in the 25-physician primary care offices.	Russell Davignon P.O. Box 547 Barre, VT 05641 802-371-4100 russell.davignon@hitchcock.org	HIE_128
VT	Improving Rural Healthcare with Technology	Utilizes existing health IT standards to integrate the current stand-alone databases and information systems of a consortium of three rural healthcare systems as the basis for creating a comprehensive electronic health record for patient care.	C. Frederick Lord, Mt. Ascutney Hospital and Health Center Windsor, VT	AHRQ_097
VT	Improving Healthcare Quality via Information Technology	Implements an integrated electronic patient medical record, electronic medication administration record, computerized physician order entry (CPOE), and clinical decision support software that will be accessible at all participating facilities which include an acute care hospital, home health care agency, ambulatory clinics, a rehab facility, and to the patient/resident from home.	Robert Pezzulich, Southwestern Vermont Health, Bennington, VT	AHRQ_098
WA	Qualis Health	Practices that participate in DOQ-IT will receive free assistance to select, implement, and optimize IT systems such as EHRs, e-prescribing, and registries. CMS has contracted with Qualis Health to provide DOQ-IT services to participating physicians in Washington, Idaho, and Alaska.	Andrea Sciaudone, RN CPHQ 800-949-7536, ext. 2030 andreas@qualishealth.org	DOQ_47
WA	e-Prescribing: Strengthening County-wide Health Information Exchange	The HIE will assist in checking for allergies, drug-drug-conflicts, duplicate drugs, and drug-disease contraindications.	Lori Nichols 715 West Orchard Drive, Suite 4 Bellingham, WA 98225 360-671-6800 lnichols@hinet.org	HIE_130* RHIO_130

WA	Community-Based Diabetes Health Information Exchange Project	This HIE is built upon an existing EMR. It will allow tracking of inpatient and outpatient data related to diabetes, which will be collected via standardized messaging from independent sources into the Electronic Medical Record (EMR) of the primary care provider. The EMR will also use a web tool to allow diabetes patients to access health education and enter health monitoring information.	Jac Davies 157 S. Howard St., Suite 500 Spokane, WA 99201 509-232-8120 daviesjc@inhs.org	HIE_131
WA	HealthKey, & the Electronic Laboratory Based Reporting System (ELBRS)	HealthKey was developed to create a replicable model for Public Key Infrastructure (PKI) and other secure infrastructure models for the health care industry. In addition to CHITA's role in HealthKey, the organization facilitates troubleshooting and assistance around HIPAA standards for data exchange, privacy and security, and hosts a number of workgroups around standards for administrative and claims data.	Michael Taylor, 206-682-2811 x10 administration@qualityhealth.org	HIE_145
WA	Kaiser Permanente and Epic Systems	The next regions to implement the patient records component will be those with previous clinical IT experience, such as Kaiser's Northwest region, where facilities have used other Epic systems for years.	Louise Liang, MD, SVP for Quality and Clinical Systems Support Kaiser Foundation Health Plan One Kaiser Plaza, Oakland, CA 94612 510 271-6317	PHIT_05d
WA	Microsoft: Digital Pharma Initiative	Microsoft Announces Digital Pharma Initiative, Providing Comprehensive Solutions Framework to Drive Business Efficiency and Speed-to-Insight in the Pharmaceutical Industry. More Than 18 Leading Companies Are Developing or Supporting Solutions Based on the Digital Pharma Initiative; Pfizer and Merck Are Among a Number of Customers That Have Deployed Microsoft-Based Solutions. The companies include Accenture, Covansys Corp., DataLabs Inc., HP, Immedient Corp., Manhattan Associates Inc., Meridio, Merit Solutions Software, Motion Computing Inc., OnSphere Corp., OSIsoft Inc., OutlookSoft Corp., ProClarity Corp., Project Assistants Inc., Proscape Technologies Inc., QUMAS, Siebel Systems Inc. and Tectura Corp.	Tim Smokoff, Managing Director Microsoft Healthcare and Life Sciences	PHIT_28
WA	Evaluating the Impact of an ACPOE/CDS System on Outcomes	Implements an ambulatory computer physician order entry (ACPOE) system with clinical decision support capabilities in an ambulatory, community-based, integrated health-system; evaluates the impact of the system both internally, on organizational processes and human factors, and externally, on patient safety as measured by medication errors and adverse drug events.	Sean Sullivan, University of Washington, Seattle, WA sdsull@u.washington.edu	AHRQ_100
WA	A Rural HIT Cooperative to Promote Clinical Improvement	Demonstrates the value of health IT in improving quality of inpatient care for community-acquired pneumonia and emergency care of acute myocardial infarctions in rural hospitals.	Elizabeth Floersheim, Rural Healthcare Quality Network, Davenport, WA 206-216-2550	AHRQ_101
WI	MetaStar	n/a	Jesi Wang, 608-441-8269 800-362-2320 jwang@metastar.com	DOQ_49
WI	Wisconsin Health Informaton Exchange	WHIE will incorporate the building blocks of an HIE from several underutilized networks to form a system that has a patient index, standards-based data storage/ transmission, security, redundancy, and consumer access.	Seth Foldy, M.D. c/o NIMI-MW 1251 Glen Oaks Lane Mequon, WI 53092-3378 414-906-0036 sfoldy@sbcglobal.net	HIE_135* RHIO_135
WI	Wellpoint eRx or Paper Reduction	WellPoint is spearheading an electronic initiative at a cost of $40 million that will reach 19,000 physicians. In California, Georgia, Missouri, and Wisconsin, physicians will be given the opportunity to choose from either of two electronic packages: a Prescription Improvement Package or a Paperwork Reduction Package.	Ron J. Ponder, PhD, EVP, Information Services, WellPoint or Nadia Leather, CGEY nadia.leather@capgemini.com 212-314-8236	PHIT_02d
WI	Planning for a Rural Prescription Medication Network	Develops a shared electronic repository for patient-level prescription medication data that enables real-time access for patients receiving healthcare services and plans a model system design to electronically link prescription medication data across hospitals and physician practices.	Robert Gribble, St. Joseph's Hospital Marshfield, WI	AHRQ_102

WI	Developing Shared EHR Infrastructure in Wisconsin	Plans the implementation of a common infrastructure for an integrated EHR and CPOE to enhance access to clinical data, develops a workable model/plan for standards-based data sharing to allow multiple providers using disparate information systems to access patient information, and creates a quality measurement and enhancement tool that would measure improvements in quality and patient care.	Tim Size Reedsburg Area Medical Center, Reedsburg, WI	AHRQ_103
WI	Improving Patient Safety/Quality with HIT Implementation	Implements an Epic health IT system and diffuses the system community-wide; identifies the prevalence of medication errors, near misses, and preventable adverse drug events; assesses costs and customer satisfaction both before and after implementation.	John Reiling St. Joseph's Community Hospital West Bend, WI	AHRQ_104
WI	CPOE Implementation in ICU's	Assesses the implementation of CPOE systems in 6 intensive care units (ICUs) and evaluates the value and outcomes of patient safety involving medication errors; quality of care; end users' job tasks, perceptions, and attitudes; and financial impact.	Pascale Carayon, University of Wisconsin, Madison, WI	AHRQ_105
WV	West Virginia Medical Institute	(No specific DOQ-IT information)	304-346-9864 800-642-8686 http://www.wvmi.org/Feedback.asp	DOQ_48
WV	West Virginia Patient Safety Project	The West Virginia Patient Safety Project is designed around a Web-based incident reporting system to enhance the hospital's capacity to detect, analyze, and correct systemic problems that could produce errors in patient care.	Patricia Ruddick, RN, MSN 3001 Chesterfield Place Charleston, WV 25304 304-346-9864 pruddick@wvmi.org	HIE_134
WV	West Virginia University School of Medicine	Dr. Julian Bailes, chairman of the Department of Neurosurgery at the West Virginia University School of Medicine, has been tapped to oversee a statewide working group studying implementation of electronic medical records technology. Will most likely include West Virginia State Medical Association, West Virginia Hospital Association, government health care providers and other health care groups.	Dr. Julian Bailes, chairman of the Department of Neurosurgery, WVU School of Medicine	PHIT_29
WV	Boone County Community Care Network	Designs a county-wide health information system that will allow health information sharing and permit real-time order placement by hospitals, health departments, private physicians' offices, clinics, and long-term care facilities.	Robert Atkins, Boone Memorial Hospital, Madison, WV	AHRQ_106
WV	Partnering to Improve Patient Safety in Rural WV	Expands the reporting of medical errors and near misses, monitors safety event reporting, and develops a learning network among small, rural hospitals and their associated ambulatory care facilities, long-term care facilities, and home health agencies.	Gail Bellamy, West Virginia Medical Institute, Charleston, WV	AHRQ_107
WY	Mountain-Pacific Quality Health Foundation	(No specific DOQ-IT information) Mountain-Pacific Quality Health Foundation is the quality improvement organization (QIO) for Montana, Wyoming, Hawaii, and the territories of Guam, the Commonwealth of the Northern Marianas and American Samoa. The Foundation operates out of offices in Helena, Montana; Cheyenne, Wyoming; and Honolulu, Hawaii. As a QIO, we receive funding from the federal government to enact programs that help ensure people with Medicare receive appropriate, high-quality care. We also hold contracts with other government agencies and private insurance companies.	307-637-8162 877-810-6248 wyoming@mpqhf.org	DOQ_50
WY	Wyoming RHIO	Wyoming is studying and planning for development of a sustainable, interoperable health care information and communication technology system to support the effective, efficient and secure exchange of health information across the spectrum of medical care stakeholders.	n/a	HIE_142

Appendix A
Commissioner Biographies

CHAIR:
Scott Wallace, J.D., M.B.A.
President & CEO
The National Alliance for Health Information Technology

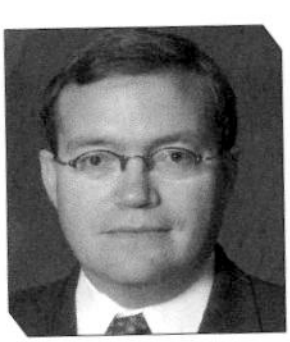

Scott Wallace was appointed as the first president and CEO of The National Alliance for Health Information Technology (Alliance) in 2003. During his time at the Alliance, the organization has made great strides in ensuring, on behalf of its members, that healthcare IT issues are addressed thoughtfully and fairly, with solutions built around the consensus positions that the Alliance has helped the field to reach.

Scott previously was the principal owner of Great Lakes Capital, a financial, commercial, and business development consulting firm with a major focus in technology. Prior to starting Great Lakes Capital, Scott led several technology-based companies. He served as president and CEO of PowerClip Co, a wireless products company; president and CEO of Eichrom Industries, an advanced materials and specialty chemical company that earned a spot on *Inc.* magazine's 1996 list of the 500 fastest growing companies in America, and vice president and general counsel for GCI, a venture capital fund.

Scott earned a jurist doctorate from the University of Chicago Law School, a master's degree with honors in business administration from the University of Chicago Graduate School of Business, and has a bachelor's degree in economics from Duke University. He started his career practicing corporate and transactional law at Kirkland & Ellis in Chicago.

He was recently named to Modern Healthcare's 100 Most Powerful.

Simon P. Cohn, M.D., M.P.H., F.A.C.E.P., F.A.C.M.I.
Associate Executive Director, Health Information Policy
Kaiser Permanente

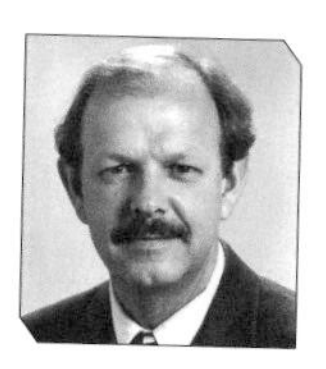

Simon P. Cohn, M.D., M.P.H. is the Associate Executive Director, Health Information Policy for Kaiser Permanente. Kaiser Permanente is the nation's largest nonprofit integrated healthcare delivery system serving 8.4 million members in nine states and the District of Columbia. Dr. Cohn is a nationally recognized expert on issues related to HIPAA Administrative Simplification, healthcare data management, clinical and administrative classifications, and the electronic transmission of healthcare data. He has been a leader in Kaiser Permanente's efforts to develop comprehensive health information systems to support both the delivery of healthcare and health research.

Dr. Cohn is Chair of the National Committee on Vital and Health Statistics (NCVHS), the main public advisory committee to U. S. Department of Health and Human Services on health information policy, HIPAA, and the national health information infrastructure. Additionally, he is a member of the AMA Common Procedural Terminology (CPT) Editorial Panel and the National Uniform Claims Committee (NUCC). He was a member of the Institute of Medicine's Committee on Data Standards for Patient Safety. In 2002, Dr. Cohn was a recipient of the President's Award from the American Medical Informatics Association for his contributions to the field and was also elected a Fellow of the American College of Medical Informatics.

He is board certified in Emergency Medicine and a Fellow of the American College of Emergency Physicians.

Don E. Detmer, M.D., M.A., F.A.C.M.I.
President and CEO
American Medical Informatics Association

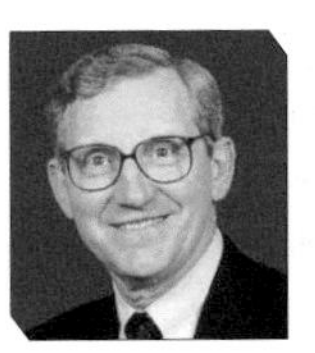

Don E. Detmer, M.D., M.A., is President and Chief Executive Officer of the American Medical Informatics Association. He is also Professor Emeritus and Professor of Medical Education in the Department of Health Evaluation Sciences at the University of Virginia and Senior Associate of the Judge Institute of Management, University of Cambridge. He is a trustee of the Nuffield Trust of London, co-chair of the Blue Ridge Academic Health Group, and research director of the J&J Centre for Advancing Health Information, based in Brussels.

Dr. Detmer is a lifetime Associate of the National Academies, and a fellow of AAAS, Academy Health, and the American Colleges of Medical Informatics, Surgeons, and Sports Medicine. From 1999-2003 he was the Dennis Gillings Professor of Health Management and Director, Cambridge University Health at the Judge Institute of Management, Cambridge's business school. Prior to the years in England, he was Vice President for Health Sciences at the Universities of Virginia and Utah and on the faculty at the University of Wisconsin-Madison. He is immediate past chairman of the Board on Health Care Services of the IOM as well as the National Committee on Vital and Health Statistics. He has also chaired the Board of Regents of the National Library of Medicine.

Dr. Detmer's education includes a medical degree from the University of Kansas with subsequent training at the National Institutes of Health, the Johns Hopkins Hospital, Duke University Medical Center, the Institute of Medicine, and Harvard Business School. His M.A. is from the University of Cambridge. Dr. Detmer's research interests include contributions to national health information policy, quality improvement, administrative medicine, vascular surgery, sports medicine, and master's level educational programs for clinician-executives.

Vicky B. Gregg
President and CEO
BlueCross BlueShield of Tennessee

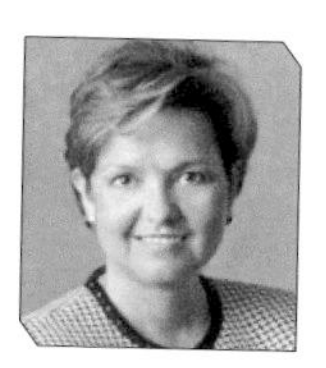

Vicky B. Gregg became CEO of BlueCross BlueShield of Tennessee in February 2003. BlueCross BlueShield headquarters is in Chattanooga, Tennessee, and is the state's largest provider of healthcare services. The company was instrumental in assisting the state in the implementation of the TennCareSM program, a Medicaid expansion program that currently provides healthcare coverage to 25 percent of the State's population. BlueCross BlueShield of Tennessee also provides Medicare intermediary services in 46 states including Part A operations in Tennessee and New Jersey. The not-for-profit company has over 4,000 employees and annualized paid claims of over $14 billion.

Before becoming CEO, Mrs. Gregg served as President and Chief Operating Officer at BlueCross BlueShield of Tennessee overseeing all aspects of the company's day-to-day operations. A nurse by education, Mrs. Gregg has over 25 years of experience in diverse healthcare environments including clinical care, hospital administration, long term care, and healthcare benefits and financing. She served as President and CEO of Volunteer State Health Plan, a subsidiary of BlueCross BlueShield of Tennessee and one of the largest Medicaid Health Maintenance Organizations in the country. Prior to joining BlueCross, Mrs. Gregg served as a Vice President for Humana with responsibility for Kentucky, Ohio, and Indiana. In her role she managed all models of managed care, including preferred provider, staff, group, and academic models. She has been a noted speaker on healthcare market evolution, implications of managed care for academic medicine, Medicaid managed care, rural healthcare delivery, and healthcare reform policy implications related to the uninsured.

Mrs. Gregg serves on numerous boards including the BlueCross BlueShield Association, Council for Affordable Quality Healthcare (CAQH), University of Tennessee Chattanooga Foundation, Chattanooga State Community College Foundation, The Enterprise Center, Nashville Healthcare Council, Tennessee Healthcare Consortium for Nursing, Allied Arts of Chattanooga, United Way of Chattanooga, the Women's Leadership Institute, and the National Institute for Health Care Management. She is an adjunct faculty member of East Tennessee State University Department of Nursing and has served on numerous appointed commissions including the Governor's Roundtable for TennCare. Mrs. Gregg was named one of two appointees by Senator Frist to be a member of the National Commission on Systemic Interoperability.

C. Martin Harris, M.D., M.B.A.
CIO
Cleveland Clinic Foundation

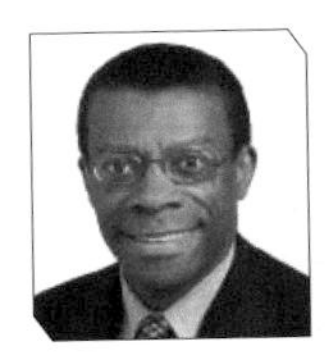

C. Martin Harris, M.D., M.B.A., is the Chief Information Officer and Chairman of the Information Technology Division of The Cleveland Clinic Foundation in Cleveland, Ohio. Additionally, Dr. Harris is Executive Director of e-Cleveland Clinic, a series of e-health clinical programs offered over the Internet.

Dr. Harris' interest and expertise in the area of improving the practice of medicine through the innovative application of information technology, is reflected in his numerous appointments to national technology organizations including:

- Chairman, Regional Health Information Organization (RHIO) Task Force of the Healthcare Information and Management Systems Society (HIMSS);

- Past Chairman, Foundation Board for the e-Health Initiative, a public policy and advocacy group established to encourage the interoperability of information technology in healthcare; and

- Advisor to the Director of the National Institutes of Health.

Dr. Harris received his undergraduate and medical degrees from the University of Pennsylvania in Philadelphia. His residency training in general internal medicine was completed at The Hospital of the University of Pennsylvania. He completed a Robert Wood Johnson Clinical Scholar fellowship in General Internal Medicine at The University of Pennsylvania School of Medicine and holds a Masters in Business Administration in Healthcare Management from The Wharton School of the University of Pennsylvania.

Gary A. Mecklenburg, M.B.A.
President and CEO
Northwestern Memorial HealthCare

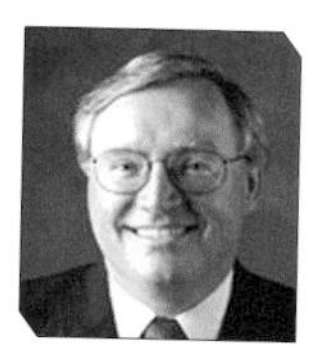

Gary A. Mecklenburg is president and CEO of Northwestern Memorial HealthCare in Chicago. He joined the organization in 1985 as President and CEO of Northwestern Memorial Hospital after five years as president of St. Joseph's Hospital and Franciscan Health Care, Inc. in Milwaukee. Mr. Mecklenburg began his career in 1970 at the University of Wisconsin Hospitals, and from 1977-1980 served as administrator of Stanford University Hospital and Clinics.

Mr. Mecklenburg is a nationally recognized leader in the healthcare field. Under his leadership, Northwestern Memorial has become one of the nation's leading teaching hospitals with a reputation for both clinical and management excellence. He is a frequent speaker and guest lecturer and serves on the Advisory Board for the Kellogg Graduate School of Management of Northwestern University.

Among his many professional activities, Mr. Mecklenburg is a past chairman of the board of trustees of the American Hospital Association and of the Illinois Hospital Association. He is currently chairman of the board of the Health Forum and of the Healthcare Research and Development Institute; and he was founding chairman of the National Alliance for Health Information Technology. Mr. Mecklenburg serves on the boards of directors of the Institute for Healthcare Improvement; the National Center for Healthcare Leadership; Becton, Dickinson and Company; Regency Hospital Company; and Cogent Healthcare.

Mr. Mecklenburg received his Bachelor of Arts degree from Northwestern University and a Master of Business Administration degree from the University of Chicago.

Herbert Pardes, M.D.
President and CEO
NewYork Presbyterian Hospital

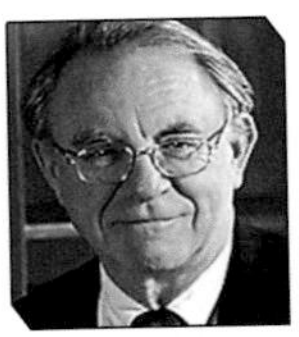

Herbert Pardes, M.D., President and CEO of NewYork-Presbyterian Hospital, has an extensive background in healthcare and academic medicine. His origins are in the field of psychiatry, and he chaired three departments of psychiatry before becoming Vice President for Health Sciences and Dean of the Faculty of Medicine at the College of Physicians & Surgeons of Columbia University. He is nationally recognized for his broad expertise in education, research, clinical care, and health policy, and as an ardent advocate of support for academic medicine. As President and CEO of NewYork-Presbyterian, Dr. Pardes has embraced a clinical mission to provide each patient with the highest quality care delivered in the most compassionate manner.

Dr. Pardes served as Director of the National Institute of Mental Health (NIMH) and U.S. Assistant Surgeon General during the Carter and Reagan Administrations (1978-84). He has also served as President of the American Psychiatric Association (1989).

Dr. Pardes left NIMH in 1984 to become Chairman of the Department of Psychiatry at Columbia University's College of Physicians & Surgeons and in 1989 was also appointed Vice President for Health Sciences for Columbia University and Dean of the Faculty of Medicine at the College of Physicians & Surgeons.

He served as Chairman of the Association of American Medical Colleges (AAMC) for 1995-96 and was Chairman of the AAMC's Council of Deans for 1994-95. In addition, he served two terms as Chairman of the New York Association of Medical Schools.

Dr. Pardes received his medical degree from the State University of New York-Downstate Medical Center (Brooklyn) in 1960. He received his Bachelor of Science degree summa cum laude from Rutgers University in 1956. He completed his internship and residency training in psychiatry at Kings County Hospital in Brooklyn and also did psychoanalytic training at the New York Psychoanalytic Institute.

Dr. Pardes chaired the Intramural Research Program Planning Committee of the NIH from 1996-1997, served on the Presidential Advisory Commission on

Consumer Protection and Quality in the Healthcare Industry, and is President of the Scientific Council of the National Alliance for Research on Schizophrenia and Depression. He serves on numerous editorial boards, has written over 130 articles and chapters on mental health and academic medicine topics, and has negotiated and conducted international collaborations with a variety of countries including India, China, and the former Soviet Union.

Dr. Pardes has earned numerous honors and awards, including election to the Institute of Medicine of the National Academy of Sciences (1997), the Sarnat International Prize in Mental Health (1997), and the U.S. Army Commendation Medal (1964) and elected to the American Academy of Arts and Sciences (2002).

Thomas M. Priselac, M.P.H.
President and CEO
Cedars-Sinai Health System

Thomas M. Priselac is President and Chief Executive Officer of the Cedars-Sinai Health System—a position he has held since January 1994.

Mr. Priselac has been associated with Cedars-Sinai since 1979. Prior to being named President and CEO, he was Executive Vice President from 1988 to 1993. Before joining Cedars-Sinai, he was on the executive staff of Montefiore Hospital in Pittsburgh.

He has served on many boards in the healthcare field over the years and currently serves as Chair-Elect of the Association of American Medical Colleges, as well as the Los Angeles Chamber of Commerce where he chairs the Health Care Committee. A past member of the American Hospital Association Board of Directors, he also formerly chaired the Hospital Association of Southern California, the California Healthcare Association, and the Association of American Medical Colleges Council of Teaching Hospitals. He also serves as an adjunct Faculty member of the UCLA School of Public Health.

A native of Pennsylvania, Mr. Priselac obtained a bachelor's degree in Biology from Washington and Jefferson College in Pennsylvania, and a master's in Public Health, Health Services Administration and Planning from the University of Pittsburgh.

Ivan Seidenberg, M.B.A.
Chairman and CEO
Verizon Communications

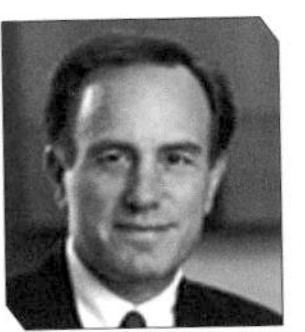

Ivan Seidenberg is chairman of the Board and chief executive officer for Verizon. On November 6, 2003, Verizon announced that Mr. Seidenberg would become chairman of the Board effective January 1, 2004. He has served as the sole CEO since April 1, 2002.

As chief executive of Bell Atlantic, and previously of NYNEX, Ivan Seidenberg was instrumental in reshaping the communications industry through two of the largest mergers in its history: the merger of Bell Atlantic and NYNEX in 1997 and the Bell Atlantic merger with GTE in 2000. He also led efforts in September 1999 to form Verizon Wireless, the nation's largest cellular business composed of the wireless assets of Bell Atlantic, GTE, and Vodafone Airtouch.

Mr. Seidenberg began his communications career more than 38 years ago as a cable splicer's assistant. His career has encompassed numerous operations and engineering assignments, including various leadership positions at AT&T and NYNEX.

He has a long-standing commitment to education and is a strong proponent of connecting students and teachers to technology. He championed a special rate for schools and libraries to connect to the Internet. Mr. Seidenberg's activism to provide electronic access to young people led to his involvement with The New York Hall of Science and Pace University, on whose boards he serves.

Mr. Seidenberg also champions diversity both within and outside the company. Under his leadership, the company has made great strides in increasing minority employment and initiated a partnership with the U.S. Small Business Administration to increase the company's purchasing from minority suppliers. Verizon's commitment to diversity has been widely recognized, with the company being cited by Fortune magazine in its list of "The 50 Best Companies for Minorities."

Besides his directorships at The Hall of Science and Pace University, Mr. Seidenberg serves on the board of directors of Honeywell, the Museum of Television and Radio, the Verizon Foundation, and Wyeth.

He earned a Bachelor of Arts degree in mathematics from City University of New York and a master's degree in business administration and marketing from Pace University.

Fredrick W. Slunecka, F.A.C.H.E.
Regional President
Avera McKennan

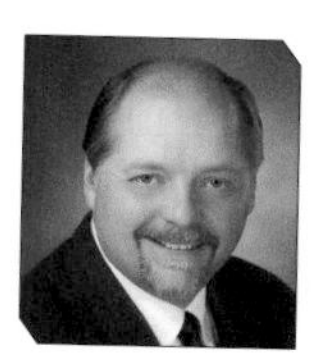

Fredrick W. Slunecka has been CEO of Avera McKennan Hospital & University Health Center, a 490-bed acute care facility affiliated with Avera Health System since 1989. He is responsible to a local board of trustees and the Avera Health Board of Directors for the operation of a $600 million organization with nearly 5,000 employees and a medical staff of 500 physicians. Major services offered include invasive cardiology, orthopedics, neurosciences, oncology including bone marrow transplant, nephrology including kidney and pancreas transplant, neonatology, obstetrics/gynecology, pediatrics, behavioral health services, inpatient rehabilitation, trauma services, helicopter and fixed wing ambulance services, home health, hospice, durable medical equipment, a 90-bed skilled nursing facility, a 100 apartment unit retirement community, and a fitness center. Residency and teaching programs in family practice, internal medicine, psychiatry, and adolescent psychiatry are offered with the University of South Dakota School of Medicine. Avera McKennan has been a national leader in telemedicine services and provides e-ICU services to several rural hospitals. Avera McKennan has received numerous accolades including Most Wired, Top 100 in Cardiology, Distinguished Hospital by Healthgrades, and Magnet Status for Nursing Care.

Mr. Slunecka is a fellow of the American College of Healthcare Executives and is involved in many civic organizations.

He received his master's degree in hospital administration from the University of Minnesota and his bachelor's degree in political science from the University of South Dakota.

William W. Stead, M.D.
Director, Informatics Center
Associate Vice-Chancellor for Health Affairs
Professor, Medicine and Biomedical Informatics
Vanderbilt University Medical Center

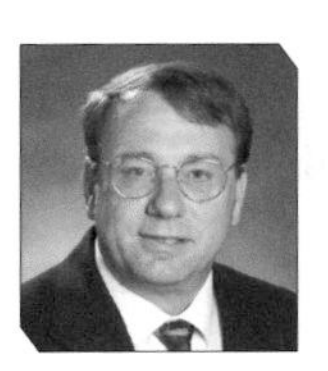

William W. Stead, M.D., is Professor of Medicine and Biomedical Informatics, Director of the Informatics Center and Associate Vice-Chancellor for Health Affairs at Vanderbilt University Medical Center. The Informatics Center brings together research and education in biomedical informatics with provision of the Medical Center's operation and decision support infrastructure. In addition to serving as the Medical Center's Chief Information Officer, Dr. Stead is Chief Information Architect for Vanderbilt University and Chairman of the Vanderbilt Center for Better Health. The Center for Better Health was established in June 2002 to help accelerate change in healthcare through optimal use of information technology.

Dr. Stead received his B.A. and M.D. from Duke University where he also served residencies in Internal Medicine and Nephrology. As an undergraduate in the 1960s, he was a member of the team that developed the Cardiology Databank, one of the first clinical epidemiology projects to change practice by linking outcomes to process. As a faculty member in Nephrology, he was the physician in the physician-engineer partnership that developed The Medical Record (TMR), one of the first practical computer-based patient record systems. He helped Duke build one of the first patient-centered hospital information systems. He has led (as PI) two prominent academic health centers, Duke in the 1980s, and Vanderbilt in the 1990s, through both planning and implementation phases of large-scale, Integrated Advanced Information Management System (IAIMS) projects. At Vanderbilt, his team has been successful in creating informatics techniques for linking information into clinical workflow, in overcoming the cultural barriers to changing practice to take advantage of these techniques, and in reducing the cost and time required to implement enterprise-wide information technology infrastructure.

Dr. Stead is a Founding Fellow of both the American College of Medical Informatics and the American Institute for Engineering in Biology and Medicine, and a member of the Institute of Medicine of the National Academies. He is currently Chairman of the Board of Regents of the National Library of Medicine and serves on the Computer Science and Telecommunication Board of the National Research Council. He was the founding Editor-in-Chief of the Journal of the American Medical Informatics Association, and served as President of the American Association for Medical Systems and Informatics and the American College of Medical Informatics.

In October 2004, Dr. Stead was appointed to the Commission on Systemic Interoperability.

In addition to his academic responsibilities, Dr. Stead is a Director of HealthStream and Director of NetSilica.

DESIGNATED FEDERAL OFFICIAL:
Donald A.B. Lindberg, M.D.
Director
National Library of Medicine

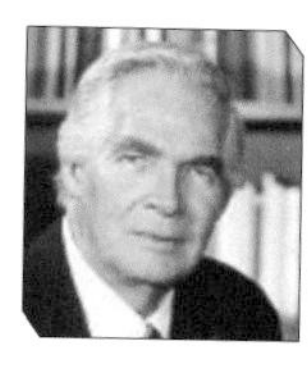

Donald A.B. Lindberg, M.D., is a scientist who has pioneered applying computer technology to healthcare beginning in 1960 at the University of Missouri. In 1984, he was appointed Director of the National Library of Medicine, the world's largest biomedical library (annual budget $275 million; 690 career staff). From 1992-1995 he served in a concurrent position as founding Director of the National Coordination Office for High Performance Computing and Communications (HPCC) in the Office of Science and Technology Policy, Executive Office of the President. In 1996, he was named by the HHS Secretary to be the U.S. Coordinator for the G-7 Global Health Applications Project.

In addition to an eminent career in pathology, Dr. Lindberg has made notable contributions to information and computer activities in medical diagnosis, artificial intelligence, and educational programs. Before his appointment as NLM Director, he was Professor of Information Science and Professor of Pathology at the University of Missouri-Columbia. He has current academic appointments as Clinical Professor of Pathology at the University ofVirginia and Adjunct Professor of Pathology at the University of Maryland School of Medicine.

Dr. Lindberg was elected the first President of the American Medical Informatics Association (AMIA). As the country's senior statesman for medicine and computers, he has been called upon to serve on many boards including the Computer Science and Engineering Board of the National Academy of Sciences, the National Board of Medical Examiners, and the Council of the Institute of Medicine of the National Academy of Sciences.

Dr. Lindberg graduated Magna cum Laude from Amherst College and received his M.D. degree from the College of Physicians and Surgeons, Columbia University. Among the honors he has received are Phi Beta Kappa, Simpson Fellow of Amherst College, Markle Scholar in Academic Medicine, Surgeon General's Medallion, recipient of the First AMA Nathan Davis Award for outstanding Member of the Executive Branch in Career Public Service, the Walter C. Alvarez Memorial Award of the American Medical Writers Association, the Presidential Senior Executive Rank Award, Founding Fellow of the American Institute of Medical and Biological Engineering, the Outstanding Service Medal of the Uniformed Services University of the Health Sciences, Federal Computer Week's Federal 100 Award, Computers in Healthcare Pioneer Award, Association of Minority Health Professions Schools Commendation, RCI High Performance Computing Industry Recognition Award, U.S. National Commission on Libraries and Information Science Silver Award, Council of Biology Editors Meritorious Award, HHS Meritorious Service Award, Medical Library Association President's Award, Fellow of the American Association for the Advancement of Science, and honorary doctorates from Amherst College, the State University of New York at Syracuse, and the University of Missouri-Columbia.

DIRECTOR:
Dana Haza
Director, Commission on Systemic Interoperability
National Library of Medicine

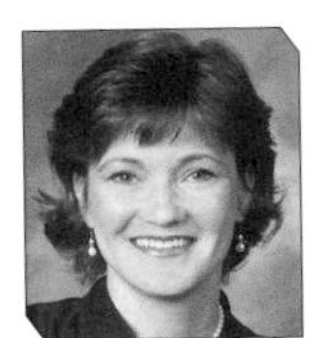

Dana Haza received a Presidential appointment to be the Director of the Commission on Systemic Interoperability early in January of 2005. It is the goal of this commission to produce a comprehensive report by the end of October, identifying the strategy necessary to foster the development of accessible electronic health information to provide optimal health and healthcare for every American. Dana is also currently co-authoring a monograph with Dr. Andy von Eschenbach, Director of the National Cancer Institute, describing the breakthroughs in cancer research that will ultimately result in much of cancer evolving into a chronic disease by 2015. Dana is passionate in her pursuit of health and wholeness for every American. This commitment is a testimony to her continual personal development and renewal as a leader in health and healthcare thinking and reform.

Prior to her appointment, Dana was the Director of Policy for Newt Gingrich at the American Enterprise Institute for Public Policy Research (AEI), one of America's largest and most respected think tanks. In her capacity as Director of Policy, Dana worked closely with a variety of federal agencies and branches of the government on such projects as the 2003 Medicare bill, patient safety issues, electronic health records, as well as with the National Cancer Institute on creating a model of eliminating suffering and death by cancer by 2015. She has co-authored the book, *Saving Lives & Saving Money*, with Newt Gingrich and Anne Woodbury. Dana has served on a congressional panel for the Academy-Health and Friend of AHRQ. She serves as a consultant to the Gingrich Group and the Center for Health Transformation. As a speaker, Dana regularly gives presentations on transformation, strategic thinking and 21st century health, and healthcare system reform to a variety of conferences, hospital boards, state health and professional societies, managed care organizations, pharmaceutical companies, as well as guest lecturing for graduate level health classes.

Dana brings to the public policy arena 15 years of healthcare experience. She was the Director of Managed Care and the Director of a 250-physician-hospital organization (PHO), an HCA facility in Augusta, GA. She has been an office manager for a variety of health specialties, and a physician recruiter. She has also served on the Boards of the Georgia Hospital Association, and Georgia Society for Managed Care, as well as in other advisory and teaching capacities. Dana formerly held the position of Special Projects Director and District Director for Georgia Congressman, Charlie Norwood. She graduated from Mercer University with a major in journalism.

After serving as the Director of the Commission on Systemic Interoperability, Dana will act as the Interim Director for the Office of Programs and Coordination in the Office of the National Coordinator for Health Information Technology.

Appendix B
American Health Information Community Charter

American Health Information Community Charter

DRAFT

1. Purpose

On April 27, 2004, the President signed Executive Order (EO) 13335 announcing his commitment to the promotion of health information technology (health IT) to lower costs, reduce medical errors, improve quality of care, and provide better information for patients and physicians. In particular, the President called for widespread adoption of electronic health records (EHRs) and for health information to follow patients throughout their care in a seamless and secure manner.

In the EO, the President enunciated a vision to provide leadership for the development and national implementation of an interoperable health IT infrastructure that: (a) ensures appropriate information to guide medical decisions is available at the time and place of care; (b) improves health care quality, reduces medical errors, and advances the delivery of appropriate, evidence-based medical care; (c) reduces health care costs resulting from inefficiency, medical errors, inappropriate care, and incomplete information; (d) promotes a more effective marketplace, greater competition, and increased choice through the wider availability of accurate information on health care costs, quality, and outcomes; (e) improves the coordination of care and information among hospitals, laboratories, physician offices, and other ambulatory care providers through an effective infrastructure for the secure and authorized exchange of healthcare information; and (f) ensures patients' individually identifiable health information is secure and protected.

The EO directed the Secretary of the Department Health and Human Services (HHS) to establish within the Office of the Secretary the position of National Health Information Technology Coordinator (National Coordinator).

Recognizing the need for public and private sector collaboration to achieve these goals, the EO charged the National Coordinator, to the extent permitted by law, to coordinate outreach and consultation by the relevant branch agencies (including Federal commissions) with public and private parties of interest, including consumers, providers, payers, and administrators.

As a part of this collaboration, the Secretary of HHS (Secretary) hereby creates the American Health Information Community (AHIC) to: 1) advise the Secretary and recommend specific actions to achieve a common interoperability framework for health IT; and 2) serve as a forum for participation from a broad range of stakeholders to provide input on achieving interoperability of health IT.

2. Authority

42 U.S.C. Sec. 217a, Sec. 222 of the Public Health Service Act, as amended. The AHIC is governed by the provisions of Public Law 92-463, as amended, (5 U.S.C. Appendix 2), which sets forth standards for the formation and use of federal advisory committees.

3. Function

The AHIC shall advise the Secretary concerning efforts to develop information technology standards and achieve interoperability of health IT so the President's health IT goals can be achieved. At the Secretary's request, the AHIC may provide advice on related matters pertaining to health IT.

The AHIC shall operate in a manner that is consistent with the EO, including not assuming or relying upon additional federal resources or spending to accomplish adoption of interoperable health information technology.

The AHIC shall, among other things, advance and develop recommendations for the following issues:

- Protection of health information through appropriate privacy and security practices;
- Ongoing harmonization of industry-wide health IT standards;
- Achievement of an Internet-based nationwide health information network that includes information tools, specialized network functions, and security protections for interoperable health information exchange;
- Acceleration of interoperable EHR adoption across the broad spectrum of health care providers;
- Compliance certification and inspection processes for EHRs, including infrastructure components through which EHRs interoperate;
- Identification of health IT standards for use by the National Institute for Standards and Technology (NIST) in a Federal Information Processing Standards (FIPS) process relevant to Federal agencies;
- Identification and prioritization of specific use cases for which health IT is valuable, beneficial and feasible, such as adverse drug event reporting, electronic prescribing, lab and claims information sharing, public health, bioterrorism surveillance, and advanced research; and
- Succession of AHIC by a private-sector health information community initiative.

4. Structure

The AHIC shall not exceed 17 voting members, including the Chair, and members shall be appointed by the Secretary. Membership shall include officials from HHS and its component agencies, and other appropriate federal agencies, including, but not limited to, the Department of Veterans Affairs, Office of Personnel Management, Department of Commerce, Department of Treasury, and the Department of Defense. The federal members may be represented by alternates. At least one member shall be an expert on matters pertaining to privacy and security protections of individually identifiable health information. The Secretary shall select other members from persons knowledgeable in the field of health IT, or in fields applicable or related thereto, including physicians, health care providers, patients, payers, purchasers, public health experts, research scientists, and a State official. Non-federal members of the AHIC will be Special Government Employees, unless classified as representatives. The Secretary shall be the Chair and may designate an Acting Chair for any meeting or portion of a meeting, as the Secretary deems appropriate.

Members shall serve 2-year terms, except that any member appointed to fill a vacancy for an unexpired term shall be appointed for the remainder of such term. A member may serve for up to 180 days after the expiration of the member's term or until a successor has taken office.

The National Coordinator shall provide management and support services for the AHIC.

Less than the full AHIC may convene to gather information; conduct research; analyze relevant issues and facts in preparation for a meeting; or draft position papers for deliberation by the AHIC.

Less than the full AHIC may convene to discuss administrative matters of the AHIC or to receive administrative information from a Federal official or agency.

5. Meetings

AHIC meetings may be held up to 12 times per year, at the call of the Chair or Acting Chair, who shall also provide the meeting agenda. A quorum shall be required for any meeting; the majority of those members appointed to the AHIC as of the date of the meeting shall constitute a quorum. Meetings shall be open to the public except when closure is specifically allowed by law, and meetings may be closed to the public only after all statutory and regulatory requirements for doing so have been met. The Secretary, or other official to whom the authority has been delegated, shall make such determinations. Notice of all meetings shall be given to the public in accordance with applicable laws.

All meetings shall be conducted, and records of the proceedings kept, as required by applicable laws and HHS regulations.

6. Compensation

Members who are not full-time Federal employees shall be paid at the rate of $250 per day, plus per diem and travel expenses in accordance with Standard Government Travel Regulations.

7. Annual Cost Estimate

Estimated annual cost for operating the AHIC, including compensation and travel expenses for members but excluding staff support, is $3 million. Estimated annual person-years of staff support required is four, at an estimated annual cost of $700,000.

8. Reports

In the event a portion of a meeting is closed to the public, a report shall be prepared which shall contain, at a minimum, a list of members and their business addresses, the committee activities, and recommendations made during the fiscal year. A copy of the report shall be provided to the Department Committee Management Office.

9. Termination Date

Unless renewed by appropriate action prior to its expiration, the AHIC shall terminate two years from the date this charter is approved. However, the maximum term of operation for the AHIC shall be five years.

Approved:

____________________	______________________________
Date	Secretary

THE SECRETARY OF HHS STATIONERY

FORMAL DETERMINATION

I determine, after appropriate consultation between this Department and General Services Administration, that formation of the American Health Information Community is in the public interest in connection with the performance of duties imposed on the Department by law, and that such duties can best be performed through the advice and counsel of such a group.

I deem that it is not feasible for the Department or any of its existing committees to perform these duties, and that a satisfactory plan for appropriate balance of committee membership has been submitted.

____________________ ______________________________

Date Secretary

Appendix C
Past Recommendations

Recommendations from Past Reports

On Healthcare, Information Technology, Patient Safety, Privacy, National Security, Computerized Medical Records, Standards, and Interoperability

Compiled May 17, 2005

Table of Contents

Recommendations from Past Reports

From ***Records, Computers and the Rights of Citizens: Report of the Secretary's Advisory Committee on Automated Personal Data Systems*** (July 1973)

RECOMMENDATIONS

Under current law, a person's privacy is poorly protected against arbitrary or abusive record-keeping practices. For this reason, as well as because of the need to establish standards of record-keeping practice appropriate to the computer age, the report recommends the enactment of a Federal "Code of Fair Information Practice" for all automated personal data systems. The Code rests on five basic principles that would be given legal effect as "safeguard requirements" for automated personal data systems.

- There must be no personal data record-keeping systems whose very existence is secret.
- There must be a way for an individual to find out what information about him is in a record and how it is used.
- There must be a way for an individual to prevent information about him that was obtained for one purpose from being used or made available for other purposes without his consent.
- There must be a way for an individual to correct or amend a record of identifiable information about him.
- Any organization creating, maintaining, using, or disseminating records of identifiable personal data must assure the reliability of the data for their intended use and must take precautions to prevent misuse of the data.

We recommend the enactment of legislation establishing a Code of Fair Information practice for all automated personal data systems.

- The Code should define "fair information practice" as adherence to specified safeguard requirements.
- The Code should prohibit violation of any safeguard requirement as an "unfair information practice."
- The Code should provide that an unfair information practice be subject to both civil and criminal penalties.
- The Code should provide for injunctions to prevent violation of any safeguard requirement.
- The Code should give individuals the right to bring suits for unfair information practices to recover actual, liquidated, and punitive damages, in individual or class actions. It should also provide for recovery of reasonable attorneys' fees and other costs of litigation incurred by individuals who bring successful suits.

Pending the enactment of a code of fair information practice, we recommend that all Federal agencies (i) apply the safeguard requirements, by administrative action, to all Federal systems, and (ii) assure, through formal rule making, that the safeguard requirements are applied to all other systems within reach of the Federal government's authority. Pending the enactment of a code of fair information practice, we urge that State and local governments, the institutions within reach of their authority, and all private organizations adopt the safeguard requirements by whatever means are appropriate.

Existing laws or regulations affording individuals greater protection than the safeguard requirements should be retained, and those providing less protection should be amended to meet the basic standards set by the safeguards. In particular, we recommend:

- That the Freedom of Information Act be amended to require an agency to obtain the consent of an individual before disclosing in personally identifiable form exempted category data about him, unless the disclosure is within the purposes of the system as specifically required by statute.
- That pending such amendment of the Act, all Federal agencies provide for obtaining the consent of individuals before disclosing individually identifiable exempted-category data about them under the Freedom of Information Act.
- That the Fair Credit Reporting Act be amended to provide for actual, personal inspection by an individual of his record along with the opportunity to copy its contents, or to have copies made; and that the exceptions from disclosure to the individual now authorized by the Fair Credit Reporting Act for medical information and sources of investigative information be omitted.

In light of our inquiry into the statistical-reporting and research uses of personal data in administrative record-keeping systems, we recommend that steps be taken to assure that all such uses are carried out in accordance with five principles:

First, when personal data are collected for administrative purposes, individuals should under no circumstances be coerced into providing additional personal data that are to be used exclusively for statistical reporting and research. When application forms or other means of collecting personal data for an administrative data system are designed, the mandatory or voluntary character of an individual's responses should be made clear.

Second, personal data used for making determinations about an individual's character, qualifications, rights, benefits, or opportunities, and personal data collected and used for statistical reporting and research, should be processed and stored separately.

Third, the amount of supplementary statistical-reporting and research data collected and stored in personally identifiable form should be kept to a minimum.

Fourth, proposals to use administrative records for statistical reporting and research should be subjected to careful scrutiny by persons of strong statistical and research competence.

Fifth, any published findings or reports that result from secondary statistical-reporting and research uses of administrative personal data systems should meet the highest standards of error measurement and documentation.

In addition, we recommend that all personal data in such systems be protected by statute from compulsory disclosure in identifiable form. Federal legislation protecting against compulsory disclosure should include the following features:

- The data to be protected should be limited to those *used exclusively for statistical reporting or research.* Thus, the protection would apply to statistical-reporting and research data derived from administrative records, and kept apart from them, but not to the administrative records themselves.
- The protection should be limited to data *identifiable with, or traceable to, specific individuals.* When data are released in statistical form, reasonable precautions to protect against "statistical disclosure" should be considered to fulfill the obligation not to disclose data that can be traced to specific individuals.
- The protection should be specific enough to qualify for non-disclosure under the Freedom of Information Act exemption for matters "specifically exempted from disclosure by statute." 5 U.S.C. 552(b)(3).

- The protection should be available for data in the custody of all statistical-reporting and research systems, whether supported by Federal funds or not.
- Either the data custodian or the individual about whom data are sought by legal process should be able to invoke the protection, but only the individual should be able to waive it.
- The Federal law should be controlling; no State statute should be taken to interfere with the protection it provides.

Use of the Social Security Number

We take the position that a standard universal identifier (SUI) should not be established in the United States now or in the foreseeable future. By our definition, the Social Security Number (SSN) cannot fully qualify as an SUI; it only approximates one. However, there is an increasing tendency for the Social Security number to be used as if it were an SUI. There are pressures on the Social Security Administration to do things that make the SSN more nearly an SUI.

We believe that any action that would tend to make the SSN more nearly an SUI should be taken only if, after careful deliberation, it appears justifiable and any attendant risks can be avoided. We recommend against the adoption of any nationwide, standard, personal identification format, with or without the SSN, that would enhance the likelihood of arbitrary or uncontrolled linkage of records about people, particularly between government and government-supported automated personal data systems.

We believe that until safeguards against abuse of automated personal data systems have become effective, constraints should be imposed on use of the Social Security number. After that the question of SSN use might properly be reopened.

As a general framework for action on the Social Security number, we recommend that Federal policy with respect to use of the SSN be governed by the following principles:

> **First**, uses of the SSN should be limited to those necessary for carrying out requirements imposed by the Federal government.
>
> **Second**, Federal agencies and departments should not require or promote use of the SSN except to the extent that they have a specific legislative mandate from the Congress to do so.
>
> **Third**, the Congress should be sparing in mandating use of the SSN, and should do so only after full and careful consideration preceded by well advertised hearings that elicit substantial public participation. Such consideration should weigh carefully the pros and cons of any proposed use, and should pay particular attention to whether effective safeguards have been applied to automated personal data systems that would be affected by the proposed use of the SSN. (Ideally, Congress should review all present Federal requirements for use of the SSN and determine whether these existing requirements should be continued, repealed, or modified.)
>
> **Fourth**, when the SSN is used in instances that do not conform to the three foregoing principles, no individual should be coerced into providing his SSN, nor should his SSN be used without his consent.
>
> **Fifth**, an individual should be fully and fairly informed of his rights and responsibilities relative to uses of the SSN, including the right to disclose his SSN whenever he deems it in his interest to do so.

In accordance with these principles, we recommend specific, preemptive Federal legislation providing:

(1) That an individual has a legal right to refuse to disclose his SSN to any person or organization that does not have specific authority provided by Federal statute to request it;

(2) That an individual has the right to redress if his lawful refusal to disclose his SSN results in the denial of a benefit, or the threat of denial of a benefit; and that, should an individual under threat of loss of benefits supply his SSN under protest to an unauthorized requestor, he shall not be considered to have forfeited his right to redress; and

(3) That any oral or written request made to an individual for his SSN must be accompanied by a clear statement indicating whether or not compliance with the request is required by Federal statute, and, if so, citing the specific legal requirement.

In addition, we recommend

(4) That the Social Security Administration undertake a positive program of issuing SSNs to ninth-grade students in schools, provided (a) that no school system be induced to cooperate in such a program contrary to its preference; and (b) that any person shall have the right to refuse to be issued an SSN in connection with such a program, and such right of refusal shall be available both to the student and to his parents or guardians.

From ***Medical Records: Problems of Confidentiality and Privacy*** (February, 1978)

RECOMMENDATIONS

- The individual's right to control, use, and access his health care records, while obtaining requisite services and benefits, requires further consideration.

From ***Health Data in the Information Age: Use, Disclosure, and Privacy*** (1994)

RECOMMENDATION 2.1 ACCURACY AND COMPLETENESS

To address these issues, the committee recommends that health database organizations take responsibility for assuring data quality on an ongoing basis and, in particular, take affirmative steps to ensure: (1) the completeness and accuracy of the data in the databases for which they are responsible and (2) the validity of data for analytic purposes for which they are used.

Part 2 of this recommendation applies to analyses that Health Database Organizations (HDOs) conduct. They cannot, of course, police the validity of data when used by others for purposes over which the HDOs have no a priori control.

RECOMMENDATION 2.2 COMPUTER-BASED PATIENT RECORD

Accordingly, the committee recommends that health database organizations support and contribute to regional and national efforts to create computer-based patient records.

RECOMMENDATION 3.1 CONDUCTING PROVIDER-SPECIFIC EVALUATIONS

The committee recommends that health database organizations produce and make publicly available appropriate and timely summaries, analyses, and multivariate analyses of all or pertinent parts of their databases. More specifically, the committee recommends that health database organizations regularly produce and publish results of provider-specific evaluations of costs, quality, and effectiveness of care.

RECOMMENDATION 3.2 DESCRIBING ANALYTIC METHODS

The committee recommends that a health database organization report the following for any analysis it releases publicly:

- general methods for ensuring completeness and accuracy of their data;
- a description of the contents and the completeness of all data files and of the variables in each file used in the analyses;
- information documenting any study of the accuracy of variables used in the analyses.

RECOMMENDATION 3.3 MINIMIZING POTENTIAL HARM

The committee recommends that, to enhance the fairness and minimize the risk of unintended harm from the publication of evaluative studies that identify individual providers, each HDO should adhere to two principles as a standard procedure prior to publication: (1) to make available to and upon request supply to institutions, practitioners, or providers identified in an analysis all data required to perform an independent analysis, and to do so with reasonable time for such analysis prior to public release of the HDO results; and (2) to accompany publication of its own analyses with notice of the existence and availability of responsible challenges to, alternate analyses of, or explanation of the findings.

RECOMMENDATION 3.4 ADVOCACY OF DATA RELEASE: PROMOTING WIDE APPLICATIONS OF HEALTH-RELATED DATA

To foster the presumed benefits of widespread applications of HDO data, the committee recommends that health database organizations should release non-person-identifiable data upon request to other entities once those data are in analyzable form. This policy should include release to any organization that meets the following criteria:

- it has a public mission statement indicating that promoting public health or the release of information to the public is a major goal;
- it enforces explicit policies regarding protection of the confidentiality and integrity of data;
- it agrees not to publish, redisclose, or transfer the raw data to any other individual or organization; and
- it agrees to disclose analyses in a public forum or publication.

The committee also recommends, as a related matter, that health database organizations make public their own policies governing the release of data.

RECOMMENDATION 4.1 PREEMPTIVE LEGISLATION

The committee recommends that the U.S. Congress move to enact preemptive legislation that will:

- establish a uniform requirement for the assurance of confidentiality and protection of privacy rights for person-identifiable health data and specify a Code of Fair Health Information Practices that ensures a proper balance among required disclosures, use of data, and patient privacy;
- impose penalties for violations of the act, including civil damages, equitable remedies, and attorney's fees where appropriate;
- provide for enforcement by the government and permit private aggrieved parties to sue;
- establish that compliance with the act's requirements would be a defense to legal actions based on charges of improper disclosure; and

- exempt health database organizations from public health reporting laws and compulsory process with respect to person-identifiable health data except for compulsory process initiated by record subjects.

RECOMMENDATION 4.2 DATA PROTECTION UNITS

The committee recommends that health database organizations establish a responsible administrative unit or board to promulgate and implement information policies concerning the acquisition and dissemination of information and establish whatever administrative mechanism is required to implement these policies. Such an administrative unit or board should:

- promulgate and implement policies concerning data protection and analyses based on such data;
- develop and implement policies that protect the confidentiality of all person-identifiable information, consistent with other policies of the organization and relevant state and federal law;
- develop and disseminate educational materials for the general public that will describe in understandable terms the analyses and their interpretation of the rights and responsibilities of individuals and the protections accorded their data by the organization;
- develop and implement security practices in the manual and automated data processing and storage systems of the organization; and
- develop and implement a comprehensive employee training program that includes instruction concerning the protection of person-identifiable data.

RECOMMENDATION 4.3 RELEASE OF PERSON-IDENTIFIED DATA

The committee recognizes that there must be release of patient-identified data related to the processing of health insurance claims. The committee recommends, however, that a health database organization *not* release person-identifiable information in any other circumstances *except* the following:

- to other HDOs whose missions are compatible with and whose confidentiality and security protections are at least as stringent as their own;
- to individuals for information about themselves;
- to parents for information about a minor child except when such release is prohibited by law;
- to legal representatives of incompetent patients for information about the patient;
- to researchers with approval from their institution's properly constituted Institutional Review Board;
- to licensed practitioners with a need to know when treating patients in life-threatening situations who are unable to consent at the time care is rendered; and
- to licensed practitioners when treating patients in all other (non-life-threatening) situations, *but only with the informed consent of the patient.*

Otherwise, the committee recommends that health database organizations not authorize access to, or release of, information on individuals with or without informed consent.

RECOMMENDATION 4.4 RESTRICTING EMPLOYER ACCESS

The committee recommends that employers not be permitted to require receipt of an individual's data from a health database organization as a condition of employment or for the receipt of benefits.

The committee recommends that an HDO report the following for any analysis it releases publicly:

- general methods for ensuring completeness and accuracy of data;
- a description of the contents and the completeness of all data files and of the variables in each file used in the analyses;
- information documenting any study of the accuracy of variables used in the analyses (Recommendation 3.2).

THE FOLLOWING IS THE SAME AS RECOMMENDATION 4.1

The committee recommends that the U.S. Congress move to enact preemptive legislation that will:

- establish a uniform requirement for the assurance of confidentiality and protection of privacy rights for person-identifiable health data and specify a Code of Fair Health Information Practices that ensures a proper balance among required disclosures, use of data, and patient privacy;
- impose penalties for violations of the act, including civil damages, equitable remedies, and attorney's fees where appropriate;
- provide for enforcement by the government and permit private aggrieved parties to sue;
- establish that compliance with the act's requirements would be a defense to legal actions based on charges of improper disclosure; and
- exempt health database organizations from public health reporting laws and compulsory process with respect to person-identifiable health data except for compulsory process initiated by record subjects (Recommendation 4.1).

From ***Standards for Medical Identifiers, Codes, and Messages Needed to Create an Efficient Computer-stored Medical Record*** (1994)

RECOMMENDATIONS

1. The American Medical Informatics Association (AMIA) recommends the use of the SSN as the patient identifier at the present time. In addition, we recommend the addition of a self-check digit to the SSN to reduce errors of identification whenever the number is hand-entered by an operator. Other options for patient identifiers should be explored for the long haul.
2. We suggest that the Health Care Financing Administration (HCFA) consider using alphanumeric codes (to reduce the number of key strokes needed to enter the identifier to a practical number), and that the Universal Physician Identifier Number (UPIN) be expanded to include all health care providers for the purpose of provider identification.
3. For the next five years, all private and government care agencies should use published health care informatics message standards as a starting point for all new applications involving applicable internal and external health care information transmissions. Different published standards would apply to different kinds of communications, depending upon the subject matter and kind of communication as described below.

4. AMIA recommends that HL7 be used for within-institution transmission of orders, clinical observations, and clinical data (including test results); admission, transfer, and discharge records; and charge and billing information.

5. ASTM E1238 should be used for most interchanges of clinical data between institutions. HL7, which is a practical superset of ASTM E1238, is an alternative when tighter linkages are desired.

6. ACR-NEMA should be used for the transmission of radiologic images and for message transmissions within PACS.

7. AMIA recommends the use of ASTM E1394 for communication of information from laboratory instruments to computer systems.

8. AMIA suggests that the NCPDP be used for communication of prescription billing information and eligibility information between the community pharmacies and third-party payers.

9. AMIA suggests the use of ASC X12's standards for billing and remittance transactions between a health care provider and a third-party payer.

10. AMIA recommends its (ASTM E1460, or "Arden Syntax") use for the transmission of medical logic modules.

11. AMIA recommends its (ASTM E1467) use for the transmission of such EEG and EMG signals.

12. ANSI Z39.50 is a draft standard for transmitting requests for bibliographic information to bibliographic retrieval systems. AMIA recommends that it be considered for all such communications.

13. AMIA recommends that during the initial five years of standards development, the federal government invest in efforts to integrate and extend these standards to all health care messages. Furthermore, we suggest that the federal government build public-domain translators between the current message systems to permit future integration of systems. The translators should be submitted as ANSI and/or IS0 standards, and would be based on the object modeling framework being developed by the joint working group created by the HISPP Message Standards Developers Subcommittee (MSDS) and coordinated by IEEE MEDIX for modeling.

14. With advice from AHCPR and CPRI, and in coordination with ANSI HISPP and the message standards developers, they should have the formal responsibility for developing these standards.

15. Codes are needed to address (at least, the following) subject domains:

    - Drugs (e.g., penicillin V)
    - Diagnoses (e.g., pneumonia, heart failure)
    - Symptoms and findings (e.g., fatigue, swollen ankle)
    - Anatomic sites (e.g., right lower lobe of lung)
    - Microbes and etiologic agents (e.g., E. coli)
    - Clinical observations (e.g., blood pressure, oral intake, physical examination of heart)
    - Patient outcome variables and functional status (e.g., SF-36, Hamilton depression score, Inter-Study TYPE variables)
    - Medical devices (e.g., hip implant, tongue blades)
    - Units of measure

- Diagnostic study results (e.g., blood glucose, chest, x-ray, cardiac MUGA)
- Procedures (e.g., triple bypass surgery, endoscopy, skin care)

From ***For the Record: Protecting Electronic Health Information*** (1997)

RECOMMENDATIONS

1. All organizations that handle patient-identifiable health care information—regardless of size—should adopt the set of technical and organizations policies, practices, and procedures described below to protect such information.

2. Government and the health care industry should take action to create the infrastructure necessary to support the privacy and security of electronic health information.

2.1 The Secretary of Health and Human Services should establish a standing health information subcommittee within the National Committee on Vital and Health Statistics to develop and update privacy and security standards for all users of health information. Membership should be drawn from existing organizations that represent the broad spectrum of users and subjects of health information.

2.2 Congress should provide initial funding for the establishment of an organization for the health-care industry to promote greater sharing of information about security threats, incidents, and solutions throughout the industry.

3. The federal government should work with industry to promote and encourage an informed public debate to determine an appropriate balance between the privacy concerns of patients and the information needs of various users of health information.

3.1 Organizations that collect, analyze, or disseminate health information should adopt a set of fair information practices similar to those contained in the federal Privacy Act of 1974.

3.2 The Department of Health and Human Services should work with state and local governments, health care researchers, and the health care industry to establish a program to promote consumer awareness of health privacy issues and the value of health information for patient care, administration, and research. It should also conduct studies that will develop a series of recommendations for improving the level of consumer awareness of health data flows.

3.3 Professional societies and industry groups (i.e., the American Hospital Association, American Medical Informatics Association, American Health Management Association, College of Health Information Management Executives, Healthcare Information and Management Systems Society, Computer-based Patient Records Institute, and American Medical Association, etc.) should continue to expand their leadership roles in educating members about privacy and security issues in their conference discussions and publications.

3.4 The Department of Health and Human Services should conduct studies to determine the extent to which—and the conditions under which—users of health information need data containing patient identities.

3.5 The Department of Health and Human Services should work with the US Office of Consumer Affairs to determine appropriate ways to provide consumers with a visible, centralized point of contact regarding privacy issues (a privacy ombudsman).

4. Any effort to develop a universal patient identifier should weigh the presumed advantages of such an identifier against potential privacy concerns. Any method used to identify patients and to link patient records in a health care environment should be evaluated against the privacy criteria listed below.

    1. The method should be accompanied by an explicit policy framework that defines the nature and character of linkages that violate patient privacy and specifies legal or other sanctions for creating such linkages. That framework should derive from the national debate advocated in Recommendation 3.

    2. It should facilitate the identification of parties that link records so that those who make improper linkages can be held responsible for their creation.

    3. It should be unidirectional to the degree that is technically feasible: it should facilitate the appropriate linking of health records given information about the patient or provided by the patient (such as the patient's identifier), but prevent a patient's identity from being easily deduced from a set of linked health records or from the identifier itself.

5. The federal government should take steps to improve information security technologies for health care applications.

5.1 To facilitate the exchange of technical knowledge on information security and the transfer of information security technology, the Department of Health and Human Services should establish formal liaisons with relevant government and industry working groups.

5.2 The Department of Health and Human Services should support research in those areas listed below that are of particular importance to the health care industry, but that might not otherwise be pursued.

- Methods of identifying and linking patient records.
- Anonymous care and pseudonyms.
- Audit tools.
- Tools for rights enforcement and management.

5.3 The Department of Health and Human Services should fund experimental testbeds that explore different approaches to access control that hold promise for being inexpensive and easy to incorporate into existing operations and that allow access during emergency situations.

From ***The Computer-Based Patient Record: An Essential Technology for Health Care*** (1991, 1997)

SUMMARY OF THE RECOMMENDATIONS OF THE INSTITUTE OF MEDICINE COMMITTEE ON IMPROVING THE PATIENT RECORD

The committee recommends the following:

1. Health care professionals and organizations should adopt the computer-based patient record (CPR) as the standard for medical and all other records related to patient care.

2. To accomplish Recommendation No. 1, the public and private sectors should join in establishing a Computer-based Patient Record Institute (CPRI) to promote and facilitate development, implementation, and dissemination of the CPR.

3. Both the public and private sectors should expand support for the CPR and CPR system implementation through research, development, and demonstration projects. Specifically, the committee recommends that Congress authorize and appropriate funds to implement the research and development agenda outlined herein. The committee further recommends that private foundations and vendors fund programs that support and facilitate this research and development agenda.

4. The CPRI should promulgate uniform national standards for data and security to facilitate implementation of the CPR and its secondary databases.

5. The CPRI should review federal and state laws and regulations for the purpose of proposing and promulgating model legislation and regulations to facilitate the implementation and dissemination of the CPR and its secondary databases and to streamline the CPR and CPR systems.

6. The costs of CPR systems should be shared by those who benefit from the value of the CPR. Specifically, the full costs of implementing and operating CPRs and CPR systems should be factored into reimbursement levels or payment schedules of both public and private sector third-party payers. In addition, users of secondary databases should support the costs of creating such databases.

7. Health care professional schools and organizations should enhance educational programs for students and practitioners in the use of computers, CPRs, and CPR systems for patient care, education, and research.

From ***To Err Is Human: Building a Safer Health System*** (2000)

RECOMMENDATIONS

4.1 Congress should create a Center for Patient Safety within the Agency for Healthcare Research and Quality. This center should

- Set the national goals for patient safety, track progress in meeting these goals, and issue an annual report to the President and Congress on patient safety; and
- Develop knowledge and understanding of errors in health care by developing a research agenda, funding Centers of Excellence, evaluating methods for identifying and preventing errors, and funding dissemination and communication activities to improve patient safety.

5.1 A nationwide mandatory reporting system should be established that provides for the collection of standardized information by state governments about adverse events that result in death or serious harm. Reporting should initially be required of hospitals and eventually be required of other institutional and ambulatory care delivery settings. Congress should

- Designate the National Forum for Health Care Quality Measurement and Reporting as the entity responsible for promulgating and maintaining a core set of reporting standards to be used by states, including a nomenclature and taxonomy for reporting;
- Require all health care organizations to report standardized information on a defined list of adverse events;
- Provide funds and technical expertise for state governments to establish or adapt their current error reporting systems to collect the standardized information, analyze it and conduct follow-up action as needed with health care organizations. Should a state choose not to implement the mandatory reporting system, the Department of Health and Human Services should be designated as the responsible entity; and

- Designate the Center for Patient Safety to:
  1) convene states to share information and expertise, and to evaluate alternative approaches taken for implementing reporting programs, identify best practices for implementation, and assess the impact of state programs; and
  2) receive and analyze aggregate reports from states to identify persistent safety issues that require more intensive analysis and/or a broader-based response (e.g., designing prototype systems or requesting a response by agencies, manufacturers or others).

5.2 The development of voluntary reporting efforts should be encouraged. The Center for Patient Safety should

- Describe and disseminate information on external voluntary reporting programs to encourage greater participation in them and track the development of new reporting systems as they form;
- Convene sponsors and users of external reporting systems to evaluate what works and what does not work well in the programs, and ways to make them more effective;
- Periodically assess whether additional efforts are needed to address gaps in information to improve patient safety and to encourage health care organizations to participate in voluntary reporting programs; and
- Fund and evaluate pilot projects for reporting systems, both within individual health care organizations and collaborative efforts among health care organizations.

6.1 Congress should pass legislation to extend peer review protections to data related to patient safety and quality improvement that are collected and analyzed by health care organizations for internal use or shared with others solely for purposes of improving safety and quality.

7.1 Performance standards and expectations for health care organizations should focus greater attention on patient safety.

- Regulators and accreditors should require health care organizations to implement meaningful patient safety programs with defined executive responsibility.
- Public and private purchasers should provide incentives to health care organizations to demonstrate continuous improvement in patient safety.

7.2 Performance standards and expectations for health professionals should focus greater attention on patient safety.

- Health professional licensing bodies should
  1) implement periodic re-examinations and re-licensing of doctors, nurses, and other key providers, based on both competence and knowledge of safety practices; and
  2) work with certifying and credentialing organizations to develop more effective methods to identify unsafe providers and take action.
- Professional societies should make a visible commitment to patient safety by establishing a permanent committee dedicated to safety improvement. This committee should
  1) develop a curriculum on patient safety and encourage its adoption into training and certification requirements;
  2) disseminate information on patient safety to members through special sessions at annual conferences, journal articles and editorials, newsletters, publications and web sites on a regular basis;

3) recognize patient safety considerations in practice guidelines and in standards related to the introduction and diffusion of new technologies, therapies and drugs;

4) work with the Center for Patient Safety to develop community-based, collaborative initiatives for error reporting and analysis and implementation of patient safety improvements; and

5) collaborate with other professional societies and disciplines in a national summit on the professional's role in patient safety.

7.3 The Food and Drug Administration (FDA) should increase attention to the safe use of drugs in both pre- and post-marketing processes through the following actions:

- Develop and enforce standards for the design of drug packaging and labeling that will maximize safety in use;
- Require pharmaceutical companies to test (using FDA-approved methods) proposed drug names to identify and remedy potential sound-alike and look-alike confusion with existing drug names; and
- Work with physicians, pharmacists, consumers, and others to establish appropriate responses to protect the safety of patients.

8.1 Healthcare organizations and the professionals affiliated with them should make continually improved patient safety a declared and serious aim by establishing patient safety programs with defined executive responsibility. Patient safety programs should

- Provide strong, clear and visible attention to safety;
- Implement non-punitive systems for reporting and analyzing errors within their organizations;
- Incorporate well-understood safety principles, such as standardizing and simplifying equipment, supplies, and processes; and
- Establish interdisciplinary team training programs for providers that incorporate proven methods of team training, such as simulation.

8.2 Healthcare organizations should implement proven medication safety practices.

From ***Networking Health: Prescriptions for the Internet*** (2000)

RECOMMENDATIONS

1.1 The health community should ensure that technical capabilities suitable for health and biomedical applications are incorporated into the testbed network being deployed under the Next Generation Internet initiative and eventually into the Internet.

1.2 To ensure that the Internet evolves in ways supportive of health needs over the long term, the health community should work with the networking community to develop improved network technologies that are of particular importance to health applications of the Internet.

- More readily scalable techniques to guarantee bandwidth on demand.
- Stronger forms of authentication.
- Symmetric or dynamically reconfigurable broadband technologies for the last mile.
- Hardened quality-of-service guarantees.
- Disaster operations.

1.3 The National Library of Medicine should forge stronger links between the health and networking research communities to ensure that the needs of the health community are better addressed in network research, development, and deployment.

1.4 The National Institutes of Health and its component agencies should fund information technology research that will develop the complementary technologies that are needed if the health community is to take advantage of the improved networking technologies that can be expected in the future.

2.1 The Department of Health and Human Services should fund pilot projects and larger demonstration programs to develop and demonstrate interoperable, scalable Internet applications for linking multiple health organizations.

2.2 Federal agencies such as the Department of Veterans Affairs, the Department of Defense, the Health Care Financing Administration, the National Institutes of Health, and the Indian Health Service should serve as role models and testbeds for the health industry by deploying Internet-based applications for their own purposes.

2.3 Health organizations in industry and academia should continue to work with the Department of Health and Human Services to evaluate various health applications of the Internet in order to improve understanding of their effects, the business models that might support them, and impediments to their expansion.

2.4 Public and private health organizations should experiment with networks based on Internet protocols and should incorporate the Internet into their future plans for new networked applications and into their overall strategic planning.

3.1 Professional associations with expertise in health issues and information technology should work with health care organizations to develop and promulgate guidelines for safe, effective use of the Internet in clinical settings.

3.2 Government, industry, and academia should work together with professional associations with experience in health and information technology to educate the broader health care communities about the ways the Internet can benefit them.

3.3 The Department of Health and Human Services should commission a study of the health information technology workforce to determine whether the supply of such workers balances the demand for them, to identify the kinds of training and education that workers at different levels will need, and to develop recommendations for ensuring an adequate supply of people with training at the intersections of information technology and health.

4.1 The Department of Health and Human Services should more aggressively address the broad set of policy issues that influence the development, deployment, and adoption of Internet-based applications in the health sector.

From ***the National Committee on Vital and Health Statistics (NCVHS) Report to the Secretary on Uniform Standards for Patient Medical Record Information*** (2000)

RECOMMENDATIONS

This Report reflects the belief that significant quality and cost benefits can be achieved in healthcare if clinically specific data are captured once at the point of care and that all other legitimate data needs are derived from those data. The standards for patient medical record information that will result from the recommendations in this Report will be consistent and compatible with the HIPAA financial and administrative transaction standards, including the upcoming claims attachment standards.

In consideration of broad industry testimony on these key issues, the NCVHS recommends that the Secretary of HHS:

1. Adopt the Guiding Principles for Selecting PMRI Standards as the criteria to select uniform data standards for patient medical record information (PMRI). These Guiding Principles are based on those published in the notice of proposed rulemaking for selecting financial and administrative transaction standards, which have been modified by adding characteristics and attributes that specifically address interoperability, data comparability, and data quality.

2. Consider acceptance of forthcoming NCVHS recommendations for specific PMRI standards. The first set of these recommendations will be delivered to the secretary eighteen months following submission of this Report and will include suggested implementation timeframes that consider industry readiness for adoption. For each recommendation for PMRI standards, NCVHS encourages the Secretary to provide an open process to give the public an opportunity to comment on the PMRI standards proposals before final rules are adopted.

3. Provide immediate funding to accelerate the development and promote early adoption of PMRI standards. This should take the form of support for:

   a. government membership and participation in standards development organizations

   b. broader participation of expert representation in standards development

   c. enhancement, distribution, and maintenance of clinical terminologies that have the potential to be PMRI standards through:

      (1) government-wide licensure or comparable arrangements so these terminologies are available for use at little or no cost.

      (2) augmentation of the national Library of Medicine's Unified Medical Language System (UMLS) to embody enhanced mapping of medical vocabularies and classifications.

      (3) development and testing of quality measures and clinical practice guidelines, such as published in the Agency for Healthcare Research and Quality (AHRQ) clearinghouses, and patient safety measures for their compatibility with existing and developing healthcare terminologies.

      (4) development and testing in multi-agency projects, such as GCPR (Government Computer-based Patient Record) framework project.

   d. coordination of data elements among all standards selected for adoption under HIPAA through the development and maintenance of an open meta-data registry and working conferences to harmonize message format and vocabulary standards.

e. improvement of drug data capture and use by:

(1) requiring the Food and Drug Administration (FDA) to make publicly available its National Drug Codes (NDC) database registry information.

(2) requiring the FDA to develop a drug classification system based on active ingredients so that all drugs that fall into a given category can be identified by the name of that category.

(3) encouraging the FDA to participate in private sector development and ongoing maintenance of a reference terminology for drugs and biologics that promotes the ability to share clinically specific information.

f. early adoption of PMRI standards within government programs to provide broadened feedback to the standards development community.

4. For each standard recommended by NCVHS, commit funding for development of a uniform implementation guide, development of conformance testing procedures, and ongoing government licensure of, or comparable arrangements for, healthcare terminology standards.

5. Support demonstration of the benefits and measurement of the costs of using uniform data standards for PMRI that provide for interoperability, data comparability, and data quality.

6. Support increases in funding for research, demonstration, and evaluation studies on clinical data capture systems and other healthcare informatics issues.

7. Accelerate development and implementation of a national health information infrastructure. HHS should work in collaboration with other federal components, state governments, and the private sector on demonstration and evaluation projects and test beds.

8. Promote United States' interest in international health data standards development through HHS participation in international healthcare informatics standards development organizations and, in cooperation with the Secretary of the Department of Commerce, through monitoring the activity of U.S. healthcare information system vendors abroad.

9. Promote the equitable distribution of the costs for using PMRI standards among all major beneficiaries of PMRI. This may take the form of incentives for submission of data using the PMRI standards that can support [[text out]]

10. Encourage enabling legislation for use and exchange of electronic PMRI, including:

a. comprehensive federal privacy and confidentiality legislation. This would ensure that all health information in any medium, used for any purpose, and disclosed to any entity receives equal privacy protection under law.

b. uniform recognition by all states of electronic health record keeping; and national standards for PMRI retention and electronic authentication (digital signatures).

From ***Crossing the Quality Chasm: A New Health System for the 21st Century*** (2001)

RECOMMENDATIONS

1. All health care organizations, professional groups, and private and public purchasers should adopt as their explicit purpose to continually reduce the burden of illness, injury, and disability, and to improve the health and functioning of the people of the United States.

2. All healthcare organizations, professional groups, and private and public purchasers should pursue six major aims; specifically, health care should be safe, effective, patient-centered, timely, efficient, and equitable.

3. Congress should continue to authorize and appropriate funds for, and the Department of Health and Human Services should move forward expeditiously with the establishment of monitoring and tracking processes for use in evaluating the progress of the health system in pursuit of the above-cited aims of safety, effectiveness, patient-centeredness, timeliness, efficiency, and equity. The Secretary of the Department of Health and Human Services should report annually to Congress and the President on the quality of care provided to the American people.

4. Private and public purchasers, healthcare organizations, clinicians, and patients should work together to redesign healthcare processes in accordance with the following rules:

    - *Care based on continuous healing relationships.* Patients should receive care whenever they need it and in many forms, not just face-to-face visits. This rule implies that the health-care system should be responsive at all times (24 hours a day, every day) and that access to care should be provided over the Internet, by television, and by other means in addition to face-to-face visits.

    - *Customization based on patient needs and values.* The system of care should be designed to meet the most common types of needs, but have the capability to respond to individual patient choices and preferences.

    - *The patient as the source of control.* Patients should be given the necessary information and the opportunity to exercise the degree of control they choose over health care decisions that affect them. The health system should be able to accommodate differences in patient preferences and encourage shared decision-making.

    - *Shared knowledge and the free flow of information.* Patients should have unfettered access to their own medical information and to clinical knowledge. Clinicians and patients should communicate effectively and share information.

    - *Evidence-based decision making.* Patients should receive care based on the best available scientific knowledge. Care should not vary illogically from clinician to clinician or from place to place.

    - *Safety as a system property.* Patients should be safe from injury caused by the care system. Reducing risk and ensuring safety require greater attention to systems that help prevent and mitigate errors.

    - *The need for transparency.* The health care system should make information available to patients and their families that allows them to make informed decisions when selecting a health plan, hospital, or clinical practice, or choosing among alternative treatments. This should include information describing the system's performance on safety, evidence-based practice, and patient satisfaction.

    - *Anticipation of needs.* The health system should anticipate patient needs, rather than simply reacting to events.

    - *Continuous decrease in waste.* The health system should not waste resources or patient time.

    - *Cooperation among clinicians.* Clinicians and institutions should actively collaborate and communicate to ensure an appropriate exchange of information and coordination of care.

5. The Agency for Health Care Research and Quality should identify not fewer than 15 priority conditions, taking into account frequency of occurrence, health burden, and resource use.

In collaboration with the National Quality Forum, the agency should convene stakeholders, including purchasers, consumers, healthcare organizations, professional groups, and others, to develop strategies, goals, and action plans for achieving substantial improvements in quality in the next 5 years for each of the priority conditions.

6. Congress should establish a Healthcare Quality Innovation Fund to support projects targeted at (1) achieving the six aims of safety, effectiveness, patient-centeredness, timeliness, efficiency, and equity; and/or (2) producing substantial improvements in quality for the priority conditions. The fund's resources should be invested in projects that will produce a public-domain portfolio of programs, tools, and technologies of widespread applicability.

7. The Agency for Healthcare Research and Quality and private foundations should convene a series of workshops involving representatives from health care and other industries and the research community to identify, adapt, and implement state-of-the-art approaches to addressing the following challenges:

    - Redesign of care processes based on best practices.
    - Use of information technologies to improve access to clinical information and support clinical decision making.
    - Knowledge and skills management.
    - Development of effective terms.
    - Coordination of care across patient conditions, services, and settings over time.
    - Incorporation of performance and outcome measurements for improvement and accountability.

8. The Secretary of the Department of Health and Human Services should be given the responsibility and necessary resources to establish and maintain a comprehensive program aimed at making scientific evidence more useful and accessible to clinicians and patients. In developing this program, the Secretary should work with federal agencies and in collaboration with professional and health care associations, the academic and research communities, and the National Quality Forum and other organizations involved in quality measurement and accountability.

9. Congress, the executive branch, leaders of health care organizations, public and private purchasers, and health informatics associations and vendors should make a renewed national commitment to building an information infrastructure to support health care delivery, consumer health, quality measurement and improvement, public accountability, clinical and health services research, and clinical educations. This commitment should lead to the elimination of most handwritten clinical data by the end of the decade.

10. Private and public purchasers should examine their current payment methods to remove barriers that currently impede quality improvement, and to build in stronger incentives for quality enhancement.

11. The Healthcare Financing Administration and the Agency for Healthcare Research and Quality, with input from private payers, healthcare organizations, and clinicians, should develop a research agenda to identify, pilot test, and evaluate various options for better aligning current payment methods with quality improvement goals.

12. A multidisciplinary summit of leaders within the health professions should be held to discuss and develop strategies for (1) restructuring clinical education to be consistent with the principles of the 21st-century health system throughout the continuum of undergraduate, graduate, and continuing education for medical, nursing, and other professional training programs; and

(2) assessing the implications of these changes for provider credentialing programs, funding, and sponsorship of education programs for health professionals.

13. The Agency for Healthcare Research and Quality should fund research to evaluate how the current regulatory and legal systems (1) facilitate or inhibit the changes needed for the 21st-century health care delivery system, and (2) can be modified to support health care professionals and organizations that seek to accomplish the six aims set forth in Chapter 2.

From the ***Final Report National Health Information Infrastructure (NHII)—Information for Health: A Strategy for Building the National Health Information Infrastructure*** (2001)

RECOMMENDATIONS FOR THE NATIONAL HEALTH INFORMATION INFRASTRUCTURE (NHII)

Federal Government

1. The Secretary of Health and Human Services should create a senior position to provide strategic national leadership for the development of the NHII and set the agenda for NHII investments, policymaking, and integration with ongoing health and healthcare activities inside and outside of Government.

2. Other HHS agencies/offices with missions and activities in NHII-related areas should designate an office or individual to participate in NHII strategic planning and ensure coordination within the agency/office and with the central NHII office.

3. Congress should provide new or expanded funding for programs that support the personal health, healthcare provider, and population health dimensions individually and jointly, with special attention to areas for which the Federal Government has a leading or exclusive role and areas already mandated by HIPAA. Examples of funding include support for

    - Development of State and local population health information capacities.
    - Professional training programs for the Federal, State, and local public health work force, and for the private healthcare work force, in information technology skills.
    - Technology centers that bring together interdisciplinary teams to explore issues related to the NHII, with an emphasis on activities that link the three dimensions.
    - Healthcare providers for investments in interoperable linked systems that support health related information flows across plans and providers.
    - Federal information technology research and development activities to stimulate research in health and healthcare applications.
    - Pilot projects that integrate data from the healthcare provider and personal health dimensions into the population health dimension at the State and local levels.

    Congress should supplement HIPAA to address standards issues related to the NHII. A "Health Information Portability and Continuity Act" should provide for the portability of health information across information systems, plans, and providers to ensure continuity of care; promote the adoption of clinical data standards; and promote consumer/patient control of personal health information.

    Congress should pass national laws and identify regulatory responsibilities for overarching issues that apply to the NHII, such as the confidentiality of personal health information, the security of health information systems, reimbursement for clinically necessary and effective electronically delivered health services, and consumer protection for misuses and abuses of health information.

4. Federal health data agencies should collaborate with State and local government agencies and standards organizations to develop common data reporting formats and standardized methods of transmission of all pertinent health data. These activities should build upon CDC NEDSS, the Health Care Service (837) Data Reporting Guide and upon efforts to develop public health data conceptual models, extending these beyond communicable diseases. This effort also should be coordinated with the United States Health Information Knowledgebase or metadata registry operated by the ANSI Healthcare Informatics Standards Board.

Other Stakeholders

Although the Committee was told that the Federal Government should assume leadership, it also heard that the Federal Government cannot build the NHII alone. Its ability to lead and coordinate rests on the assumption that many other stakeholders in the public and private sectors will play key roles within their own areas and will work together.

State and Local Government

1. Each State should establish a mechanism to provide strategic leadership and coordination of activities related to the NHII. This mechanism, which may be a new office, preferably located in the Office of the Governor, Office of the State Health Officer, or other combined health and human services agency, should have broad oversight of the integration of NHII components into the public health and healthcare programs in their States. The functions of the leadership would be to solicit input from all relevant stakeholders, including consumers, about the development and uses of the NHII and to oversee personal health information privacy issues and activities.

2. State and local data agencies should collaborate with Federal agencies and standards organizations to develop common data reporting formats and standardized methods of transmission for all pertinent health data.

3. State and local health agencies should invest in the collection and analysis of population health data to permit real-time, small-area analysis of acute public health problems and to understand health issues related to new or rapidly growing populations and health disparities, and they should combine health data sources for population analysis.

Healthcare Providers

1. Each healthcare professional and provider membership and trade organization should establish a mechanism to provide strategic leadership on issues related to NHII development and implementation. The functions of the leadership would include representing the membership or trade organization in meetings convened by HHS and collaborative activities with other stakeholders, promoting internal review of organizational practices and systems for consistency with the NHII and developing timetables for needed revisions and enhancements, and overseeing personal health information privacy issues and activities.

2. Healthcare provider organizations. Each individual healthcare provider organization should establish a mechanism to provide strategic leadership and coordination on issues related to NHII development and implementation. The leadership would be responsible for overseeing personal health information privacy and security issues and activities and ensuring that stakeholders from the personal health and population health dimensions can provide appropriate input into plans and decisions. The leadership should identify representatives with diverse backgrounds to participate actively in the work of standards development organizations.

Healthcare Plans and Purchasers

1. Each healthcare plan and purchaser should establish a mechanism to provide strategic leadership and coordination on issues related to NHII development and implementation. These responsibilities could be assigned to the Chief Information Officers of their organizations. A designated

individual should represent the organization in meetings convened by HHS and collaborative activities with other stakeholders and oversee personal health information issues and activities.

2. Healthcare plans and purchasers should examine their practices and systems for consistency with the NHII and set timetables for needed revisions and enhancements. They should ensure that stakeholders from the personal health and population health dimensions provide appropriate input into NHII plans and decisions.

3. Healthcare plans and purchasers should identify representatives with diverse backgrounds to participate actively in the work of standards development organizations.

Standards Development Organizations

1. Standards development organizations should develop new or modified standards as requirements become known.

2. Standards development organizations should ensure participation by consumer representatives.

3. Standards development organizations should identify mechanisms to accelerate the standards development process and improve the coordination of standards development across standard setting bodies and consistent with the direction of the NHII.

4. Standards development organizations should promote cooperation with standards being developed internationally for population health, patient care, or data-security purposes.

Information Technology Industry

1. Information technology organizations and trade groups should designate internal representatives to provide strategic leadership and coordination on issues related to NHII development and implementation. Representatives should participate in meetings convened by HHS and collaborative activities with other stakeholders.

2. The information technology industry should develop and promote cost-effective healthcare software and technologies that comply with national standards so that they can support the appropriate sharing of electronic information for healthcare providers, consumers/patients, and public health agencies and the improved delivery of clinical and public health services.

Consumer and Patient Advocacy Groups

1. Consumer and patient advocacy groups should promote policies that encourage the use of electronic technologies in healthcare organizations and by healthcare providers to improve the quality of services, to decrease rates of adverse effects, and to increase access to on-line/wireless health information and services for consumers, patients, and clients. They should advocate for privacy protections for consumers, patients, and clients when they exchange health information electronically and for equal access to technology and information by all population groups.

2. Consumer and patient advocacy groups should participate in NHII-related committees organized by national and State agencies, and by health plan and provider organizations, and in standards development efforts.

3. Consumer and patient advocacy groups should collaborate with healthcare provider organizations, health plans and purchasers, and public health organizations to promote and facilitate the use of information technologies by healthcare providers, health plans, and public health entities.

Community Organizations

1. Community organizations should help identify community health data needs.

2. Community organizations should identify necessary partnerships to exchange health data. They also should identify and help reduce barriers to community level collection and exchange of health data.

3. Community organizations should develop local laypersons' capacities to collect and apply health data to individual and community health improvements.

4. Community organizations should develop programs that address the "digital divide" and promote equal access to technology and information by all population groups.

Academic and Research Organizations

1. Academic and research organizations should develop research proposals that integrate health information infrastructure and applications with other types of information infrastructure development (e.g., NGI and Internet2).

2. Academic and research organizations should develop collaborations with service providers, standards development organizations, and their communities to take innovations from research to implementation.

From ***Fostering Rapid Advances in Health Care: Learning from System Demonstrations*** (2002)

RECOMMENDATIONS

In response to a request from the Secretary of the Department of Health and Human Services, the Institute of Medicine convened a committee to identify possible demonstration projects that might be implemented in 2003, with the hope of yielding models for broader health system reform within a few years. The committee is recommending a substantial portfolio of demonstration projects: 10-12 chronic care demonstrations, a primary care demonstration with 40 participating sites, 8-10 information and communications technology infrastructure demonstrations, 3-5 state health insurance coverage demonstrations, and 4-5 state liability demonstrations. As a set the demonstrations address key aspects of the healthcare delivery system and the financing and legal environment in which healthcare is provided. The launching of a carefully crafted set of demonstrations is viewed as a way to initiate a "building block" approach to health system change.

These demonstrations should lead to a health care system in which patients' experiences would be very different from today's norm. For a typical patient with one or more chronic conditions requiring ongoing management, as well as preventive and acute care needs, the system should provide a continuous relationship with a personal clinician who functions with the support of a multidisciplinary team. Patients should be able to access care over the Internet, by telephone, and by other means in addition to face-to-face visits. There should be few concerns about safety, but in the event that a patient is harmed, the clinician should inform the patient immediately, apologize, and take action to mitigate the consequences. Care should not vary illogically from clinician to clinician or place to place. Each patient should receive the best that science has to offer, whether for ongoing treatment of a chronic condition or care for an acute episode. This does not imply one-size-fits-all care. Patients will have different preferences (e.g., watchful waiting versus surgical intervention for prostate cancer), differing needs for education and support, and differing constraints (e.g., a need for home care with family support versus short-term rehabilitative care).

For many people, chronic disease could have been avoided or delayed had educational and other supportive interventions been provided to assist them in modifying health behaviors. These demonstration projects would involve the following components:

- Coordinating structure—During the first year, the grant recipient would be responsible for establishing a broad-based coordinating structure with participation from all stakeholders.

- Chronic care management programs—Each demonstration site would establish chronic care management programs that would provide evidence-based treatment of chronic diseases, services to detect and minimize the consequences of common geriatric syndromes, services to meet the preventive and acute care needs of the enrolled chronically ill population, and extended outreach and coordination with social and environmental services.

- Information and communications technology—A major component of these demonstrations should be the expanded use of Information and Communications Technology (ICT) to improve care for the chronically ill.
- Benefits, Co-payments, Provider Payments, and Accountability—Demonstration sites should be given the flexibility under Medicare and other insurance programs to innovate in such areas as benefits coverage, beneficiary co-payments, provider payments, and accountability.
- Learning collaboratives and community-wide educational efforts—Each demonstration site, with assistance from the National Library of Medicine and the Agency for Healthcare Research and Quality (AHRQ), should engage in efforts to assist clinicians and patients in gaining access to scientific knowledge, practice guidelines, certified protocols, identified best practices, and decision support tools.

The 21st-century healthcare system should deliver far greater value than is currently the case. Patients have a right to demand—and healthcare leaders have an obligation to act now to ensure that they receive—care that is safe, effective, patient-centered, timely, efficient, and equitable. The committee believes the proposed demonstration projects would represent a substantial step in that direction.

From ***The Future of the Public's Health in the 21st Century*** (2002)

RECOMMENDATIONS

1. The Secretary of the Department of Health and Human Services (DHHS), in consultation with states, should appoint a national commission to develop a framework and recommendations for state public health law reform. In particular, the national commission would review all existing public health law as well as the Turning Point Model State Public Health Act and the Model State Emergency Health Powers Act; provide guidance and technical assistance to help states reform their laws to meet modern scientific and legal standards; and help foster greater consistency within and among states, especially in their approach to different health threats.
2. All federal, state, and local governmental public health agencies should develop strategies to ensure that public health workers who are involved in the provision of essential public health services demonstrate mastery of the core public health competencies appropriate to their jobs. The Council on Linkages between Academia and Public Health Practice should also encourage the competency development of public health professionals working in public health system roles in for-profit and nongovernmental entities.
3. Congress should designate funds for the Centers for Disease Control and Prevention (CDC) and the Health Resources and Services Administration (HRSA) to periodically assess the preparedness of the public health workforce, to document the training necessary to meet basic competency expectations, and to advise on the funding necessary to provide such training.
4. Leadership training, support, and development should be a high priority for governmental public health agencies and other organizations in the public health system and for schools of public health that supply the public health infrastructure with its professionals and leaders.

5. A formal national dialogue should be initiated to address the issue of public health workforce credentialing. The Secretary of DHHS should appoint a national commission on public health workforce credentialing to lead this dialogue. The commission should be charged to determine if a credentialing system would further the goal of creating a competent workforce and, if applicable, the manner and time frame for implementation by governmental public health agencies at all levels. The dialogue should include representatives from federal, state, and local public health agencies, academia, and public health professional organizations who can represent and discuss the various perspectives on the workforce credentialing debate.

6. All partners within the public health system should place special emphasis on communication as a critical core competency of public health practice. Governmental public health agencies at all levels should use existing and emerging tools (including information technologies) for effective management of public health information and for internal and external communication. To be effective, such communication must be culturally appropriate and suitable to the literacy levels of the individuals in the communities they serve.

7. The Secretary of DHHS should provide leadership to facilitate the development and implementation of the National Health Information Infrastructure (NHII). Implementation of NHII should take into account, where possible, the findings and recommendations of the National Committee on Vital and Health Statistics (NCVHS) working group on NHII. Congress should consider options for funding the development and deployment of NHII (e.g., in support of clinical care, health information for the public, and public health practice and research) through payment changes, tax credits, subsidized loans, or grants.

8. DHHS should be accountable for assessing the state of the nation's governmental public health infrastructure and its capacity to provide the essential public health services to every community and for reporting that assessment annually to Congress and the nation. The assessment should include a thorough evaluation of federal, state, and local funding for the nation's governmental public health infrastructure and should be conducted in collaboration with state and local officials. The assessment should identify strengths and gaps and serve as the basis for plans to develop a funding and technical assistance plan to assure sustainability. The public availability of these reports will enable state and local public health agencies to use them for continual self-assessment and evaluation.

9. DHHS should evaluate the status of the nation's public health laboratory system, including an assessment of the impact of recent increased funding. The evaluation should identify remaining gaps, and funding should be allocated to close them. Working with the states, DHHS should agree on a base funding level that will maintain the enhanced laboratory system and allow the rapid deployment of newly developed technologies.

10. DHHS should develop a comprehensive investment plan for a strong national governmental public health infrastructure with a timetable, clear performance measures, and regular progress reports to the public. State and local governments should also provide adequate, consistent, and sustainable funding for the governmental public health infrastructure.

11. The federal government and states should renew efforts to experiment with clustering or consolidation of categorical grants for the purpose of increasing local flexibility to address priority health concerns and enhance the efficient use of limited resources.

12. The Secretary of DHHS should appoint a national commission to consider if an accreditation system would be useful for improving and building state and local public health agency capacities. If such a system is deemed useful, the commission should make recommendations on how it would be governed and develop mechanisms (e.g., incentives) to gain state and local government participation in the accreditation effort. Membership on this commission should include representatives from CDC, the Association of State and Territorial Health Officials, the National Association of County and City Health Officials, and nongovernmental organizations.

13. CDC, in collaboration with the Council on Linkages between Academia and Public Health Practice and other public health system partners, should develop a research agenda and estimate the funding needed to build the evidence base that will guide policy making for public health practice.

14. The Secretary of DHHS should review the regulatory authorities of DHHS agencies with health-related responsibilities to reduce overlap and inconsistencies, ensure that the department's management structure is best suited to coordinate among agencies within DHHS with health-related responsibilities, and, to the extent possible, simplify relationships with state and local governmental public health agencies. Similar efforts should be made to improve coordination with other federal cabinet agencies performing important public health services, such as the Department of Agriculture and the Environmental Protection Agency.

15. Congress should mandate the establishment of a National Public Health Council. This National Public Health Council would bring together the Secretary of DHHS and state health commissioners at least annually to

    1. Provide a forum for communication and collaboration on action to achieve national health goals as articulated in *Healthy People 2010*;
    2. Advise the Secretary of DHHS on public health issues;
    3. Advise the Secretary of DHHS on financing and regulations that affect governmental public health capacity at the state and local levels;
    4. Provide a forum for overseeing the development of an incentive-based federal–state-funded system to sustain a governmental public health infrastructure that can assure the availability of essential public health services to every American community and can monitor progress toward this goal (e.g., through report cards);
    5. Review and evaluate the domestic policies of other cabinet agencies for their impact on national health outcomes (e.g., through health impact reports) and on the reduction and elimination of health disparities; and
    6. Submit an annual report on their deliberations and recommendations to Congress.

The Council should be chaired by the Secretary of DHHS and co-chaired by a state health director on a rotating basis. An appropriately resourced secretariat should be established in the Office of the Secretary to ensure that the Council has access to the information and expertise of all DHHS agencies during its deliberations.

Community

16. Local governmental public health agencies should support community-led efforts to inventory resources, assess needs, formulate collaborative responses, and evaluate outcomes for community health improvement and the elimination of health disparities. Governmental public health agencies should provide community organizations and coalitions with technical assistance and support in identifying and securing resources as needed and at all phases of the process.

17. Governmental and private-sector funders of community health initiatives should plan their investments with a focus on long-lasting change. Such a focus would include realistic time lines, an emphasis on ongoing community engagement and leadership, and a final goal of institutionalizing effective project components in the local community or public health system as appropriate.

Health Care Delivery System

18. Adequate population health cannot be achieved without making comprehensive and affordable health care available to every person residing in the United States. It is the responsibility of the federal government to lead a national effort to examine the options available to achieve stable health care coverage of individuals and families and to assure the implementation of plans to achieve that result.

19. All public and privately funded insurance plans should include age-appropriate preventive services as recommended by the U.S. Preventive Services Task Force and provide evidence-based coverage of oral health, mental health, and substance abuse treatment services.

20. Bold, large-scale demonstrations should be funded by the federal government and other major investors in health care to test radical new approaches to increase the efficiency and effectiveness of health care financing and delivery systems. The experiments should effectively link delivery systems with other components of the public health system and focus on improving population health while eliminating disparities. The demonstrations should be supported by adequate resources to enable innovative ideas to be fairly tested.

Businesses and Employers

21. The federal government should develop programs to assist small employers and employers with low-wage workers to purchase health insurance at reasonable rates.

22. The corporate community and public health agencies should initiate and enhance joint efforts to strengthen health promotion and disease and injury prevention programs for employees and their communities. As an early step, the corporate and governmental public health community should:

    a. Strengthen partnership and collaboration by:

        - developing direct linkages between local public health agencies and business leaders to forge a common language and understanding of employee and community health problems and to participate in setting community health goals and strategies for achieving them; and
        - developing innovative ways for the corporate and governmental public health communities to gather, interpret, and exchange mutually meaningful data and information, such as the translation of health information to support corporate health promotion and health care purchasing activities.

    b. Enhance communication by

        - developing effective employer and community communication and education programs focused on the benefits of and options for health promotion and disease and injury prevention; and
        - using proven marketing and social marketing techniques to promote individual behavioral and community change.

    c. Develop the evidence base for workplace and community interventions through greater public, private, and philanthropic investments in research to extend the science and improve the effectiveness of workplace and community interventions to promote health and prevent disease and injury.

    d. Recognize business leadership in employee and community health by elevating the level of recognition given to corporate investment in employee and community health. The Secretaries of DHHS and the Department of Commerce, along with business leaders (e.g., chambers of commerce and business roundtables), should jointly sponsor a Corporate Investment in Health Award. The award would recognize private-sector entities that have demonstrated exemplary civic and social responsibility for improving the health of their workers and the community.

Media

23. An ongoing dialogue should be maintained between medical and public health officials and editors and journalists at the local level and their representative associations nationally. Furthermore, foundations and governmental health agencies should provide opportunities to develop and evaluate educational and training programs that provide journalists with experiences that will

deepen their knowledge of public health subject matter and provide public health workers with a foundation in communication theory, messaging, and application.

24. The television networks, television stations, and cable providers should increase the amount of time they donate to public service announcements (PSAs) as partial fulfillment of the public service requirement in their Federal Communications Commission (FCC) licensing agreements.
25. The FCC should review its regulations for PSA broadcasting on television and radio to ensure a more balanced broadcasting schedule that will reach a greater proportion of the viewing and listening audiences.
26. Public health officials and local and national entertainment media should work together to facilitate the communication of accurate information about disease and about medical and health issues in the entertainment media.
27. Public health and communication researchers should develop an evidence base on media influences on health knowledge and behavior, as well as on the promotion of healthy public policy.

Academia

28. Academic institutions should increase integrated interdisciplinary learning opportunities for students in public health and other related health science professions. Such efforts should include not only multidisciplinary education but also interdisciplinary education and appropriate incentives for faculty to undertake such activities.
29. Congress should increase funding for Health Resources and Services Administration (HRSA) programs that provide financial support for students enrolled in public health degree programs through mechanisms such as training grants, loan repayments, and service obligation grants. Funding should also be provided to strengthen the Public Health Training Center program to effectively meet the educational needs of the existing public health workforce and to facilitate public health worker access to the centers. Support for leadership training of state and local health department directors and local community leaders should continue through funding of the National and Regional Public Health Leadership Institutes and distance-learning materials developed by HRSA and the Centers for Disease Control and Prevention (CDC).
30. Federal funders of research and academic institutions should recognize and reward faculty scholarship related to public health practice research.
31. The committee recommends that Congress provide funds for CDC to enhance its investigator-initiated program for prevention research while maintaining a strong Centers, Institutes, and Offices (CIO)-generated research program. CDC should take steps that include:
    - expanding the external peer review mechanism for review of investigator-initiated research;
    - allowing research to be conducted over the more generous time lines often required by prevention research; and
    - establishing a central mechanism for coordination of investigator-initiated proposal submissions.
32. CDC should authorize an analysis of the funding levels necessary for effective Prevention Research Center functioning, taking into account the levels authorized by P.L. 98–551 as well as the amount of prevention research occurring in other institutions and organizations.
33. NIH should increase the portion of its budget allocated to population- and community-based prevention research that:

- addresses population-level health problems;
- involves a definable population and operates at the level of the whole person;
- evaluates the application and impacts of new discoveries on the actual health of the population; and
- focuses on the behavioral and environmental (social, economic, cultural, physical) factors associated with primary and secondary prevention of disease and disability in populations.
- furthermore, the committee recommends that the Director of NIH report annually to the Secretary of DHHS on the scope of population- and community-based prevention research activities undertaken by the NIH centers and institutes.

34. Academic institutions should develop criteria for recognizing and rewarding faculty scholarship related to service activities that strengthen public health practice.

From ***Information Technology for Counterterrorism: Immediate Actions and Future Possibilities*** (2003)

Short-Term Recommendation 1: The nation should develop a program that focuses on the communications and computing needs of emergency responders. Such a program would have two essential components:

- Ensuring that authoritative, current-knowledge expertise and support regarding IT are available to emergency-response agencies prior to and during emergencies, including terrorist attacks.
- Upgrading the capabilities of the command, control, communications, and intelligence (C3I) systems of emergency-response agencies through the use of existing technologies. Such upgrades might include transitioning from analog to digital systems and deploying a separate emergency-response communications network in the aftermath of a disaster.

Short-Term Recommendation 2: The nation should promote the use of best practices in information and network security in all relevant public agencies and private organizations.

- *For IT users on the operational level*: Ensure that adequate information-security tools are available. Conduct frequent, unannounced red-team penetration testing of deployed systems. Promptly fix problems and vulnerabilities that are known. Mandate the use of strong authentication mechanisms. Use defense-in-depth in addition to perimeter defense.
- *For IT vendors*: Develop tools to monitor systems automatically for consistency with defined secure configurations. Provide well-engineered schemes for user authentication based on hardware tokens. Conduct more rigorous testing of software and systems for security flaws.
- *For the federal government*: Position critical federal information systems as models for good security practices. Remedy the failure of the market to account adequately for information security so that appropriate market pro-security mechanisms develop.

From ***Patient Safety: Achieving a New Standard for Care*** (2004)

RECOMMENDATIONS

Recommendation 1. Americans expect and deserve safe care. Improved information and data systems are needed to support efforts to make patient safety a standard of care in hospitals, in doctors' offices, in nursing homes, and in every other health care setting. All health care organizations should establish comprehensive patient safety systems that:

- Provide immediate access to complete patient information and decision support tools (e.g., alerts, reminders) for clinicians and their patients.
- Capture information on patient safety—including both adverse events and near misses—as a by-product of care, and use this information to design even safer care delivery systems.

Recommendation 2. A national health information infrastructure—a foundation of systems, technology, applications, standards, and policies—is required to make patient safety a standard of care.

- The federal government should facilitate deployment of the national health information infrastructure through the provision of targeted financial support and the ongoing promulgation and maintenance of standards for data that support patient safety.
- Health care providers should invest in electronic health record systems that possess the key capabilities necessary to provide safe and effective care and to enable the continuous redesign of care processes to improve patient safety.

Recommendation 3. Congress should provide clear direction, enabling authority, and financial support for the establishment of national standards for data that support patient safety. Various government agencies will need to assume major new responsibilities, and additional support will be required. Specifically:

- The Department of Health and Human Services (DHHS) should be given the lead role in establishing and maintaining a public–private partnership for the promulgation of standards for data that support patient safety.
- The Consolidated Health Informatics (CHI) initiative, in collaboration with the National Committee on Vital and Health Statistics (NCVHS), should identify data standards appropriate for national adoption and gaps in existing standards that need to be addressed. The membership of NCVHS should continue to be broad and diverse, with adequate representation of all stakeholders, including consumers, state governments, professional groups, and standards-setting bodies.
- The Agency for Healthcare Research and Quality (AHRQ) in collaboration with the National Library of Medicine and others should

  (1) provide administrative and technical support for the CHI and NCVHS efforts; (2) ensure the development of implementation guides, certification procedures, and conformance testing for all data standards; (3) provide financial support and oversight for developmental activities to fill gaps in data standards; and (4) coordinate activities and maintain a clearinghouse of information in support of national data standards and their implementation to improve patient safety.
- The National Library of Medicine should be designated as the responsible entity for distributing all national clinical terminologies that relate to patient safety and for ensuring the quality of terminology mappings.

Recommendation 4. The lack of comprehensive standards for data to support patient safety impedes private-sector investment in information technology and other efforts to improve patient safety. The federal government should accelerate the adoption of standards for such data by pursuing the following efforts:

- *Clinical data interchange standards*. The federal government should set an aggressive agenda for the establishment of standards for the interchange of clinical data to support patient safety. Federal financial support should be provided to accomplish this agenda.
    - After ample time for provider compliance, federal government health care programs should incorporate into their contractual and regulatory requirements standards already approved by the secretaries of DHHS, the Veterans Administration, and the Department of Defense (i.e., the HL7 version 2.x series for clinical data messaging, DICOM for medical imaging, IEEE 1073 for medical devices, LOINC for laboratory test results, and NCPDP Script for prescription data).
    - AHRQ should provide support for (1) accelerated completion (within 2 years) of HL7 version 3.0; (2) specifications for the HL7 Clinical Document Architecture and implementation guides; and (3) analysis of alternative methods for addressing the need to support patient safety by instituting a unique health identifier for individuals, such as implementation of a voluntary unique health identifier program.
- *Clinical terminologies*. The federal government should move expeditiously to identify a core set of well-integrated, nonredundant clinical terminologies for clinical care, quality improvement, and patient safety reporting. Revisions, extensions, and additions to the codes should be compatible with, yet go beyond, the federal government's initiative to integrate all federal reporting systems.
    - AHRQ should undertake a study of the core terminologies, supplemental terminologies, and standards mandated by the Health Insurance Portability and Accountability Act to identify areas of overlap and gaps in the terminologies to address patient safety requirements. The study should begin by convening domain experts to develop a process for ensuring comprehensive coverage of the terminologies for the 20 IOM priority areas.
    - The National Library of Medicine should provide support for the accelerated completion of RxNORM for clinical drugs. The National Library of Medicine also should develop high-quality mappings among the core terminologies and supplemental terminologies identified by the CHI and NCVHS.
- *Knowledge representation*. The federal government should provide support for the accelerated development of knowledge representation standards to facilitate effective use of decision support in clinical information systems.
    - The National Library of Medicine should provide support for the development of standards for evidence-based knowledge representation.
    - AHRQ, in collaboration with the National Institutes of Health, the Food and Drug Administration, and other agencies, should provide support for the development of a generic guideline representation model for use in representing clinical guidelines in a computer-executable format that can be employed in decision support tools.

Recommendation 5. All healthcare settings should establish comprehensive patient safety programs operated by trained personnel within a culture of safety. These programs should encompass (1) case finding—identifying system failures, (2) analysis—understanding the factors that contribute to system failures, and (3) system redesign—making improvements in care processes to prevent errors in the future. Patient safety programs should invite the participation of patients and their families and be responsive to their inquiries.

Recommendation 6. The federal government should pursue a robust applied research agenda on patient safety, focused on enhancing knowledge, developing tools, and disseminating results to maximize the impact of patient safety systems. AHRQ should play a lead role in coordinating this research agenda among federal agencies (e.g., the National Library of Medicine) and the private sector. The research agenda should include the following:

- Knowledge generation
  - High-risk patients—Identify patients at risk for medication errors, nosocomial infections, falls, and other high-risk events.
  - Near-miss incidents—Test the causal continuum assumption (that near misses and adverse events are causally related), develop and test a recovery taxonomy, and extend the current individual human error/recovery models to team-based errors and recoveries.
  - Hazard analysis—Assess the validity and efficiency of integrating retrospective techniques (e.g., incident analysis) with prospective techniques.
  - High-yield activities—Study the cost/benefit of various approaches to patient safety, including analysis of reporting systems for near misses and adverse events.
  - Patient roles—Study the role of patients in the prevention, early detection, and mitigation of harm due to errors.
- Tool development
  - Early detection capabilities—Develop and evaluate various methods for employing data-driven triggers to detect adverse drug events, nosocomial infections, and other high-risk events (e.g., patient falls, decubitus ulcers, complications of blood product transfusions).
  - Prevention capabilities—Develop and evaluate point-of-care decision support to prevent errors of omission or commission.
  - Data mining techniques—Identify and develop data mining techniques to enhance learning from regional and national patient safety databases. Apply natural language processing techniques to facilitate the extraction of patient safety–related concepts from text documents and incident reports.
- Dissemination—Deploy knowledge and tools to clinicians and patients.

Recommendation 7. AHRQ should develop an event taxonomy and common report format for submission of data to the national patient safety database. Specifically:

- The event taxonomy should address near misses and adverse events, cover errors of both omission and commission, allow for the designation of primary and secondary event types for cases in which more than one factor precipitated the adverse event, and be incorporated into SNOMED CT.
- The standardized report format should include the following:
  - A standardized minimum set of data elements.
  - Data necessary to calculate a risk assessment index for determining prospectively the probability of an event and its severity.
  - A free-text narrative of the event.
  - Data necessary to support use of the Eindhoven Classification Model—Medical Version for classifying root causes, including expansions for (1) recovery factors associated with near-miss events, (2) corrective actions taken to recover from adverse events, and (3) patient outcome/functional status as a result of those corrective actions.

  - A free-text section for lessons learned as a result of the event.
  - Clinical documentation of the patient context.
- The taxonomy and report format should be used by the federal reporting system integration project in the areas for basic domain, event type, risk assessment, and causal analysis but should provide for more extensive support for patient safety research and analysis (Department of Health and Human Services, 2002c).

From ***Letter to HHS Secretary Tommy G. Thompson from John R. Lumpkin, Chairman, National Committee on Vital and Health Statistics: First Set of Recommendations on E-Prescribing Standards*** (2004)

RECOMMENDED ACTIONS:

Recommended Action 1.1: HHS should ensure that e-prescribing standards are not only appropriate for Medicare Part D but also for all types of prescribers, dispensers, and public and private sector payers.

Recommended Action 1.2: HHS should ensure that e-prescribing standards are compatible with those adopted as HIPAA and CHI standards, and with those recommended in November 2003 by NCVHS for clinical data terminologies.

Recommended Action 2.1: HHS should work with the industry in its rulemaking process to determine how best to afford flexibility in keeping standards in pace with the industry, including standards for HIPAA and e-prescribing. For example, HHS might consider recognizing new versions of standards, without a separate regulation, if they are backward compatible.

Recommended Action 3.1: HHS should recognize as a foundation standard the most current version of NCDPDP SCRIPT for new prescriptions, prescription renewals, cancellations, and changes between prescribers and dispensers. The National Council for Prescription Drug Programs (NCPDP) SCRIPT Standard would include its present code sets and various mailbox and acknowledgement functions, as applicable.

Recommended Action 3.2: HHS should include the fill status notification function of the NCPDP SCRIPT Standard in the 2006 pilot tests. These pilot tests should assess the business value and clinical utility of the fill status notification function, as well as evaluate privacy issues and possible mitigation strategies.

Recommended Action 4.1: HHS should financially support the acceleration of coordination activities between Health Level 7 (HL7) and NCPDP for electronic medication ordering and prescribing. HHS should also support ongoing maintenance of the HL7 and NCPDP SCRIPT coordination.

Recommended Action 4.2: HHS should recognize the exchange of new prescriptions, renewals, cancellations, changes, and fill status notification within the same enterprise [[delete bracketed number?]][10] as outside the scope of MMA e-prescribing standard specifications.

Recommended Action 4.3: HHS should require that any prescriber that uses an HL7 message within an enterprise convert it to NCPDP SCRIPT if the message is being transmitted to a dispenser outside of the enterprise. HHS also should require that any retail pharmacy within an enterprise be able to receive prescription transmittals via NCPDP SCRIPT from outside the enterprise.

Recommended Action 5.1: HHS should actively participate in and support the rapid development of an NCPDP standard for formulary and benefit information file transfer, using the RxHub protocol as a basis.

Recommended Action 5.2: NCVHS will closely monitor the progress of NCPDP's developing a standard for a formulary and benefit information file transfer protocol, and provide advice to the Secretary in time for adoption as a foundation standard and/or readiness for the 2006 pilot tests.

Recommended Action 6.1: HHS should recognize the ASC X12N 270/271 Health Care Eligibility Inquiry and Response Standard Version 004010X092A1 as a foundation standard for conducting eligibility inquiries from prescribers to payers/PBMs.

Recommended Action 6.2: HHS should support NCPDP's efforts to create a guidance document to map the pharmacy information on the Medicare Part D Pharmacy ID Card to the appropriate fields on the ASC X12N 270/271 in further support of its use in e-prescribing.

Recommended Action 6.3: HHS should work with ASC X12 to determine if there are any requirements under MMA with respect to how situational data elements are used in the ASC X12N 270/271, especially concerning the quality of information needed for real-time drug benefits. Use of these situational data elements could be addressed in trading partner agreements. Specifications of use of situational data elements, as well as proper usage of the functional acknowledgments, should be included in the 2006 pilot tests.

Recommended Action 6.4: HHS should ensure that the functionality of the ASC X12N 270/271, as adopted under HIPAA, keeps pace with requirements for e-prescribing and that new versions to the Standard be pilot tested.

Recommended Action 7.1: HHS should support ASC X12 in their efforts to incorporate functionality for real-time prior authorization messages for drugs in the ASC X12N 278 Health Care Services Review Standard Version 004010X094A1for use between the prescriber and payer/PBM.

Recommended Action 7.2: HHS should support standards development organizations and other industry participants in developing prior authorization work flow scenarios to contribute to the design of the 2006 pilot tests.

Recommended Action 7.3: HHS should evaluate the economic and quality of care impacts of automating prior authorization communications between dispensers and prescribers and between payers and prescribers in its 2006 pilot tests.

Recommended Action 7.4: HHS should ensure that the functionality of the ASC X12N 278, as adopted under HIPAA, keeps pace with requirements for e-prescribing and that new versions to the Standard be pilot tested.

Recommended Action 8.1: HHS should actively participate in and support rapid development of an NCPDP standard for a medication history message for communication from a payer/PBM to a prescriber, using the RxHub protocol as a basis.

Recommended Action 8.2: NCVHS will closely monitor the progress of NCPDP's developing a standard medication history message for communication from a payer/PBM to a prescriber, and provide advice to the Secretary in time for adoption as a foundation standard and/or readiness for the 2006 pilot tests.

Recommended Action 9.1: HHS should include in the 2006 pilot tests the RxNorm terminology in the NCPDP SCRIPT Standard for new prescriptions, renewals, and changes. RxNorm is being included in the 2006 pilot tests to determine how well the RxNorm clinical drug, strength, and dosage information can be translated from the prescriber's system into an NDC at the dispenser's system that represents the prescriber's intent. This translation will require the participation of intermediary drug knowledge base vendors until the RxNorm is fully mapped.

Recommended Action 9.2: HHS should accelerate the promulgation of the Food & Drug Administration's (FDA) Drug Listing rule and hence the ability to support the correlation of National Drug Code (NDC) with RxNorm (e.g., for passing daily updates of the SPL to NLM for inclusion in the DailyMed). Timely rulemaking is critical to sustain the daily use of RxNorm beyond the 2006 pilot tests.

Recommended Action 9.3: HHS should ensure that, if the Medicare Part D Model Guidelines and NDF-RT differ, an accurate mapping exists so they both can be used successfully.

Recommended Action 10.1: HHS should support NCPDP, HL7, and others (especially including the prescriber community) in addressing SIG components in their standards. This should include preserving the ability to incorporate free text whenever necessary (e.g., for complex dosing instructions, and to address special cultural sensitivities, language, and literacy requirements).

Recommended Action 10.2: HHS should include in the 2006 pilot tests the structured and codified SIGs as developed through standards development organization efforts.

Recommended Action 11.1: HHS should ensure that the NPI, when it becomes available, is incorporated as the primary identifier for dispensers in the NCPDP SCRIPT and other e-prescribing standards.

Recommended Action 11.2: HHS should accelerate the enumeration of all dispensers to support transition to the NPI for e-prescribing.

Recommended Action 11.3: HHS should permit the industry to use the NCPDP Provider Identifier Number in the event that the NPS cannot enumerate dispensers in time for Medicare Part D implementation.

Recommended Action 11.4: HHS should evaluate how mass enumeration of dispensers for the NPI can occur using the NCPDP Provider Identifier Number database.

Recommended Action 11.5: HHS, when requiring the NPI as the primary identifier for dispensers, should protect the ability to maintain linkages to the NCPDP Provider Identifier Number database for current claims processing purposes.

Recommended Action 12.1: HHS should ensure that the NPI, when it becomes available, is incorporated as the primary identifier for prescribers in the NCPDP SCRIPT and other e-prescribing standards. It should be noted that the NPI must be at the individual prescriber level, because a prescription cannot be written at a group level.

Recommended Action 12.2: HHS should accelerate the enumeration of all prescribers to support transition to the NPI for e-prescribing.

Recommended Action 12.3: HHS should permit the industry to use the NCPDP HCIdea in the event that the NPS cannot enumerate prescribers in time for Medicare Part D implementation.

Recommended Action 12.4: HHS should work with the industry to identify issues and possible solutions that deal with all elements of the prescriber location and include those solutions in the 2006 pilot tests.

Recommended Action 12.5: HHS should evaluate how mass enumeration of prescribers for the NPI can occur using the NCPDP HCIdea database.

Recommended Action 12.6: HHS, when requiring the NPI as the primary identifier for prescribers, should protect the ability to maintain linkages to the NCPDP HCIdea database for e-prescribing routing functions.

Recommended Action 13:1: HHS should support the efforts of standards development organizations to incorporate in the foundation standards as many as possible of the additional functions required for MMA, as identified in these recommendations.

Recommended Action 13.2: HHS should include foundation standards with as many as possible of the additional functions required for MMA in the 2006 pilot tests.

Recommended Action 13.3: HHS should immediately begin to work with the vendors to ensure readiness for the pilot tests on January 1, 2006.

Recommended Action 13.4: HHS should identify and widely publicize specific goals, objectives, timelines, and metrics to guide the design and assessment and increase industry awareness of the 2006 pilot tests. HHS should include metrics that address economic, quality of care, patient safety, and patient and prescriber satisfaction factors.

Recommended Action 13.5: After the pilot tests, HHS should develop and widely disseminate information concerning any economic and quality of care benefits of e-prescribing, provide comprehensive education on implementation strategies, describe how e-prescribing can be implemented consistent with the privacy protections under HIPAA, and address other elements that contribute to successful and widespread prescriber adoption and patient acceptance.

Recommended Action 14.1: HHS should financially support standards coordination activities to ensure a seamless e-prescribing process across provider domains (e.g., physician office, hospital, long term care), dispensers, and payers/PBMs.

Recommended Action 14.2: HHS should encourage standards development organizations to adopt a change management process that permits versions to maintain interoperability.

Recommended Action 15.1: HHS should ensure that regulations define the parameters of safe harbor, ensure preservation of provider/patient choice, and require that e-prescribing messages received through e-prescribing applications be free from commercial bias.

Recommended Action 16.1: HHS should support standards development organizations in their development of conformance tests for the e-prescribing standards and their implementation guides.

Recommended Action 16.2: HHS should require that e-prescribing system vendors validate the conformance of their e-prescribing messages.

Recommended Action 16.3: The HHS Office of the National Coordinator for Health Information Technology should investigate how e-prescribing applications might best be certified.

From: ***Letter to HHS Secretary Mike Leavitt from Simon P. Cohn, Chairman, National Committee on Vital and Health Statistics: Second Set of Recommendations on E-Prescribing Standards*** (2005)

Recommended Action 1.1: HHS, Drug Enforcement Administration (DEA), and state boards of pharmacy should recognize the current e-prescribing network practices that are in compliance with HIPAA security and authentication requirements as a basis for securing electronic prescriptions. These security practices are discussed in the background and illustrated in Appendix A. In addition, these practices are applied in conjunction with the dispensers' responsibility to use their professional judgment in determining the validity of prescriptions. Different requirements may be needed for transmission of electronic prescriptions that do not go through such networks.

Recommended Action 1.2: HHS and Department of Justice (DOJ) should work together to reconcile different agency mission requirements in a manner that will address DEA needs for adequate security of prescriptions for all controlled substances, without seriously impairing the growth of e-prescribing in support of patient safety as mandated by MMA.

Recommended Action 2.1: HHS should evaluate emerging technologies such as biometrics, digital signature, and PKI for higher assurance authentication, message integrity, and non-repudiation in a research agenda for e-prescribing and all other aspects of health information technology.

Recommendations Relative to Progress on NCVHS Recommendations from the September 2, 2004 Letter:

Recommended Action 3.1: NCVHS will continue to monitor the progress of the development of the NCPDP Formulary and Benefit Coverage Message Standard and will report any further recommendations to HHS based upon this progress.

Recommended Action 4.1: NCVHS will continue to monitor the progress of the development of the NCPDP Medication History Message Standards and will report any further recommendations to HHS based upon this progress.

Recommended Action 5.1: HHS should include the fill status notification function of the NCPDP SCRIPT Standard in the 2006 pilot tests, consistent with NCVHS recommendations of September 2, 2004.

Recommended Action 6.1: HHS should include evaluation of structured and codified SIGs in the 2006 pilot tests, consistent with NCVHS recommendations of September 2, 2004.

Recommended Action 7.1: HHS should include evaluation of RxNorm in the e-prescribing pilots. The pilots should evaluate the use of RxNorm codes as the primary identifiers of orderable drugs in prescription messages. This would assess how well the RxNorm codes capture the intent of the prescriber and whether a dispenser can accurately fill the prescription based on the Rxnorm code. RxNorm should also be evaluated for use where a proprietary code is used for the orderable drug and the RxNorm code is included in the message to provide interoperability with other proprietary coding systems from drug knowledge bases.

Recommended Action 7.2: HHS should take immediate steps to accelerate the promulgation and implementation of FDA's Drug Listing Rule in order to make the inclusion of RxNorm in the 2006 pilot tests as comprehensive as possible. Delayed promulgation may jeopardize the success of the 2006 pilot tests. This is also necessary to achieve the patient safety objectives of MMA.

Recommended Action 8.1: HHS should support the standards development organizations (NCPDP, HL7, and ASC X12) in their efforts to incorporate functionality for real-time prior authorization messages for medications in the ASC X12N 278 Health Care Services Review Standard and ASC X12N 275 Claims Attachment Standard.

Recommended Action 8.2: HHS should include the evaluation of the interaction of standards related to the flow of prior authorization in the 2006 e-prescribing pilot tests.

Recommended Action 9.1: HHS should recognize the exchange of prescription messages within the same enterprise as outside the scope of MMA e-prescribing standard specifications.

Recommended Action 9.2: HHS should require that any prescriber that uses an HL7 message within an enterprise convert it to NCPDP SCRIPT if the message is being transmitted to a dispenser outside of the enterprise. HHS also should require that any retail pharmacy within an enterprise be able to receive prescription transmittals via NCPDP SCRIPT from outside the enterprise.

Recommended Action 9.3: HHS should financially support the acceleration of coordination activities between HL7 and NCPDP for electronic medication ordering and prescribing. HHS should also support ongoing maintenance of the HL7 and NCPDP SCRIPT coordination.

Recommended Action 10.1: HHS should identify and evaluate any privacy issues (within the context of the HIPAA Privacy Rule and health records laws) that arise during the 2006 pilot tests of e-prescribing. Special attention should be placed on issues regarding individuals' rights to request restrictions on access to their prescription records.

Recommended Action 10.2: HHS should use experience gained from the e-prescribing pilot tests to develop appropriate actions for handling privacy issues.

From ***Quality Through Collaboration: The Future of Rural Health*** (2005)

RECOMMENDATIONS

1. Congress should provide appropriate direction and financial resources to assist rural providers in converting to electronic health records over the next 5 years. Working collaboratively with the Office of the National Coordinator for Health Information Technology:

    - The Indian Health Service should develop a strategy for transitioning all of its provider sites (including those operated by tribal governments under the Self-Determination Act) from paper to electronic health records.
    - The Health Resources and Services Administration should develop a strategy for transitioning community health centers, rural health clinics, critical access hospitals, and other rural providers from paper to electronic health records.
    - The Centers for Medicare and Medicaid Services and the state governments should consider providing financial rewards to providers participating in Medicare or Medicaid programs that invest in electronic health records. These two large public insurance programs should work together to re-examine their benefit and payment programs to ensure appropriate coverage of telehealth and other health services delivered electronically.

2. The Agency for Healthcare Research and Quality's Health Information Technology Program should be expanded. Adequate resources should be provided to allow the agency to sponsor developmental programs for information and communications technology in five rural areas. Communities should be selected from across the range of rural environments, including frontier areas. The 5-year developmental programs should commence in fiscal year 2006 and result in the establishment of state-of-the-art information and communications technology infrastructure that is accessible to all providers and all consumers in those communities.

3. The National Library of Medicine, in collaboration with the Office of the National Coordinator for Health Information Technology and the Agency for Healthcare Research and Quality, should establish regional information and communications technology/telehealth resource centers that are interconnected with the National Network of Libraries of Medicine. These resource centers should provide a full spectrum of services, including the following:

    - Information resources for health professionals and consumers, including access to on-line information sources and technical assistance with on-line applications, such as distance monitoring.
    - Lifelong educational programs for health care professionals.
    - An on-call resource center to assist communities in resolving technical, organizational, clinical, financial, and legal questions related to information and communications technology.

Summary of Nationwide Health Information Network (NHIN) Request for Information (RFI) Responses (2005)

RECOMMENDATIONS

Drawn from the respondents' unique perspectives, the comments offered a wide range of thoughtful suggestions. Among the many opinions expressed, the following concepts emerged from the majority of RFI respondents:

- A NHIN should be a decentralized architecture built using the Internet linked by uniform communications and a software framework of open standards and policies.
- A NHIN should reflect the interests of all stakeholders and be a joint public/private effort.
- A governance entity composed of public and private stakeholders should oversee the determination of standards and policies.
- A NHIN should be patient-centric with sufficient safeguards to protect the privacy of personal health information.
- Incentives will be needed to accelerate deployment and adoption of a NHIN.
- Existing technologies, federal leadership, prototype regional exchange efforts, and certification of EHRs will be the critical enablers of a NHIN.
- Key challenges will be the need for additional and better-refined standards; addressing privacy concerns; paying for the development and operation of, and access to the NHIN; accurately matching patients; and addressing discordant inter- and intra-state laws regarding health information exchange.

Health Information Technology (HIT) Leadership Panel Final Report (2005)

RECOMMENDATIONS

The HIT Leadership Panel identified three key imperatives for HIT:

1. Widespread adoption of interoperable HIT should be a top priority for the U.S. health care system.
2. The federal government should use its leverage as the nation's largest health care payer and provider to drive adoption of HIT.
3. Private sector purchasers and health care organizations can and should collaborate alongside the federal government to drive adoption of HIT.

Rather than attempting to implement HIT all at once through a "big bang," implementation should occur through a well-planned sequence of steps and incentives to promote widespread HIT adoption.

Both carrots (i.e., incentives) and, when necessary, sticks (i.e., mandates, other requirements) should be used to promote the widespread adoption of HIT.

The HIT Leadership Panel also suggested that mechanisms be created to incentivize or otherwise assist providers to install HIT and reengineer health care processes to take full advantage of its potential benefits.

The national HIT vision must be communicated clearly and directly to enlist consumer support for the widespread adoption of HIT, including the necessary investment to achieve this vision. This vision should convey how the American consumer has the most to gain from adoption of HIT, including more safe and effective health care in a more efficient, personalized, and secure system.

The federal government and other HIT proponents must specifically address the protections to privacy and confidentiality afforded by the Health Insurance Portability and Accountability Act (HIPAA) and continue to promote and enforce related standards and safeguards accordingly.

The federal government should monitor progress and impact of widespread HIT adoption to ensure that no population group is left out or disadvantaged by this transition in HIT.

Appendix D
Bibliography

BIBLIOGRAPHY

"Reducing and Preventing Adverse Drug Events To Decrease Hospital Costs." *Research in Action: Issue 1* Agency for Healthcare Research and Quality. March 2001.

"At a Tipping Point: Transforming Medicine with Health Information Technology, A Guide for Consumers." April 1 2005. MedStar eHealth Initiative, Verizon. August 2005. <http://ccbh.ehealthinitiative.org/communities/community.aspx?Section=100&Category=211&Document=621>

"Many Nationwide Believe in the Potential Benefits of Electronic Medical Records and Are Interested in Online Communications with Physicians." HarrisInteractive. March 2 2005. August 2005. <http://www.harrisinteractive.com/news/allnewsbydate.asp?NewsID=895>

"Thedacare, Inc. –Touchpoint Health Plan". 2005. *Center for Health Transformation*. August 15 2005. <http://www.healthtransformation.net/Transforming_Examples/Transforming_Examples_Resource_Center/139.cfm>

2002 Himss/Astrazeneca Clinician Survey. Healthcare Information and Management Systems Society, AstraZeneca, 2002. < http://www.himss.org/content/files/surveyresults/Final%20Final%20Report.pdf >

2005 Tax Filing Season Sets Records. Internal Revenue Service IRS.gov. July 2005. <http://www.irs.gov/newsroom/article/0,,id=138112,00.html>

A guide to the National Program for Information Technology. NHS Connecting for Health. United Kingdom Department of Health. <http://www.connectingforhealth.nhs.uk/>

A Nation's Health At Risk. National Association of Community Health Centers. 2004.

About Infoway. Canada Health Infoway, 2004. August 2005. <http://www.infoway-inforoute.ca/aboutinfoway/index.php?lang=en>

Adler, Kenneth. "Why It's Time to Purchase an Electronic Health Record System." *American Academy of Family Physicians: News & Publications*, November/December 2004. <http://www.aafp.org/fpm/20041100/43whyi.html>

Advanced Studies in Medicine 4.8 (2004): 439.

American Bankers Association. *2004 ABA Issue Summary: ATM Fact Sheet*. 2004. <http://www.aba.com/NR/rdonlyres/80468400-4225-11D4-AAE6-00508B95258D/34469/ATMfacts.pdf>

American Society of Health-System Pharmacists. "IOM Sets Strategy for Improving Rural Health Care Quality." December 15 2004. < http://www.ashp.org/news/showArticle.cfm?cfid=19987294&CFToken=93416380&&id=8935>

Associated Press (2005). "Update 5: Polo Ralph Lauren Customers' Data Stolen." *Forbes*. June 2005. <http://www.forbes.com/business/feeds/ap/2005/04/14/ap1947570.html>

Baldwin, Fred. "Nine Tech Trends." *Healthcare Informatics Online*. February 2005: p. 13.

Blendon, Robert J. "Views of Practicing Physicians and the Public on Medical Errors." *New England Journal of Medicine* 347.24 (2002): 1933-40.

Brewer, T. and G. Colditz. "Postmarketing Surveillance and Adverse Drug Reactions: Current Perspectives and Future Needs." *Journal of the American Medical Association* 281.9 (1999): 824-29.

Burt, C. and E. Hing. *Use of Computerized Clinical Support Systems in Medical Settings: United States, 2001-03* Division of Health Care Statistics of the National Center for Health Statistics. 2005.

Chronic Disease Prevention. National Center for Chronic Disease Prevention and Health Promotion. <http://www.cdc.gov/nccdphp/>

Commonwealth of Massachusetts. Group Insurance Commission. *Patient Safety.* 2005. <http://www.mass.gov/gic/safety.htm#top_of_page >

Comprehensive Computerised Primary Care Records Are An Essential Component Of Any National Health Information Strategy: Report From An International Consensus Conference. British Computer Society. Informatics in Primary Care 2004; 12:255–64.

Electronic Prescribing Can Reduce Medication Errors. Institute for Safe Medication Practices. August 2005 <http://www.ismp.org/msaarticles/whitepaper.html>

Erisman, Gary. *Rural Emergency Response - the Safety and Health Safety Net.* National Ag Safety Database. 2001. <http://www.cdc.gov/nasd/docs/d001701-d001800/d001781/d001781.pdf >

Eschenbach, Andrew C. von. "Director's Update: Clinical Trial System of Future." *NCI Cancer Bulletin.* October 26 2004: 2.

Evans, Bruce. "Rural Health Care's Missing Link." *Fire Chief.* June 2002.

Fell, Daniel. "Seven Steps: Using Marketing in Healthcare Technology Planning." *HealthLeaders News.* May 23 2005.

Financial, Legal and Organizational Approaches to Achieving Electronic Connectivity in Healthcare. Connecting for Health Collaborative of the Markle Foundation, 2004.

Finerfrock, Bill. "Presentation on Electronic Medical Records in Rural Health Clinics (Teleconference Transcript)." *Health Resources and Services Administration* 2005. <http://ruralhealth.hrsa.gov/RHC/March16Transcript.htm>

Florida State. Agency for Health Care Administration. "Florida Medicaid Nominated For National Award." Press Release. August 3 2004. <http://www.fdhc.state.fl.us/Executive/Communications/Press_Releases/archive/2004/08_03_2004.shtml>

Fox, Susannah. *Eight in Ten Internet Users Have Looked For Health Information Online, With Increased Interest in Diet, Fitness, Drugs, Health Insurance, Experimental Treatments, and Particular Doctors and Hospitals.* Health Information Online. May 17 2005. <http://www.pewinternet.org/PPF/r/95/report_display.asp>

Frank, Peggy. Testimony before the Commission on Systemic Interoperability. March 15 2005.

Global Technology Centre. *Reactive to Adaptive: Transforming Hospitals with Digital Technology.* 2005.

Harris Interactive. *2004 Commonwealth Fund International Health Policy Survey of Adults' Experiences with Primary Care*The Commonwealth Fund. 2004. <http://www.cmwf.org/surveys/surveys_show.htm?doc_id=245240>

Hearing before the Subcommittee on Oversight and Investigations of the House Veterans' Affairs Committee. 108th Congress, Second Session. March 17, 2004. 108-32. "Hearing VI on the department of Veterans' Affairs Information Technology Programs." Written testimony of John D Halamka, MD, MS. 59-68.

Hill, Michael. "Moving Creates Boom in Long Distance Care." *The Washington Post.* March 17, 2005.

Horrigan, John. "Pew Internet Project Data Memo." *Pew Internet & American Life Project.* April 2004.

Increasing use of electronic prescriptions in Sweden. European eGovernment News. April 27 2005; <www.europa.eu.int/idabc/en/document/4221/353>

Information from The Commonwealth Fund, 2004.

Information from the Harris Interactive Survey, 2001.

Information from the Medistat 2004, Published by Espicom Business Intelligence.

In-Hospital Deaths from Medical Errors at 195,000 per Year, HealthGrades' Study Finds. HealthGrades. July 27 2004. <http://www.healthgrades.com/aboutus/index.cfm?fuseaction=mod&modtype=content&modact=Media_PressRelease_Detail&&press_id=135 >

Internet Medical Records for Migrant Workers. Local Frontiers - Sonoma Medicine. 55.2 (Spring 2004) <http://www.vwsvia.org/>

Internet Travel: Abstract. September 1 2003. Mintel International Group Ltd. August 2005. <http://www.marketresearch.com/product/print/default.asp?g=1&productid=931785>

InterSystems Corporation Press Release. "CareGroup Healthcare System Expects System Projects Multi-million Dollar ROI from CareWeb Application Built on Caché e-DBMS Technology." April 10, 2000.

Kerr, Karolyn. "The Electronic Health Record in New Zealand-Part 1." *Health Care and Informatics Review Online.* 8.1 March 2004. <http://www.enigma.co.nz/hcro/website/index.cfm?fuseaction=articledisplay&featureid=040304 >

Kohn, L., J. Corrigan, and M. Donaldson. *To Err is Human: Building a Safer Health System.* Committee of Health Care in America, Institute of Medicine; 2000.

Komando, Kim. *Online Banking's Best Lure: Online Bill Paying.* 2005. Microsoft: Small Business Center. <http://www.microsoft.com/smallbusiness/resources/technology/business_software/online_bankings_best_lure_online_bill_paying.mspx>

Larson, Ruth. "Medical Advances Can Outpace Doctors: Retraining Not Enforced, Critics Say." *Washington Times* March 21, 1999.

Lenard, Jeff. Commission on Systemic Interoperability Staff Interview. May 2005.

Living Will – Health Care Proxy. United States Living Will Registry. July 2005. <http://www.uslivingwillregistry.com/info-english.shtm>

McGrady, J. "May Sales Report." Retail Ventures. June 2005. <http://www.retailventuresinc.com/index.jsp>

Mearian, Lucas. "Data Snafus Spur IT Action: Bank Mishap Prompts Call for Network Backup." *COMPUTERWORLD.* March 7 2005. < http://www.computerworld.com/?source=nav_tab>

Menachemi, N., and R. Brooks. "Exploring the Return on Investment Associated with Health Information Technologies." *Florida State University College of Medicine.* February 2005: 36.

Miller, Donald. "Prenatal Care: A Strategic First Step Toward EMR Acceptance." *Journal of Healthcare Information Management* 17.2 (2003): 47-50.

Morrow, Dr. James. Commission on Systemic Interoperability, Staff Interview. February 2005.

Morrow, Dr. James. Commission on Systemic Interoperability Staff Interview. July 2005.

National Center for Health Statistics. *Health, United States, 2004: With Chartbook on Trends in the Health of Americans.* Hyattsville, Maryland: 2004.

Office of the National Coordinator for Health Information Technology of the United States Department of Health and Human Services. "American Health Information Community (the Community)." 2005. August 2005. <http://www.os.dhhs.gov/healthit/ahic.html >

Pan, E., D. Johnston, and J. Walker. *The Value of Healthcare Information Exchange and Interoperability*: Center for Information Technology Leadership, 2004.

Patton, Susannah. "Sharing Data, Saving Lives." *CIO Magazine* 2005.

Pearlstein, Steven. "Innovation Comes From Within." *The Washington Post* March 4 2005.

Perez, E., and R. Brooks. "File Sharing: For Big Vendor of Personal Data, A Theft Lays Bare the Downside." *Wall Street Journal*. May 3, 2005.

Pew Internet. "More Internet Users do 'Health Homework' Online." Press Release. May 17 2005. <http://www.pewinternet.org/press_release.asp?r=106>

Physician Characteristics and Distribution in the U.S., 2005 Edition and Prior Editions. American Medical Association < http://www.ama-assn.org/ama/pub/category/12912.html>

Rx: Healthcare FYI #17. Congressman Tim Murphy. August 2005. <http://murphy.house.gov/News/DocumentSingle.aspx?DocumentID=29510>

Skinner, Sandra. Commission on Systemic Interoperability Staff Interview. July 2005.

Smith, Peter. Et. al. "Missing Clinical Information During Primary Care Visits," *The Journal of the American Medical Association* 2005.

Some laws such as the Health Information Portability and Accountability Act of 1996 (HIPAA) (Public Law 104-191 from the 104th Congress) may need revision in light of the benefits and concerns that arise under an electronic and interoperable system.

Stark II Analysis and Summary: Introduction. American Academy of Physical Medicine & Rehabilitation. 2005 <http://www.aapmr.org/hpl/pmrprac/starkb.htm>

Statement of Mike Leavitt Secretary of Department of Health and Human Services before the Committee on the Budget, United States Senate, July 20, 2005.

Stuart, Stephen A. "HIPAA/State Law Preemption Fact Sheet." *State of California Office of HIPAA Implementation* January 9 2003.

Tang, P.C, D. Fafchaps, and E.H. Shortliffe. "Traditional Hospital Records as a Source of Clinical Data in the Outpatient Setting." *Eighteenth Annual Symposium on Computer Applications in Medical Care*. Washington DC, 1994: 575-79.

The Commonwealth Fund 2003 National Survey of Physicians and Quality of Care. Harris Interactive, 2003 <http://www.cmwf.org/surveys/surveys_show.htm?doc_id=278869>

The cost of electronic patient referrals in Denmark summary report: ACCA and Medcom in collaboration with the European Commission Information Society Directorate-General. 2004.

The Personal Health Working Group: Final Report. Connecting for Health Collaborative. Markle Foundation, July 1, 2003.

The Value of Computerized Provider Order Entry in Ambulatory Settings. Center for Information Technology Leadership. March 2003.

This Summer's Blockbuster Hit: The Internet. July 20 2004. Freelance Writing. July 2005. <http://www.freelancewriting.com/survey-072004-01.html>

TouchScript Medication Management System: Financial Impact Analysis on Pharmacy Risk Pools. Cap Gemini Ernst & Young. October 2000.

Trude, Sally. *So Much to Do, So Little Time: Physician Capacity Constraints, 1997-2001.* Center for Studying Health System Change, 2003.

United States Department of Health and Human Services. Office of the National Coordinator for Health Information Technology. *Summary of Nationwide Health Information Network (NHIN) Request for Information (RFI) Responses.* June 2005.

United States Department of Health and Human Services. Office of the Assistant Secretary for Planning and Evaluation. *Effects of Health Care Spending on the U.S. Economy* 2005. August 2005 <http://aspe.hhs.gov/health/costgrowth/report.pdf>

United States Department of Veterans Affairs. *Facts About the Department of Veterans Affairs.* June 2005. <http://www1.va.gov/opa/fact/vafacts.html >

United States White House. "Broadband Rights-of-Way Memorandum." Memo to the Heads of Executive Departments and Agencies. April 26, 2004.

United States White House. Office of the Press Secretary. *President Discusses Health Care Information Technology Benefits.* January 27, 2005. <http://www.whitehouse.gov/news/releases/2005/01/20050127-7.html>

United States. Cong. Senate. *The Identity Theft and Assumption Deterrence Act.* 105th Cong., 2nd sess. Washington: GPO, 1998: Title 19 U.S. Code § 1028.

United States. Office of Inspector General. Office of Public Affairs. *Fact Sheet: Federal Anti-Kickback Law and Regulatory Safe Harbors.* November 1999.

Westin, Alan. *How the Public Views Health Privacy: Survey Findings From 1978 to 2005.* PrivacyExchange. February 23 2005. <http://privacyexchange.org/>

What's Different About Rural Health Care? National Rural Health Association. July 2005. <http://www.nrharural.org/about/sub/different.html>

Wooley, Mary. *Research for Health: The Power of Advocacy.* January 14 2005. Research!America. PowerPoint. August 2005. <http://www.nlm.nih.gov/csi/research_america_011405.pdf>

Woolhandler, S., T. Campbell, and D. U. Himmelstein. "Costs of Health Care Administration in the United States and Canada." *New England Journal of Medicine 349* (2003): 768-75.

Young, Scott. *The Role of Health IT in Reducing Medical Errors and Improving Healthcare Quality & Patient Safety.* September 22 2004. AHRQ. PowerPoint. August 2005. <http://www.ehealthinitiative.org/assets/documents/Capitol_Hill_Briefings/Young9-22-04.PPT>

Zahn, Evan. Commission on Systemic Interoperability Staff Interview. July 2005.

Appendix E
Index

INDEX

A

B

C

I

J

K

L

M

N

O

P

Q

R

S

T

U

V

W

Z